Essential Public Health
Theory and Practice

T0075254

Essential
Public Health

Theory and Practice
Third Edition

Edited by

Kirsteen Watson

University of Cambridge and NHS England

Jan Yates

NHS England

Stephen Gillam

University of Cambridge

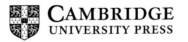

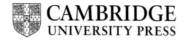

Shaftesbury Road, Cambridge CB2 8EA, United Kingdom

One Liberty Plaza, 20th Floor, New York, NY 10006, USA

477 Williamstown Road, Port Melbourne, VIC 3207, Australia

314–321, 3rd Floor, Plot 3, Splendor Forum, Jasola District Centre, New Delhi – 110025, India

103 Penang Road, #05-06/07, Visioncrest Commercial, Singapore 238467

Cambridge University Press is part of Cambridge University Press & Assessment,
a department of the University of Cambridge.

We share the University's mission to contribute to society through the pursuit of
education, learning and research at the highest international levels of excellence.

www.cambridge.org
Information on this title: www.cambridge.org/9781009378291

DOI: 10.1017/9781009378260

First Edition 2007
Second Edition 2012
Third Edition 2024

Printed in the United Kingdom by CPI Group Ltd, Croydon CR0 4YY

A catalogue record for this publication is available from the British Library.

Library of Congress Cataloging-in-Publication Data
Names: Watson, Kirsteen, 1980- editor. | Gillam, Stephen, editor. | Yates, Jan, editor.
Title: Essential public health : theory and practice / edited by Kirsteen Watson, Stephen Gillam,
    Jan Yates.
Description: 3. | Cambridge, United Kingdom ; New York, NY : Cambridge University Press,
    2023. | Includes bibliographical references and index.
Identifiers: LCCN 2023024101 (print) | LCCN 2023024102 (ebook) | ISBN 9781009378291
    (paperback) | ISBN 9781009378260 (epub)
Subjects: MESH: Public Health Practice | Community Health Services | Needs Assessment |
    Delivery of Health Care | Health Status
Classification: LCC RA418 (print) | LCC RA418 (ebook) | NLM WA 100 | DDC 362.1–dc23/eng/
    20230626
LC record available at https://lccn.loc.gov/2023024101
LC ebook record available at https://lccn.loc.gov/2023024102

ISBN 978-1-009-37829-1 Paperback

Contents

**Additional resources can be found at
https://www.cambridge.org/essentialpublichealth**

Contributors

JENNY AMERY
Chair of Joseph Rowntree Charitable Trust
Formerly Chief Professional Officer Health and Education, UK Department for
International Development (DFID), and NHS Consultant in Public Health

PADMANABHAN BADRINATH
Assistant Professor, Department of Public Health and Primary Care, University of
Cambridge, and Interim Consultant in Public Health Medicine

JOHN BATTERSBY
Head of East of England School of Public Health, NHS England

PETER BRADLEY
Director of Public Health/Medical Officer of Health, Government of Jersey, Jersey

SUE COHEN
Independent Public Health Consultant

MARY FORTUNE
Senior Teaching Associate in Medical Statistics and Assessment, University of
Cambridge

STEPHEN GILLAM
General practitioner and public health specialist, University of Cambridge

SARA GODWARD
Training Programme Director, East of England School of Public Health, NHS
England

BEVERLEY GRIGGS
Consultant in Health Protection, Public Health Wales, Cardiff

LOUISE LAFORTUNE
Principal Research Associate, Cambridge Public Health, University of Cambridge

RAJALAKSHMI LAKSHMAN
Senior Clinician Scientist, MRC Epidemiology Unit, University of Cambridge
Consultant in Public Health Medicine, Cambridgeshire & Peterborough

RICHARD LEWIS
Visiting Senior Fellow, Nuffield Trust, London

REBECCA ROBERTS
Public Health Registrar, East of England Public Health Training Programme

LINCOLN SARGEANT
Director of Public Health, Torbay Council

JAMES SMITH
Assistant Director, Public Health Education Group, Department of Public Health and
Primary Care, University of Cambridge
Sustainability Lead, Cambridge Public Health Interdisciplinary Research
Centre, University of Cambridge

NICHOLAS STEEL
Professor of Public Health, University of East Anglia

ANNE SWIFT
Consultant in Public Health Medicine and Director, Public Health Education
Group, Department of Public Health and Primary Care, University of Cambridge

GILLIAN TURNER
Health Systems Consultant, Reading
Formerly Senior Health Adviser at the UK Department for International
Development (DFID)

KIRSTEEN WATSON
Training Programme Director, East of England School of Public Health, NHS England
Assistant Director, Public Health Educaiton Group, Department of Public Health and
Primary Care, University of Cambridge

JAN YATES
Regional Head of Screening Quality Assurance, NHS England
Independent Consultant, Bernache Leadership

Foreword

A management consultant once told me that he had been brought in by a major city to develop a public health strategy. I asked him what he had recommended. 'Anti-smoking and statins', was the answer. 'Did you get paid a lot for that?', I asked.

Both the management consultant and the person who commissioned him would have done well to read this book. They might then have realised that their approach can be characterised as narrowly conceived preventive medicine – treating individuals to alter disease risk (statins) or attempting to change individual behaviours (anti-smoking). Both are worthy and necessary, but only part of public health.

When at the UCL Institute of Health Equity we have been asked by cities what they can do to improve health, we start with the goals of addressing health inequalities and sustainability. My own starting position is the Marmot Reviews: *Fair Society Healthy Lives* and *Health Equity in England: The Marmot Review 10 Years On*. Our findings and recommendations are based on a comprehensive review of evidence as synthesised, for example, by the Commission on Social Determinants of Health. Our domains of recommendations are not a world apart from chapters in this book: give every child the best start in life; education; employment and working conditions; minimum income for healthy living; healthy and sustainable places; taking a social determinants approach to prevention and lifestyle. We have characterised this as addressing the causes of the causes.

Even before working with local organisations and people to work out a strategy, and tactics, it is worth asking how we would know if we were making any difference. To do that, we need an assessment of where we are with health, health inequalities and the social determinants of health. In other words, we need a monitoring framework of the sort described here that shows whether the causes of the causes, health and health inequalities, are moving in the right direction.

We might well have been following the chapters in this book. As a community group said to me: our values determine what we want to measure. Getting the goals right, and then pursuing the steps necessary to achieve them, are essential components of public health.

If anyone doubted the importance of public health, such doubts were dispelled by the COVID-19 pandemic. Managing the pandemic should have been public health in action. In Britain, we were not well prepared, not least because public health budgets had been sharply reduced, and then the main public health agency was dismantled in the middle of the pandemic.

It was predictable that the pandemic would expose the underlying inequalities in society, and amplify them – so it proved. The pandemic emphasised the absolute necessity of following the principles and practical steps laid out in this excellent book. A well-resourced health-care system is absolutely vital, but public health, too, is essential. The more people have the knowledge and understanding contained in this book, the better off we will be as a society.

Michael Marmot

Acknowledgements

The editors would like to formally thank all of the authors for their thoughtful and knowledgeable contributions to this textbook, without which this third edition would not have been possible.

The editors and authors would like to thank family, friends and colleagues for their encouragement and ideas – and, of course, to thank our students.

Special thanks from the editors to our families for their patience and support: KW to Agnes, Callum, Stuart, Moi, Bill and Pat; JY to Rick; and SG to Val.

We are also grateful to Professor Nick Mays and Professor David Pencheon for their comments on Chapters 15 and 16 respectively.

Introduction

Kirsteen Watson, Jan Yates and Stephen Gillam

Historical Background

Public health cannot be understood or fully appreciated without some knowledge of its history. Conventionally, this begins with the large body of work associated with Hippocrates (c. 460–370 BC). In these writings, health was viewed as resulting from a sound balance of the humours. Therapy included diet, exercise and other interventions tailored to the individual – akin to today's emphasis on healthy living and lifestyle. The Hippocratics were, in addition, early exponents of environmentalism. In 'Airs, Waters, Places', the occurrence of disease was linked to such factors as climate, soil and water quality. Proposals for disease prevention were related to specific social and economic circumstances.

Until recently, it was a commonly held view that improvements in health were the result of scientific medicine. This view was based on experience of the modern management of sickness by dedicated health workers able to draw on an ever-growing range of diagnostics, medicines and surgical interventions. The demise of epidemics and infectious disease (until the manifestation of AIDS), the dramatic decline in maternal and infant mortality rates and the progressive increase in the proportion of the population living into old age coincided in Britain with the development of the National Health Service (NHS, established in 1948). Henceforth, good-quality medical care was available to most people when they needed it at no immediate cost. Clearly, there have been advances in scientific medicine with enormous benefit to humankind, but have they alone or even mainly been responsible for the dramatic improvements in mortality rates evident in developed countries in the last 150 years? What lessons can we learn from how these improvements have been brought about?

Public health has been defined as 'the science and art of preventing disease, prolonging life and promoting health through the organised efforts of society' [1]. In Europe and North America, four distinct phases of activity in relation to public health over the last 200 years can be identified. The first phase began in the industrialised cities of Northern Europe in response to the appalling toll of death and disease among working-class people who were living in abject poverty. Large numbers of people had been displaced from the land by landlords seeking to take advantage of the agricultural revolution. They had been attracted to growing cities as a result of the industrial revolution and produced massive changes in population patterns and the physical environment in which people lived [2].

The first Medical Officer of Health in the UK, William Duncan (1805–1863), was appointed in Liverpool. Duncan surveyed housing conditions in the 1830s and discovered that one-third of the population was living in the cellars of back-to-back houses with earth floors, no ventilation or sanitation and as many as 16 people to a room. It was no surprise to him that fevers were rampant. The response to similar situations in large industrial towns was the development of a public health movement based on the activities of medical officers of health and sanitary inspectors, and supported by legislation.

The public health movement, with its emphasis on environmental change, was eclipsed in the 1870s by an approach at the level of the individual, ushered in by the development of the 'germ theory' of disease and the possibilities offered by immunisation and vaccination. Action to improve the health of the population moved on first to preventive services targeted at individuals, such as immunisation and family planning, and later to a range of other initiatives, including the development of community and school nursing services. The introduction of school meals was part of a package of measures to address the poor nutrition among working-class people, which had been brought to public notice by the poor physical condition of recruits to the army during the Boer War at the turn of the twentieth century.

This second phase also marked the increasing involvement of the state in medical and social welfare through the provision of hospital and clinic services [2]. It was in turn superseded by a 'therapeutic era' dating from the 1930s, with the advent of insulin and sulphonamides. Until that time, there was little that was effective in doctors' therapeutic arsenal. The beginning of this era coincided with the apparent demise of infectious diseases on the one hand and the development of ideas about the welfare state in many developed countries on the other. Historically, it marked a weakening of departments of public health and a shift of power and resources to hospital-based services.

By the early 1970s, the therapeutic era was itself being challenged by those such as Ivan Illich (1926–2002), who viewed the activities of the medical profession as part of the problem rather than the solution. Illich was a Catholic priest who had come to view the medical establishment as a major threat to health. His radical critique of industrialised medicine is simply summarised [3]. Death, pain and sickness are part of human experience and all cultures have developed means to help people cope with them. Modern medicine has destroyed these cultural and individual capacities, through its misguided attempts to deplete death, pain and sickness. Such 'social and cultural iatrogenesis' has shaped the way that people decipher reality. People are conditioned to 'get' things rather than do them. 'Well-being' has become a passive state rather than an activity.

The most influential body of work belonged to Thomas McKeown (1911–1988). He demonstrated that dramatic increases in the British population could only be accounted for by a reduction in death rates, especially in childhood. He estimated that 80–90% of the total reduction in death rates from the beginning of the eighteenth century to the present day had been caused by a reduction in those deaths due to infection – especially tuberculosis, chest infections and water- and food-borne diarrhoeal disease [4].

Most strikingly, with the exception of vaccination against smallpox (which was associated with nearly 2% of the decline in the death rate from 1848 to 1971), immunisation and therapy had an insignificant effect on mortality from infectious diseases until well into the twentieth century. Most of the reduction in mortality from TB, bronchitis, pneumonia, influenza, whooping cough and food- and water-borne diseases had already occurred before effective immunisation and treatment became available. McKeown placed particular emphasis on raised nutritional standards as a consequence of rising living standards. This thesis was challenged in turn by those who stress the importance of public health measures [5].

The birth of a 'new public health' movement dated from the 1970s [6]. This approach brought together environmental change and personal preventive measures with appropriate therapeutic interventions, especially for older and disabled people. Educational approaches to health promotion have proved disappointingly ineffective. Contemporary health problems are therefore seen as being societal rather than solely individual in their origins, thereby avoiding the trap of 'blaming the victim'.

The intriguing truth is that the role of knowledge as a determinant of health is as yet ill defined. Scientific advances in our understanding of how to improve health are embodied in the evolving panoply of medical interventions – new drugs, vaccines, diagnostics, etc. These new insights are, in turn, assimilated more informally by health professionals and the general public. How to harness new knowledge more effectively, for example, through the exploitation of new information technologies and marketing techniques, is a topic of growing interest to students of public health [7].

In the early twentieth century, the decline of childhood mortality was powerfully determined by the propagation to parents of new bacteriological knowledge [8]. Over the last three decades, increased access to knowledge and technology has accounted for as much as two-thirds of the annual decline in under-5 mortality rates in low- and middle-income countries [9]. Knowledge – or rather wilful ignorance – was an important determinant of political responses to the COVID-19 pandemic. The practices of isolation, quarantine and personal protection evolved in the Middle Ages in response to the Black Death. Delays in 'locking down' and ineffective systems for tracing disease fatally hampered early control in the UK [10]. Yet the pandemic also showcased extraordinary technical advances in drug and vaccine development and evidenced remarkable societal compliance with restrictions on individual freedom and risk-reduction measures.

In any event, what is needed to address society's health problems are rational health-promoting public policies with a sound basis in epidemiology: the study of the distribution and determinants of disease in human populations.

Health-Care's Contribution in Context

Health professionals have long lived with the ambiguities of their portrayal in literature and the media: on the one hand as compassionate modern miracle-workers, on the other as self-interested charlatans. The implications of McKeown and Illich's work were largely ignored by clinicians. However, powerful counter-arguments have been mounted in their defence.

Attempts have been made to estimate the actual contribution of medical care to life extension or quality of life [11]. Estimating the increased life expectancy attributable to the treatment of a particular condition involves a three-step procedure:

- calculating increases in life expectancy resulting from a decline in disease-specific death rates;
- estimating increases in life expectancy when therapy is provided under optimal conditions (using the results of clinical trials, using life tables); and
- estimating how much of the decline in death rates can be attributed to medical care provided in routine practice.

Twenty years ago, Bunker credited 5 of the 30-year increase in life expectancy since 1900, and half the 7 years of increase since 1950, to clinical services (preventive as well as therapeutic) [12]. In other words, compared with the large improvements in life expectancy gained from advancing public health, the contribution of medical care was relatively small, but is now a more significant determinant of life expectancy. The continuing inequalities in health point to further potential for improvement.

There are thus three main approaches to improving the health of the population as a whole and national policy must take into account their strengths and limitations.

- Increasing investment in medical care may make the most predictable contribution to reducing death and suffering, but its impact is limited.
- The benefits of health promotion and changing lifestyles are less predictable.
- Redistribution of wealth and resources addresses determinants of glaring health inequalities, but is of still more uncertain benefit.

Domains of Public Health

Public health in the UK NHS has undergone dramatic changes in recent years. All health professionals require some generalist understanding in this field. Rather fewer will need more advanced skills in support of aspects of their jobs (e.g. health visitors, general practitioners, commissioning managers). This group also includes non-medical professions such as environmental health and allied agencies such as charities and voluntary groups. A small number of individuals will specialise in public health, but this group is expanding. Specialists in public health increasingly hail from non-medical backgrounds.

Nowadays, public health is seen as having three core domains: health improvement, health protection and improving services, with three functions of public health intelligence, academic public health and workforce development underpinning each domain (Figure 1) [13]. All these domains are covered within this book. Each has its own chapter and examples from all three are used to demonstrate how the skills underpinning public health are put into practice.

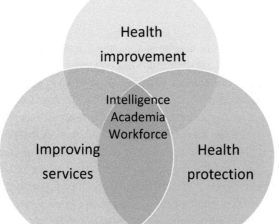

Figure 1 Domains of public health practice [13].

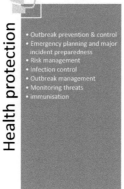

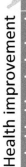

Health improvement
- Strategically assess the health and wellbeing needs of the local population
- Interpret intelligence about health outcomes
- Conduct health equity audits and health impact assessments
- Commission appropriate and effective health and wellbeing initiatives
- Partnership working
- Enable and support communities
- Act as advocates for health
- Build sustainable capacity and resources
- Develop evidence and evaluate programmes

Health protection
- Outbreak prevention & control
- Emergency planning and major incident preparedness
- Risk management
- Infection control
- Outbreak management
- Monitoring threats
- Immunisation

Health services
- Health service commissioning
- Health and social care service prioritisation
- Ensure equity of provision
- Ensure clinical governance and quality improvement
- Provide healthcare audit, evaluation and research
- Ensure patient safety
- Healthcare development and planning
- Leadership for healthcare

The disciplines that underpin public health include medicine and other clinical fields, epidemiology, demography, statistics, economics, sociology, psychology, ethics, leadership, policy and management. Public health specialists typically work with many other disciplines whose activities impact on the population's health. These might, for example, include health-service managers, environmental health officers or local political representatives.

The science of public health is concerned with using these disciplines to make a diagnosis of a population's, rather than an individual's, health problems, establishing the causes and effects of those problems, and determining effective interventions. The art of public health is to create and use opportunities to implement effective solutions to population health and health-care problems. This book intends to capture both the art and the science.

Throughout their careers, health-care and allied professionals are presented with opportunities to help prevent disease and promote health. Doctors and nurses, for example, need to look beyond their individual patients to improve the health of the population and later in their careers, many will be involved in health-service management. Health professionals with a clear understanding of their role within the wider context of health and social care can influence the planning and organisation of services. They can help to ensure that the development of health services really benefits patients.

This book seeks to develop for its readers a 'public health perspective', asking such questions as:

- What are the basic causes of this disease and can it be prevented?
- What are the most cost-effective approaches to its clinical management?
- Can health and other services be better organised to deliver the best models of practice, such as health-care delivery?
- What strategies could be adopted at a population level to ameliorate the burden of this disease?

As we have seen, population approaches to health improvement can be portrayed as in opposition to clinical care. This dichotomy is overstated and, in many respects, clinical and epidemiological skills serve complementary functions. There are parallels between the activities of health professionals caring for individuals and public health workers tending populations (Table 1).

Table 1 Individual and population health – parallels in practice

Individual	Population
Examination of a patient	Community health surveys
Drawing up diagnostic possibilities	Assessing health-care needs: setting priorities
Treatment of a patient	Preventive programmes, service organisation
Continuing observation	Continuing monitoring and surveillance
Evaluation of treatment	Evaluation of programmes/services

Public Health and Today's NHS

In 2012, Directors of Public Health and their teams moved from within the health sector to the local authorities from whence they originally evolved. (The first Medical Officers of Health began discharging their responsibilities from municipalities in the middle of the nineteenth century.) This placed them closer to those responsible for upstream influences on health (e.g. in housing, transport, leisure and the environment).

The NHS has been the focus for frequent reorganisation, but public health teams continue to play a significant role in the commissioning and management of health-care services. Under the Health and Care Act 2022, 42 Integrated Care Boards were set up as statutory organisations responsible for arranging the provision of local health services and managing the local NHS budget.

In response to the COVID-19 pandemic, the health improvement, prevention and health-care functions of Public Health England moved into the new Office for Health Improvement and Disparities. Health protection functions moved to a new UK Health Security Agency established to strengthen emergency preparedness and protect people from infectious diseases and other health threats (see Chapter 10). The rationale for recent reforms is described further in Chapter 15.

As well as specialised public health practitioners within these settings, the roles of many other professionals involve elements of public health within their role, including, for example (although not limited to):

- Environmental health officers – tackling food safety, communicable disease control, healthy environments.
- Health visitors and school nurses – child health-care includes important public health work such as encouraging breastfeeding and promoting smoking cessation.
- District nurses – care of the elderly includes areas such as ensuring adequate heating and safety in the home.
- Voluntary organisations – for example, mental health charities carry out mental health promotion.
- Information analysts, epidemiologists, researchers and librarians – these people are key to the ability of public health specialists to use information and evidence to measure and improve health.
- Occupational health officers – essential to manipulating the risks to health from our working environments and making individual and structural changes to minimise these.

This book is aimed at *all* who engage in public health practice, be they a public health practitioner, manager or registrar. Health professionals from medicine, nursing and allied professions, colleagues in local government and those in the voluntary sector will also find useful material applicable to their practice. This book is for anyone who wishes to promote health and well-being, understand wider determinants and societal influences on health, tackle inequalities and improve the quality, coordination and communication of services.

The Structure of This Book

The first section focuses on core skills in public health as outlined in Figure 2. For each step in this process, a chapter offers insight into key concepts and skills required for these disciplines or topics.

Chapter 1 focuses on how to assess needs and this is built on in Chapter 2, which outlines sources of health information to inform this. Chapter 3 provides an introduction to the discipline of epidemiology (also the subject of a companion book in this series), and Chapter 4 describes how to use evidence in practice.

The next three chapters build on these fundamental skills and translate them into action: Chapter 5 considers the processes and considerations involved in decision-making and priority setting; Chapter 6 describes methods for evaluation and improving quality of care; and Chapter 7 considers the role of public health practitioners as leaders and managers, and how to widen their influence and deployment of expertise to best effect.

Some specific areas of care are seen as coming under the remit of public health, so the final three chapters in Part 1 offer an introduction to improving population

Figure 2 Core skills described in Part 1 of the book.

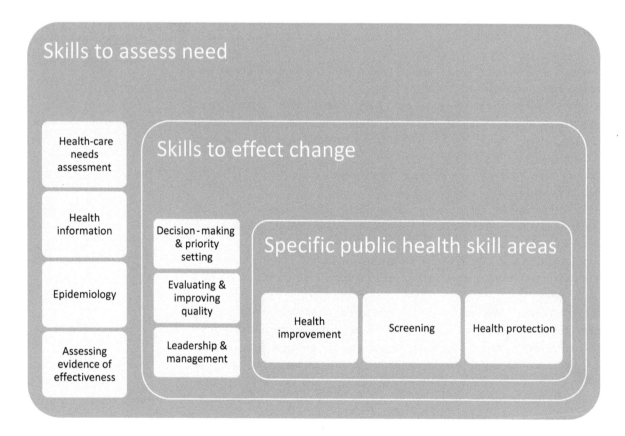

health (Chapter 8), screening (Chapter 9) and health protection (Chapter 10). The toolkit of public health skills a practitioner needs to acquire are added to at each stage and are rarely useful in isolation.

The second half of the book considers the main challenges that public health practitioners are facing and the contexts within which they work. A life-course approach is adopted in Chapters 11, 12 and 13, considering first the specific challenges of child public health before moving on to the health of adults and then older people.

Chapter 14 considers the impact of working in public health on the narrowing of health inequalities; and Chapter 15 covers the role and impact of policy development. Finally, Chapter 16 focuses on international development and Chapter 17 on the crucial role of sustainability and 'planetary health'.

Figure 3 demonstrates how these public health challenges are connected.

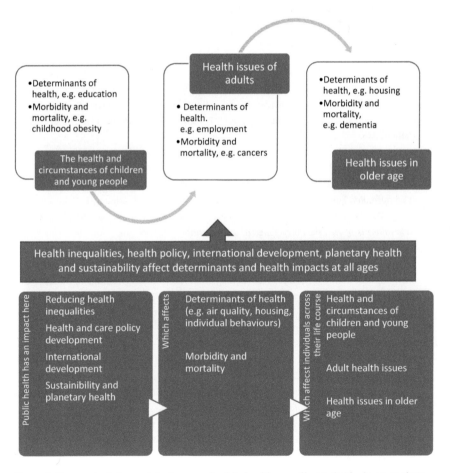

Figure 3 How contexts for and challenges of public health can affect individuals across their whole life course.

Throughout the book, there are questions in the margin to engage the reader, prompt reflection on core material and to encourage you to consider how this knowledge and these skills might be applied to different situations in your own practice. Alongside this book, there is also an Internet Companion (www .cambridge.org/9781107601765), where you will find suggestions for further reading, additional material, interactive exercises and self-assessment questions.

REFERENCES

1. Department of Health, Public health in England: Report of the Committee of Inquiry into the Future Development of the Public Health Function, London, 1988.
2. C. Hamlin, The history and development of public health in high-income countries. In R. Detels, R. Beaglehole, M. A. Lansang and M. Gulliford (eds.), *Oxford Textbook of Public Health*, 5th ed., Oxford, Oxford University Press, 2009, ch. 1.2.
3. I. Illich, *The Limits to Medicine: Medical Nemesis: The Expropriation of Health*, London, Penguin, 1976.
4. T. McKeown, *The Modern Rise of Population*, London, Edward Arnold, 1976.
5. S. Szereter, The importance of social intervention in Britain's mortality decline 1850–1914: A re-interpretation of the role of public health. In B. Davey, A. Gray and C. Seale (eds.), *World Health and Disease: A Reader*, 3rd ed., Milton Keynes, Open University Press, 2002.
6. J. Ashton, Public health and primary care: Towards a common agenda, *Public Health* **104**(6), 1990, 387–98.
7. National Social Marketing Centre for Excellence, *Social Marketing: Pocket Guide*, London, Department of Health, 2005.
8. D. C. Ewbank and S. H. Preston, Personal health behaviour and the decline in infant and child mortality: The United States, 1900–1930. In J. C. Caldwell, S. Findley, P. Caldwell *et al.* (eds.), *What We Know about Health Transition; The Cultural, Social and Behavioural Determinants of Health: Proceedings of an International Workshop, Canberra, May 1989*, Canberra, Australian National University, 1989, pp. 116–49.
9. D. T. Jamison, Investing in health. In D. T. Jamison, J. G. Breman, A. R. Measham *et al.* (eds.), *Disease Control Priorities in Developing Countries*, 2nd ed., Washington, DC and New York, NY, The World Bank and Oxford University Press, 2006, pp. 3–36.
10. G. Scaly, B. Jacobson and K. Abbasi, UK's response to covid-19 'too little, too late, too flawed', *British Medical Journal* 369, 2020, m1932.
11. J. Powles, Public health policy in developed countries. In R. Detels, R. Beaglehole, M. A. Lansang and M. Gulliford (eds.), *Oxford Textbook of Public Health*, 5th ed., Oxford, Oxford University Press, 2009, ch. 3.2.
12. J. Bunker, The role of medical care in contributing to health improvement within society, *International Journal of Epidemiology* **30**(6), 2001, 1260–3.
13. Faculty of Public Health, Functions and standards of a public health system, 2nd ed. Available at: www.fph.org.uk/media/3031/fph_systems_and_function-final-v2.pdf.

Part 1

The Public Health Toolkit

Health Needs Assessment
Stephen Gillam and Padmanabhan Badrinath

Key points

- Health-care needs assessment is central to the planning process.
- Health needs should be distinguished from the need for health-care; the latter is nowadays defined in terms of the ability to benefit from care.
- There are three commonly contrasted approaches to needs assessment: corporate, comparative and epidemiological.
- Many toolkits and other resources have been developed to assist those undertaking health-care needs assessments.

1.1 Introduction

As is outlined in Figure 3 in the Introduction, the first element of understanding how to improve the health and well-being of a population relies on a thorough assessment of the needs of the specified population, be it a local population defined by geography, a specific age group or those with certain characteristics.

This chapter begins by considering how 'health need' can be conceptualised; the distinction between need, demand and supply; and the difference between health needs and the need for health-care. Secondly, the wider determinants of health are introduced and their relation to health needs discussed. Finally, the steps involved in a systematic assessment of the health needs of a defined population are explained, including tools and resources used to achieve this. Practical challenges are considered.

1.2 How Can Health 'Needs' of the Population Be Conceptualised?

Health professionals spend much time learning to assess the needs of individuals; many know less about defining the needs of a population. The need for health underlies, but does not wholly determine, the need for health-care. Health-care needs are often measured in terms of 'demand' – what patients ask for – but demand is to a great extent 'supply-induced' – determined by what care is on offer. For example, variations in general practice referral or consultation rates have less to do with the health status of the populations served than with differences between doctors, such as their skills or referral thresholds [1].

There is no generally accepted definition of 'need'. Last's notion of a 'clinical iceberg' of disease [2] whereby we see or identify only a small tip of what might be occurring in the population has been supported by various community studies indicating much illness is unknown to health professionals (see Figure 1.1). Public health specialists have responsibility for the whole population, and it is important to consider the needs of those who do not contact the health service with symptomatic disease, including those who are at risk of health problems, have early stages of disease or have opted not to seek treatment or advice – the submerged part of the disease 'iceberg'.

Needs can be classified in terms of diseases, priority groups, geographical areas, services or using a lifecycle approach (children/teenagers/adults/older people). Bradshaw's often-quoted taxonomy highlighted four types of need [3]:
- expressed needs (needs expressed by action, for instance visiting a doctor or seeking social care);
- normative needs (defined by 'experts');
- comparative needs (comparing one group of people with another);
- felt needs (those needs people say they have, for instance in a survey).

What might be expressed, normative, comparative and felt needs for an example such as diabetes care?

Figure 1.1 The iceberg of disease [2].

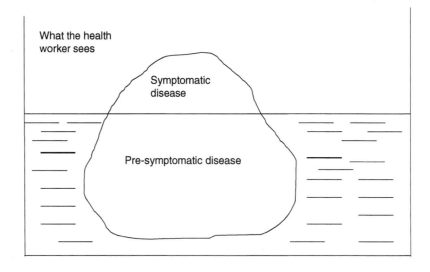

What the health worker sees

Symptomatic disease

Pre-symptomatic disease

1.2.1 Health or Health-care?

Health is famously difficult to define. The World Health Organization's definition of health embraces the physical, social and emotional well-being of an individual, group or community and emphasises health as a positive resource of life, not just the absence of disease [4]. Health needs accordingly encompass education, social services, housing, the environment and social policy.

The need for health-care is the population's ability to benefit from health-care, which is in turn the sum of many individuals' ability to benefit [5]. As well as treatment, health-care includes prevention, diagnosis, continuing care, rehabilitation and palliative care. The ability to benefit does not mean that all outcomes will be favourable, but implies outcomes that will, on average, be effective. Some benefits may be manifest in changes of clinical status; others, such as the benefits of reassurance or the support of carers, are difficult to measure. Diagnosis and reassurance form an important part of primary care when many people may require no more than a negative diagnosis. Health needs assessment thus requires knowledge of the incidence of the health or social problem (risk factor, disease, disability), its prevalence and the effectiveness of interventions to address it.

1.2.2 Individual or Population?

Health and social care services focus on the individual and need is defined in terms of what can be done for the patients, carers or families they see. However, this may neglect the health needs of people not receiving care (e.g. attending outpatient departments, attending a vaccination hub or known to social care services). Traditionally, the clinical view enshrined in such notions as 'clinical freedom' has taken little account of treatment cost. Services of doubtful efficacy may have been provided if they may be even remotely beneficial to patients. In contrast, the view of public health professionals who adopt a population approach seeks to prioritise within finite budgets. Individual clinical decisions may be made without considering the opportunity costs of treatment, while at a population level such opportunity costs must be minimised if the health of the population is to be maximised.

How could needs be assessed for those individuals 'underneath the clinical iceberg' or not accessing services?

The ethical conflicts raised are not easily resolved. Health professionals will only reluctantly withhold interventions of minor benefit for the greater good of potential patients. Tension between what is best for the individual and what may be best for society will always present a dilemma for clinicians. In reality, a complex range of considerations (of which cost-effectiveness is but one) will always determine both clinical and strategic decision-making. This is explored further in Chapter 5 on decision-making and priority setting.

1.2.3 Need, Supply or Demand?

Health-care is never organised as a 'pure' market in economic terms. Its products are heavily subsidised and regulated in all countries. The main reason for this is asymmetry of information whereby patients lack knowledge of their own treatment needs and depend on health-care providers to make appropriate decisions. The clinician acts as the patient's 'agent' to translate demands into needs. However, the literature on variation in referrals, prescribing and other activity rates reveals that this agency relationship is complex.

Professional perceptions of need may differ from those of consumers [6]. The latter are more likely to be influenced by external factors such as media coverage and the opinions of relatives and friends. Consumers' priorities also vary with age, health status and previous experience of health-service use.

The health problems considered to constitute need may change over time. Much universal screening activity, for example in the field of child health surveillance, is no longer supported by research evidence. New needs accrue with the development of new technology. There is usually a time lag before lay demand (for health) reflects scientific evidence of need (for health-care). Unfortunately, an even longer time lag distorts the provision of health services. Their supply is affected by historical factors, and by public and political pressures. The closure of hospital beds is ever politically charged. Health services tend to be regarded as untouchable even when their usefulness has been outlived, while medical innovations are generally implemented before they have been fully evaluated. The pharmaceutical industry, the professions themselves and the media are among interested parties that can manipulate demand. (For instance, how would you assess the need for treatments for Pre-diabetes or Hypoactive Sexual Desire Disorder?)

The relationship between need, demand and supply is illustrated in Figure 1.2. It shows seven fields of services divided into those for which there is a need but no demand or supply (segment 1), those for which there is a demand but no need or supply (segment 2), those for which there is a supply but no need or demand (segment 3) and various other degrees of overlap. Any intervention can be fitted into one of these fields. For example, rehabilitation after myocardial infarction may be needed but not supplied or demanded. Antibiotics for upper-respiratory-tract infection may be demanded but not needed or supplied, and so on. Much effort is required on behalf of patients, providers and purchasers to make the three cycles more confluent. Much is known about how to change professional behaviour through financial incentives, protocols, education, audit and even contracts (see Chapter 6): the factors influencing patient preferences are less well understood.

From Figure 1.2, seven types of service can be identified.

1. Services where there is a need but no demand or supply – for example, family-planning and contraceptive services are needed in many parts of the developing world to improve women's reproductive health. They are frequently neither *demanded* nor *supplied*.

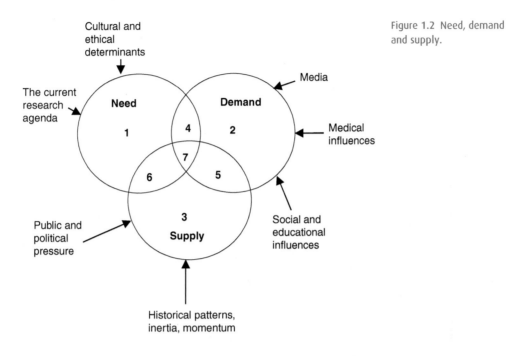

Figure 1.2 Need, demand and supply.

2. Services for which there is a demand but no need or supply – for example, patients may ask for (*demand*) expectorants for coughs and colds. However, cough mixtures are ineffective (no *need*) and seldom prescribed (no *supply*).

3. Services for which there is a supply but no need or demand – for example, with respect to the provision of routine health checks in people over 75 years of age, most people do not request these (no *demand*), but in some practices they are provided (*supply*). Research suggests that the benefits of such checks do not outweigh the costs (no *need*).

4. Services for which there is a need and demand but no supply – for example, substance misuse is a common and dangerous affliction. Methadone maintenance programmes can reduce the physical risks of heroin addiction (*demand*) and may increase the chances of drug misusers giving up (*need*), but they are not always available (no *supply*). Much social care is in short supply.

5. Services for which there is a demand and supply but no need – for example, people may request (*demand*) and be prescribed (*supply*) long-acting benzodiazepines for insomnia. In the long term, this is not effective (no *need*).

6. Services for which there is a need and supply but no demand – for example, even when it is offered, not all health-care staff take up the opportunity of hepatitis B immunisation (*supply* but no *demand*). Yet they are at risk of hepatitis B infection and immunisation is effective at preventing it (*need*).

7. Services for which there is a need, demand and supply – for example, people with insulin-dependent diabetes ask for (*demand*) insulin, it is effective at maintaining their health (*need*) and the UK National Health Service, unlike many others, can afford to provide it (*supply*).

Can you identify other examples for these seven types of service?

1.3 Understanding Determinants of Health

Another important aspect of understanding health needs is to appreciate the factors and determinants which contribute to the health and well-being of the population. Health and care services must address not only health needs, but act to try to promote health and well-being, prevent ill health and tackle underlying causes of health and inequality (see Chapter 8 for further consideration of approaches to improve the health of the population and Chapter 14 for further detail on inequalities).

The 'rainbow' model of determinants of health created by Dahlgren and Whitehead is a useful and often-cited model to consider the wider determinants of health, which work at different levels (see Figure 1.3) [7]. These are:

- **Individual lifestyle factors**, which can be grouped into fixed factors such as age, sex and genetics, and modifiable factors such as diet, physical activity, cigarette smoking and alcohol consumption.
- **Social and community networks** (interactions between friends, family and other members of the community) play an important role in maintaining people's health and are particularly important in maintaining good mental health.

Figure 1.3 Determinants of health by Dahlgren and Whitehead [7].
Reproduced with permission.

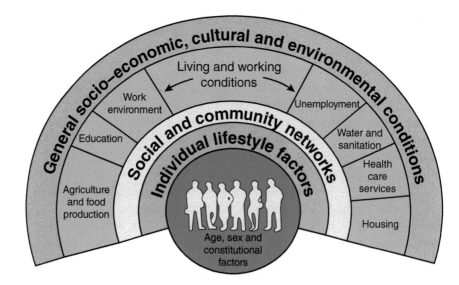

- **Living and working conditions** such as education, agriculture and food production, work environment, housing, water and sanitation, and unemployment also have a role.
- **General socioeconomic, cultural and environmental conditions** such as standard of living, mean income levels, the rights of women in society, employment rates, levels of deprivation and inequalities prevalent in society as a whole have an impact on adult health.

Pencheon and Bradley's model for the driving forces for health and well-being also broadens this to consider avenues for improving health and well-being (see Chapter 8).

1.3.1 Health Needs Assessment (HNA) in Practice

In the UK, after the so-called 'internal market' between health-care purchasers and providers was introduced in the early 1990s, purchasing decisions based on the needs of the population to achieve 'health gain' came into focus (see also Chapter 15). Commissioning organisations with the responsibility to purchase care have been required to assess the needs of their population and to use these needs to set priorities and improve health. Public health practitioners, with their training in epidemiology, disease control and health promotion, have developed a number of techniques to assess population needs. Clinicians are nowadays closer to the commissioning process, in order to incorporate their practical experience of service provision. At the same time, it is essential to involve the general public in shaping services and a number of techniques have been developed to assess health needs from the user's perspective.

Why is assessing needs and priorities important?

There is a gradual move towards integrated commissioning of health and social care, and integration across providers of services to generate greater efficiency and reduce duplication. At present, most health-care is commissioned by Integrated Care Boards, comprising health, social care and public health representatives, which place contracts with providers of care, such as acute hospital trusts, community services and the voluntary sector. Central to commissioning in the UK remain strategic needs assessments undertaken jointly between health and social care in local government to define the current and future health and social care needs of local populations. The information produces a shared view across local government, health services and other relevant organisations, and is used to jointly plan health and care services for those populations.

What additional information could be sourced to understand wider determinants of health needs?

The aim of a health needs assessment is therefore to describe health and well-being problems in a population and detect differences within and between different groups in order to determine health priorities and unmet need (see Box 1.1). It

> **Box 1.1 Five objectives of a health-care needs assessment**
>
> 1. **Planning.** This is the central objective of needs assessment; to help decide what services are required; for how many people; the effectiveness of these services; the benefits that will be expected; and at what cost.
> 2. **Intelligence.** Gathering information to get an overview and an increased understanding of the existing health or social care service, the population it serves and the population's health needs.
> 3. **Equity.** Improving the allocation of resources between and within different groups and reducing inequalities.
> 4. **Target efficiency.** Having assessed needs, measuring whether or not resources have been appropriately directed: i.e. Do those who need a service get it? Do those who get a service need it? This is related to audit.
> 5. **Involvement of stakeholders.** Carrying out a health needs assessment can stimulate the involvement and ownership of the various partners in the process, particularly patient and carer groups, to ensure commissioned services are fit for purpose.

should look at the wider factors that influence health, including health behaviours such as smoking and social determinants such as housing, transport and employment. It should also look at inequalities within the population and compare local populations with other areas to understand relative need. It should identify where people are able to benefit either from health-service care or from wider social and environmental change and balance any potential change against clinical, ethical and economic considerations: that is, what should be done, what can be done and what can be afforded [8]. Assessment of health-care provision should specify:

- the quantity of care activity required (e.g. numbers of operations, admissions, attendances at emergency departments, in-/outpatients, individual social care packages, supported discharge beds, etc.); and
- the quality of care required, by specifying and monitoring standards (with measures such as infections, readmissions within 30 days of discharge and measures of patient care and family satisfaction).

Health needs assessment is thus a method that:

- is objective, valid and takes a systematic approach;
- involves a number of professionals and the general public;
- involves using different sources and methods of collecting and analysing information, described further in Chapter 2;
- involves epidemiological analysis and qualitative and comparative methods, described further in Chapter 3;

- seeks to identify needs, evidence-based treatments or services (see Chapter 4);
- recommends changes to optimise the delivery of health services (see Chapter 5); and
- identifies opportunities for quality improvement (see Chapter 6).

The NHS and health systems across the world face similar pressures. These include the rising cost of health-care due to continuing scientific advances, increasing life expectancy and rising public expectations. At the same time, most countries face similar dilemmas: health-service resources are limited and people face inequitable access to existing care. People whose health needs are greatest are least likely to have access to health-care (the 'inverse care law' referred to several times throughout this book). Finally, there are concerns about the appropriateness, effectiveness and quality of that care. The challenge is to make decisions that maximise the benefit for the population, taking into account the resources available. Needs assessment helps this decision-making and involves at least three steps.

1.3.1.1 Step 1: Identifying Health Priorities by Defining the Population under Scrutiny and Collecting and Analysing Routine Data – 'Comparative' Needs Assessment

Routine data indicate what it is that people are dying from, why they consult general practices, hospitals and social services or what care they may not be receiving that could improve their health, well-being and independence. This will help to prioritise topics for local discussion (Step 2) with a range of other local agencies and professionals. These data allow comparisons to be drawn between local services and those available in other geographical areas. It is also possible to compare these data with previously set standards. For example, one might compare hospital rates of health-care-acquired infections with government standards.

Much data are already available and provide information to 'start the ball rolling'.

Chapter 2 gives an indication of routinely available information, which may be accessed from health-care organisations. Discussions about the data will help lead to a consensus on what areas are priorities. It can also be a starting point to involve the public.

There are some disadvantages. The data may be quite old (it often takes up to two years for routine data to become available), some ill health may have been misdiagnosed or not reported, and hospital data may reflect different admission policies for the same condition. Nevertheless, data collection does help to start the process and is a means to approaching others who have a contribution to make.

1.3.1.2 Step 2: Agreeing Local Priorities by Involving Other Agencies, Users and the Public – Corporate Needs Assessment

There are a confusing number of terms for this process, including community appraisals, rapid appraisals and community surveys. Many of the techniques have been pioneered in developing countries by researchers using qualitative methods [9] – semi-structured interviews, for example. These approaches to understanding behaviours and beliefs may reduce the distorting effect of measuring needs through the eyes of health professionals.

Professionals from other agencies, including local government and the voluntary sector, may have differing ideas from health professionals and it is vital to take these ideas into account. It is important to be aware of the limitations of professional knowledge. In England, the Health and Social Care Act 2012 established 'Healthwatch', an independent organisation with branches in each locality to represent the views of service users. It is also important to directly seek and include the ideas of users and carers about what improves their health and well-being. These factors may include, for example, acceptable employment, adequate housing, better choice of food, access to green spaces or a bus route.

Can you find high-quality examples of including the views of individuals and communities in health needs assessment and commissioning processes?

There are a number of ways of getting the public involved, including:

- **Citizens' juries**. Representatives of the public or local opinion leaders are selected. Experts give evidence and jurors have an opportunity to ask questions and debate.
- **User consultation panels**. Local people are selected as representatives of the locality. Typically, members are rotated to include a broad range of views. Topics are considered in advance and members are presented with relevant information. A moderator facilitates the meeting.
- **Focus groups**. Semi-structured discussion groups of six to eight people led by a moderator.
- **Questionnaire surveys**. These can be postal, or distributed by hand or electronically. This is often most appropriate when the issues behind questions are well known.
- **Panels**. These are large sociologically representative samples (around 100) of a population in a primary care trust, a clinical commissioning group or a health board, which are surveyed at intervals.
- **Interviews**. For example, with patients after a clinic visit on the quality of care, or with health workers on what they know of people's perceptions of local needs.
- **Rapid appraisal**. This involves the public directly in the assessment and definition of local needs through a series of face-to-face interviews with local informants who have a knowledge of the community. From these interviews and from appraisal of local documents about the neighbourhood or community, a list of priorities is drawn up. This is then assessed collectively by means of a public meeting. Working groups develop action plans. The approach is 'bottom-up' and the key philosophy is not only of public involvement, but of a collective response to health needs.

1.3.1.3 Step 3: Undertaking an Epidemiological Needs Assessment

This stage involves examining specific priorities in more detail (Box 1.2). An epidemiological approach to assessing health needs involves three kinds of measurement. It measures:

> **Box 1.2 Priorities for the purposes of HNA may comprise:**
>
> - a whole speciality, e.g. mental health;
> - a disease, e.g. coronary heart disease or diabetes;
> - a client group, e.g. substance misusers;
> - groups waiting for interventions, e.g. those waiting for hip operations, families waiting for special educational needs and disabilities (SEND) assessment;
> - potentially disadvantaged or vulnerable groups such as ethnic minorities;
> - socially deprived groups, e.g. tenants of particular housing estates, isolated vulnerable older people.

1. **The size of the problem**. It looks at how much illness or ill health there is in the community by assessing the incidence and prevalence.
2. **The current services that exist to meet this burden**. It examines how local provision compares with other areas, whether the services meet the needs or whether they are over- or under-provided.
3. **Whether the services are effective**. If new services are required to meet unmet need, it looks at what is known about what works or will make a difference.

Resources for health-care are always finite, so the purpose of this type of needs assessment is to identify health improvements which can be achieved by reallocating resources to remedy over-provision (sometimes) and unmet need. Recommendations are then made on necessary service changes. Chapter 3 describes core principles of epidemiology to assist in the analysis of such data. Toolkits are also available to help undertake needs assessment at a local level [8].

1.3.1.4 Policy, Planning and Strategy Development

The cycle of planning for health-care delivery should originate in an assessment of needs: where are we now and where do we want to get to? The rest of the process is mostly concerned with how to get there (Figure 1.4). Comprehensive needs assessment will generate a bewildering array of possible needs. There are many ways of identifying priorities and this issue is discussed in Chapter 5. The assessment of health impact can help compare how different proposals affect health and inequity [10], a topic which is further explored in Chapter 14.

At whatever level in the system priorities are being agreed, the process should involve as many of the people who will be affected by the choice as reasonably possible (see Chapter 5). Teams need to take careful stock of their current workload when making a decision. In many important areas, work may already be on-going (e.g. falls prevention). There is little point in setting grandiose objectives that cannot realistically be attained. Audit and evaluation (to see whether we have got to where we want to go) is

Figure 1.4 The planning cycle.

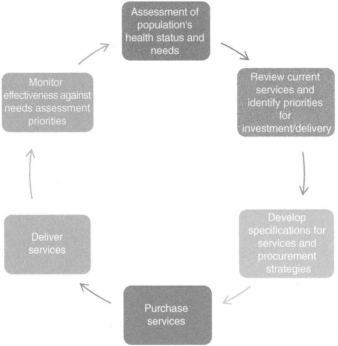

therefore integrally related to needs assessment (see Chapter 6). Indeed, the selection of topics for evaluation should be framed by systematic assessment of priority needs.

A description of the planning process may falsely imply an orderly sequence. Few practitioners with experience of policy-making will subscribe to this myth of rational planning (see Chapter 15). In real life, it is rarely possible to maintain forward progress around the cycle for long. The process is iterative rather than cyclical. The commonest causes of disruption, other than shortage of finance, are vague objectives, lack of information and changing circumstances, people and politics. The COVID-19 pandemic graphically illustrated the need to be able to plan coherently at pace – even with partial information. Public health advice must remain transparent and autonomous [11].

 Use the stages in Figure 1.4 and the example in Table 1.1 to work through the planning cycle for another service or public health intervention.

An understanding of the contingent nature of much planning is important in effecting change. However, consideration of both the planning process and policy-making process as a cycle is helpful when working at a local level within the NHS or partner organisations such as local authorities or voluntary sector organisations. Devising services to reduce the harm caused by alcohol can be used as an example to consider how the planning cycle could work in practice (see Table 1.1). Alcohol

Table 1.1 An example of local policy and planning

Stage	Possible local actions
Assessment of health status and need	Local needs assessment is carried out and identifies high levels of adolescent drinking and local 'hot spots' such as town-centre venues. Police enforcement activity levels are high in specific locations and public perception of street safety has been worsening. Local emergency departments report disorder issues and levels of alcohol-related admissions are higher than the national average. General practitioners are surveyed and low levels of awareness of the effectiveness of brief interventions to address excess alcohol use are found.
Review current services and prioritise	Stakeholder engagement takes account of the local context (e.g. local consumption levels, the ease of availability, views of local health professionals, views of local schools, the level of enforcements, local political imperatives, local commercial interests and the views of the public). This identifies a need to share information between health and the police, to provide additional capacity in emergency departments, to provide brief intervention training to GPs and support and education in secondary schools, and to adjust policing policies in certain locations.
Develop service specifications and procurement plans	A specification is drawn up for an alcohol specialist nurse to be based in the emergency department, an information system to enable data sharing and the provision of brief intervention training in general practice. A business case for an additional community safety officer capacity is drawn up. Key decision-making forums approve additional resources based on a cost-effectiveness analysis.
Purchase services	Local procurement guidance is followed and potential service providers assessed to determine which are the most appropriate.
Deliver services	Funding is provided, staff are employed, services commence delivery.
Monitor and evaluate services	Key performance indicators on which to assess outcomes have been specified to enable service monitoring and evaluation. These are collected on an on-going basis and any issues they highlight are reviewed.

harm reduction has been a UK government priority for several years and the local translation of this into action will depend on local needs.

1.4 Conclusions

Health needs assessment is the first and, arguably, most important step in planning and evaluating the delivery of care. It is not possible to tell how cost-effective care is if we do not know what our population needs, i.e. what services they will benefit from. Certainly in UK health policy this is increasingly recognised and assessment of both health needs (e.g. the needs of a specific minority population, not restricted simply to the need for NHS services) and health-care needs (e.g. the needs of a locality for mental health-care) are prerequisites for the assignment of resources.

REFERENCES

1. M. Roland and A. Coulter, *Hospital Referrals*, Oxford, Oxford University Press, 1993.

2. J. M. Last, The iceberg: Completing the clinical picture in general practice. *The Lancet* **2**, 1963, 28–31.

3. J. S. Bradshaw, A taxonomy of social need. In G. McLachlan (ed.), *Problems and Progress in Medical Care: Essays on Current Research, 7th series*, London, Oxford University Press, 1972, pp. 71–82.

4. World Health Organization, *The First Ten Years of the World Health Organization*, Geneva, WHO, 1958.

5. A. Stevens, J. Raftery, J. Mant and S. Simpson. *Health Care Needs Assessment: The Epidemiologically Based Needs Assessment Reviews*, Oxford, Radcliffe Medical Press, 2004, vols. 1 and 2.

6. A. O'Shaughnessy, J. Wright and B. Cave, Assessing health needs. In I. Kawachi, I. Lang and W. Ricciardi (eds.), *Oxford Handbook of Public Health Practice*, 4th ed., Oxford, Oxford University Press, 2020, ch. 1.4, pp. 42–53.

7. G. Dahlgren and N. Whitehead, *Policies and Strategies to Promote Social Equity in Health*, Stockholm, Institute of Futures Studies, 1991.

8. C. Cavanagh and K. Chadwick, *Summary: Health Needs Assessment at a Glance*, London, National Institute of Health and Clinical Excellence, 2005. Available at: https://ihub.scot/media/1841/health_needs_assessment_a_practical_guide.pdf.

9. H. Annett and S. Rifkin, *Guidelines for Rapid Participatory Appraisal to Assess Community Health Needs: A Focus on Health Improvements for Low Income Urban and Rural Areas*, Geneva, World Health Organization, 1995.

10. M. Douglas and B. Cave, Assessing health impacts. In I. Kawachi, I. Lang and W. Ricciardi (eds.), *Oxford Handbook of Public Health Practice*, 4th ed., Oxford, Oxford University Press, 2020, ch. 1.5, pp. 54–65.

11. J. Jarman, S. Rozenblum, M. Falkenbach *et al.*, Role of scientific advice in covid-19 policy, *British Medical Journal* **378**, 2022, e070572.

Health Information

John Battersby

Key points

- Understanding the demography and the health status of a population is essential before planning effective interventions and services to improve health and to prevent disease.
- Public health practitioners will draw on a variety of health information to help them determine the health status of their populations of interest:
  - demographic data, including population estimates and projections;
  - mortality data (e.g. all deaths, deaths from specific causes, in specific subsets of the population standardised to account for different population structures, deaths in and around childbirth, years of life lost);
  - objectively measured morbidity data (e.g. infectious disease rates, hospital activity, primary care data, registered diseases);
  - data on behaviours and the social determinants of health and well-being (e.g. smoking, unemployment, deprivation);
  - analysis of health inequalities; and
  - data collated at regional or national level by statistical organisations or national public health organisations.

2.1 Introduction

To effectively target public health interventions for greatest impact, it is essential that public health practitioners have a clear understanding of the populations they work with. As described in Chapter 1, understanding these populations, their health status and health needs draws on skills from several disciplines, including demography, epidemiology and statistics. Brought together, these skills allow the practitioner to understand the characteristics of the population of interest, the key health issues that it faces and the broader factors that have a particular influence on the health of that population. These broader factors are generally referred to as the wider determinants of health or the social determinants of health. Information is also vital in allowing practitioners to assess the impact of public health interventions.

2.2 Understanding and Measuring Populations

Populations can be defined at various levels from small geographic or administrative areas right up to whole countries or even the global population. The population of interest may be a specific group within a broader population, for example people below or above a specific age, people who share characteristics or behaviours, or people resident in specific settings such as the population of a prison. It is particularly useful to be able to understand the characteristics of populations at a granular level. In the UK, this could be administrative areas such as local authority ward level or middle or lower super output areas. Super output areas are small geographical areas in the UK that have been designed to improve reporting of small area statistics by providing a more stable set of geographies.

2.2.1 Size and Structure

The first step in understanding a population is to determine its size and age-sex structure. At a country level, this can be achieved in two main ways:
- collecting information on births, deaths and migration to estimate the population size and age-sex structure; and
- periodically counting the whole population – this generally takes the form of a population census.

In practice, countries may use a combination of the two approaches; using a periodic census to provide an accurate baseline and then estimating the impact of changes in the intervening years. Both approaches require significant infrastructure and resource, and the availability and quality of information will vary between countries. Most developed countries have systems in place for registering births and deaths and some will also undertake a periodic census of their populations. This takes place every 10 years in the case of the UK.

Once collected, the size and age-sex structure of a population is typically presented in the form of a population pyramid. Pyramids provide a simple way of comparing population structures and can give a considerable amount of information about the underlying population and some potential health needs. At country level, comparing population pyramids can indicate the state of development of each country (see Figures 2.1 and 2.2 as an example).

Population pyramids can indicate the likely health issues with a population. The pyramid for Mauritania shows a stepped reduction in the population at each 5-year age band from birth. This is strongly suggestive of high infant and child mortality rates and in fact other data show that the under-5 mortality rate in Mauritania is 78 per 1,000 (compared with 4.3 in the UK). The health needs in Mauritania will,

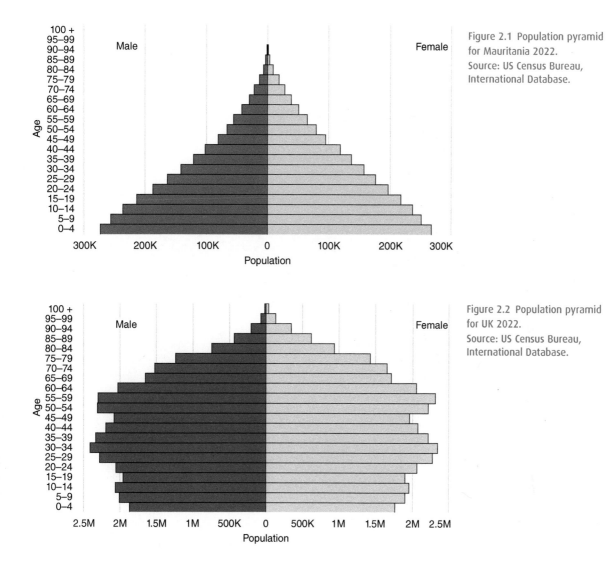

Figure 2.1 Population pyramid for Mauritania 2022.
Source: US Census Bureau, International Database.

Figure 2.2 Population pyramid for UK 2022.
Source: US Census Bureau, International Database.

therefore, be very different from those in the UK, where the population pyramid indicates that there is a large population of people over the age of 65, so one can expect that chronic diseases such as diabetes, cardiovascular disease and cancers will be a major issue. The pyramid is also reflective of the life expectancy at various ages. In high-income countries such as the UK, life expectancy is much higher than in countries with a lower income. In the UK, the life expectancy at birth is 81.9 years, whereas in Mauritania it is 65.2 years.

Use the two pyramids in Figures 2.1 and 2.2 to describe in words the population structures of Mauritania and the UK.

Box 2.1 Epidemiologic transition

Epidemiologic (sometimes referred to as demographic) transition describes the change in birth and death rates from high fertility and high mortality rates in lower-income societies to low fertility and low mortality rates in high-income societies. Five stages can be identified during a country's demographic transition, as shown in Figure 2.3:

1. High stationary: high birth rate and high mortality, so population remains stable.
2. Early expanding: death rate begins to decline but birth rate remains high.
3. Late expanding: death rate declines further and birth rate starts to fall.
4. Low stationary: low birth and death rates, so population remains stable.
5. Declining: birth rate starts to decline but death rate remains stable, so population declines.

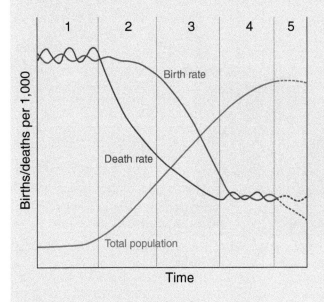

Figure 2.3 The five stages of epidemiologic transition.

2.2.2 Population Trends

The global population continues to increase, having more than tripled since the middle of the twentieth century [1]. Populations are growing fastest in the poorest countries, particularly sub-Saharan Africa. Populations in many European countries are falling and fertility in all European countries is now below the level required for full replacement of their populations in the long run (around 2.1 children per woman) [2].

These population trends are determined by three key components:

- fertility;
- mortality; and
- migration.

2.2.3 Fertility

In demography, fertility refers to the bearing of children, as opposed to the ability to have children. There are various measures of fertility:

$$\text{Birth rate} = \frac{number\ of\ births\ \in\ a\ year}{mid\text{-}year\ population} \times 1{,}000 \tag{2.1}$$

$$\text{Fertility rate} = \frac{number\ of\ live\ births\ \in\ year}{mid\text{-}year\ population\ of\ women\ aged\ 15{-}44} \times 1{,}000 \tag{2.2}$$

Fertility rates can be standardised to account for differences in the age structures of populations. Standardisation allows calculation of the *total fertility rate in a specific year*, which is defined as the total number of children that would be born to each woman if she were to live to the end of her child-bearing years and give birth to children in alignment with the prevailing age-specific fertility rates.

There is more detail on age standardisation in the section on mortality.

2.2.4 Mortality

Mortality describes death rates due to a range of causes. There are various measures of mortality, the key ones being:

$$\text{Crude mortality rate} = \frac{number\ of\ deaths\ \in\ a\ year}{mid\text{-}year\ population} \times 1{,}000 \tag{2.3}$$

$$\text{Age} - \text{(sex-)specific mortality rate} = \frac{number\ of\ deaths\ during\ year\ \in\ a\ particular\ age(sex)\ group}{mid\text{-}year\ population\ of\ age(sex)\ group} \times 1{,}000 \tag{2.4}$$

$$\text{Cause} - \text{specific mortality rate} = \frac{number\ of\ deaths\ \in\ year\ due\ to\ a\ particular\ cause}{mid\text{-}year\ population} \times 1{,}000 \tag{2.5}$$

$$\text{Proportional mortality rate } (\%) = \frac{number\ of\ deaths\ \in\ year\ due\ to\ a\ particular\ cause}{total\ number\ of\ deaths\ \in\ year} \times 100 \tag{2.6}$$

Explore local data on cause-specific mortality for your local population. How do rates compare with other areas and how might this inform your practice? For example, mortality from road traffic accidents?

Mortality rates will be influenced by the age structure of a population. For example, the greater the proportion of elderly people in a population, the higher one would expect the mortality rate to be. To allow for this, comparing mortality rates between different populations requires adjustments to be made. These adjustments are known as age standardisation. There are two approaches to age standardisation which are typically used [3]:

- **Direct age standardisation**. The age-specific rates of the subject population are applied to each stratum in the age structure of the standard population. This gives the overall rate that would have occurred in the subject population if it had the standard age-profile.

- **Indirect age standardisation**. The age-specific rates of a chosen standard population (usually the relevant national or regional population) are applied to the age structure of the subject population to give an expected number of events. The observed number of events is then compared to that expected and is usually expressed as a ratio (observed/expected). A common example is the *standardised mortality ratio* (SMR).

Deaths in and around the time of childbirth are important indicators of the scale of issues such as infectious disease, malnutrition and quality of maternity services. The main indicators for these deaths include:

$$\text{Infant mortality rate} = \frac{number\ of\ deaths \in year\ under\ 1\ year\ of\ age}{number\ of\ live\ births \in year} \times 1{,}000 \tag{2.7}$$

$$\text{Neonatal mortality rate} = \frac{number\ of\ deaths \in year\ under\ 28\ days\ of\ age}{number\ of\ live\ births \in year} \times 1{,}000 \tag{2.8}$$

$$\text{Perinatal mortality rate} = \frac{number\ of\ stillbirths + deaths\ under\ 7\ days\ of\ age \in year}{total\ number\ of\ births(live + stll) \in year} \times 1{,}000 \tag{2.9}$$

$$\text{Maternal mortality rate} = \frac{number\ of\ deaths \in year\ due\ to\ complications\ of\ pregnancy,\ childbirth\ \&\ puerperal\ causes\ within\ 42\ days}{number\ of\ live\ births \in year} \times 100{,}000 \tag{2.10}$$

$$\text{Stillbirth rate} = \frac{stillbirths \in year}{number\ of\ total\ births \in year} \times 1{,}000 \tag{2.11}$$

2.2.5 Migration

Populations may change in both size and structure because of migration. There are many factors that influence migration: economics, political instability, conflict and the consequences of global warming are some of the key drivers of migration. These are also facilitated by advances in transport, communication and trade.

It is estimated that in 2020 there were around 281 million international migrants living in countries other than where they were born – an increase of 128 million from 1990 [4].

Migration occurs not only from lower-income countries to high-income countries, but also from one lower-income country to another, as well as between high-income countries. There are benefits and risks to increasing migration, which can:

- increase or decrease educational levels as young people take up unskilled positions abroad or those educated abroad fail to return home;
- have a positive effect on income (e.g. through remittances as migrants send funds home to families);
- potentially increase socioeconomic inequity as some individuals, communities or countries benefit more than others; or it may have a negative effect on an economy by potentially reducing external competitiveness;
- increase poverty and inequity within countries where rural-to-urban migration is high (e.g. China); in rural areas, the poorest cannot afford to move and those who move into cities tend to be the more educated;
- increase personal vulnerability due to the potential for illegal migration and 'human trafficking' (e.g. women recruited as domestic labour may be vulnerable to sexual exploitation);
- lead to racism and isolation;
- lead to a reduction in the human capital needed to deliver key services at home; and/or
- lead to population structural imbalances (e.g. as those unable to move, such as the elderly, concentrate in one place).

Information on migration may be derived from censuses, surveys and other administrative-record systems. However, these vary in accuracy across the world.

With declining fertility rates and ageing populations, many high-income countries use managed migration as a way of meeting their demographic, economic-development and labour-market needs. Migration that increases population sizes or alters patterns of infectious diseases may result in changing needs for health-care. Public health professionals need to ensure that local health services are culturally sensitive and accessible to migrants (e.g. through appropriate translation services). Many countries have migrant health screening in place to protect the Indigenous population from communicable diseases.

2.3 Population Estimates and Projections

Determining the size and age-sex structure of a population can be done by counting or estimating changes to a baseline population based on what is known about births, deaths and migration.

How can local population projections inform planning of services?

There are two approaches to estimation of future population size and structure [5]:

- **Population estimates**. An estimate is a calculation of the size or structure of a population or another characteristic of the current or past population. Population estimates start with a known baseline, usually taken from a census of the population, and then add in the numbers of births, subtract the numbers of deaths and make an adjustment for known migration.
- **Population projections**. A projection forecasts population characteristics into the future. Population projections also start with a known baseline, but then adjust this based on known fertility and mortality rates, as well as predicted migration rates.

2.4 Civil Registration and Vital Statistics

The calculation of the fertility and mortality rates that have been described earlier depends on an effective civil registration function for the collection of the data on births and deaths. Such systems may also collect data about other life events such as marriage and divorce.

Most countries have systems in place that require registration of births and deaths with the appropriate government authority. As well as the legal requirement to register, the need to appear in government records to access services acts as an incentive to registration and in most high-income countries, registration data are very accurate. However, these systems are complex and resource-intensive and in some lower-income countries systems may be less reliable or, occasionally, non-existent.

As well as recording that a death has occurred, civil registration systems usually collect additional information about the cause of death, contributing factors and, sometimes, details of occupation. Information on cause of death is then coded using an internationally recognised coding system, the International Classification of Diseases [6], which, since January 2022, is in its eleventh version (ICD-11). Despite the use of a standardised classification, differences in recording and application of the classification means that comparisons between countries need to be undertaken carefully. In the UK, the coding of death certificates is automated and mortality data are published by the Office for National Statistics. Data feeds are also provided to Directors of Public Health, giving them details of deaths within the populations that they cover. Public health teams will undertake further analysis of mortality data, including generating standardised rates and calculating life expectancy for their populations.

The International Classification of Disease is not the only classification system in use. Clinical terminologies such as SNOMED CT (systematised nomenclature of medicine – clinical terms) [7] are used to support information systems in primary and secondary care. Terminologies such as SNOMED allow for the recording of additional information, for example about symptoms and investigations, as well as diagnoses, and are mapped to international standards such as ICD.

2.5 Life Expectancy and Years of Life Lost

Mortality rates alone give only a partial picture of the public health impact of diseases. The significance of common causes of death (e.g. pneumonia at the end of life) may eclipse rarer but devastating causes of death earlier in life (e.g. road traffic fatalities). Life expectancy [8] provides an estimate of the average expected life span of a population based on current patterns of mortality. It is calculated from a life table and is usually calculated separately for males and females because of their different mortality patterns. Life expectancy can be calculated for defined populations and used as a high-level indicator of health.

Life expectancy can be calculated from birth, from specific ages, typically life expectancy at age 60 or 65, or it can be calculated as *healthy life expectancy* or *Disability Free Life Expectancy*. Globally, life expectancy has increased by more than 6 years between 2000 and 2019 [9]. Healthy life expectancy has also increased, but at a slower rate than life expectancy. In some high-income countries such as the UK, the rate of increase in life expectancy has slowed down in recent years.

Years of potential life lost relate to the average age at which deaths occur and the expected life span of the population, so provides a measure of the relative importance of conditions in causing mortality.

Years of life lost (YLL) are calculated for each person who died before age 75. For example, a person who died at age 30 would contribute 45 potential years of life lost. (Deaths in individuals aged 75 or older are not included in the calculation.) YLL are the sum of the YLL contributed by each individual. They can be expressed as a rate where the total years of life lost by the total population less than 75 years of age are divided by the population count.

In addition to the use of YLL, the use of life expectancy as a measure of a population's health status can be modified by using adjustments such as those used in developing quality-adjusted life years (QALYs) [10]. These measures give an indication of the quality of life expected rather than just the extent. QALYs are calculated by estimating the years of life remaining for a person following a particular treatment or intervention and weighting each year with a quality-of-life score (on a 0 to 1 scale). It is often measured in terms of the person's ability to carry out the activities of daily life, and freedom from pain and mental disturbance. A disability-adjusted life year or DALY is a measure of the impact of a disease or injury in terms of healthy years lost. DALYs for a disease take into account the years of life lost and the years spent with a disability. These are further described in the economics section in Chapter 5.

When might it be useful to consider YLL rather than mortality?

Box 2.2 International comparisons

Comparing the health status of populations across countries provides useful information about the scope for improvement and the possible reasons for differences. However, comparing both demographic and other health data between countries is not straightforward.

- Demographic comparisons are hampered by the fact that not all countries carry out a regular census and, if they do, they may not be repeated at a similar frequency.
- Many lower-income countries do not have the resources to maintain accurate registration systems for births and deaths.
- The information collected on death certificates, and the way it is coded, may differ between countries.
- Differing health systems will vary in their emphasis on the collection of health data and the way that it can be used for understanding the health status of a population.
- Information about health behaviours and the social determinants of health is often drawn from surveys which may not be generalisable to other settings.

2.6 Measuring Morbidity

Morbidity is defined as 'any departure, subjective or objective, from a state of physiological or psychological well-being. In this sense, sickness, illness, and disease are similarly defined and synonymous' [11]. Morbidity statistics will be described (with the UK as an example) under the following headings:

1. infectious diseases;
2. hospital data;
3. primary care data; and
4. disease registers.

With any data, it is important to consider whether it is fit for purpose and what are the strengths and weaknesses of the source (see Box 2.3).

Box 2.3 Are the data you have fit for purpose?

You should ask the following questions of any data obtained:

1. Are the data **related clearly to specific ages and sexes**? If the disease or determinant in which you are interested varies by age or sex, you may need to standardise rates to allow comparisons.
2. Are the data clearly **related to a specific time period**? Time trends are helpful in supporting the planning of health-care or other public health interventions.

Data often take time to collate, and it is important to use the most up-to-date information available.

3. Are the data clearly **related to specific geographical locations**? You need to ensure that the data you have are related to your population and take care in extrapolating information from other populations to your own.

4. Are the data **complete**? Are there any population groups missing? Some causes of death may be more easily identified and recorded more frequently than others and some may carry stigma (e.g. HIV) and be less well recorded. Population surveys of self-reported health have variable uptake rates and may not be representative of the whole population. Are the same data collected across geographical areas? Data coverage in rural areas may be less complete than urban ones.

5. Are the data **accurate**? What do the definitions of data fields mean? For example, what clinical indications would a field called 'CHD' include? Has it been transcribed from original data, allowing the introduction of errors? Are the data coded and are the codes used in the same way by everyone? Have the definitions or codes changed over time if you are looking at time trends?

6. Are the data **relevant** to the question you have? It is often tempting to use readily available routine data without real thought as to whether they are right for the job!

2.6.1 Infectious Diseases and Surveillance

In the UK and many other countries, certain communicable diseases are notifiable by law. The most recent example of this is COVID-19, which was added to the list of notifiable diseases in the UK in 2020 during the Coronavirus pandemic. The notification system provides a rich source of information on communicable disease, one aspect of the health of a population. Other data on communicable diseases are available from laboratories and elsewhere and are helpful in determining public health policy such as vaccination requirements, sexual health-service needs and likely sources of communicable disease outbreaks for a population.

The collection of data about infectious disease is a form of disease surveillance (see Chapter 10 on health protection). Surveillance is the systematic ongoing collection, collation and analysis of data and the timely dissemination of information to ensure appropriate action can be taken. Infectious disease surveillance allows the identification of patterns of infectious disease that are different from those that are expected. In some cases, this could be an increase in cases of a disease that appears to be linked in time, place or person (e.g. a food-borne outbreak which requires investigation), or it could be a single case of an unusual disease (e.g. a single case of rabies in the UK would trigger action). Surveillance systems can operate across countries to provide early warning of threats to population health and health-care systems.

The concept of surveillance can be applied equally well to non-communicable diseases (e.g. heart disease and diabetes). Changes in patterns of these diseases trigger further investigation and then dissemination of information to those in a position to take the appropriate action.

Despite legal requirements to notify some infectious diseases, and reporting systems that are often automated, data may be incomplete. Nevertheless, surveillance systems provide valid information that is relatively consistent and can be used as a crude indicator of change in prevalence of diseases in the community. The surveillance system will usually trigger an alert that something doesn't look right, and then additional analysis can be undertaken to identify whether the alert needs further investigation or action.

2.6.2 Hospital Data

The recording of hospital activity can be traced to the eighteenth century and an early proponent in the UK was Florence Nightingale. However, it was not until after the founding of the NHS in 1948 that a system for collecting these data was introduced. Today in the NHS, hospital episode statistics (HES) data [12] are collected on patient administration systems (PAS) and diagnostic/intervention coding is added at hospital trust level (see below). The following data are recorded:

- demographic, e.g. age, sex, marital status, residence, ethnic codes;
- administrative, e.g. length of stay, waiting list and source of admission;
- clinical speciality, main condition and operation details.

Hospital activity data are only a proxy measure of morbidity and represent process data on those treated by the hospital system. They also reflect the more severe end of the spectrum of morbidity as many conditions do not often lead to a hospital admission. However, data about utilisation by speciality, principal diagnosis and operation can provide indices of morbidity. Emergency department and outpatient data are also available in HES; however, these data are generally less reliable than inpatient admissions data.

What type of hospital data might help to inform a health needs assessment for a local population of older people over 65 years of age, for example?

Coding of the clinical elements of HES allows linkage to the international classification of disease (ICD-11) coding, SNOMED CT and international comparisons. In the UK, there is also a separate coding system for classifying clinical interventions and procedures known as OPCS-4. A combination of diagnostic (ICD-11) and intervention (OPCS-4) codes is used to administer the payment by results system [13], which is an important mechanism for funding secondary care activity.

2.6.3 Primary Care Data

The focus for medical care outside hospitals in the UK is general medical practice. Data can be collected via relatively infrequent patient surveys or through clinical information systems which support the day-to-day care of patients, and which also allow the establishment of disease registers to support the management of chronic conditions (e.g. coronary heart disease, diabetes, epilepsy). This source of data is useful as, although not always complete, it is available at very small population levels and can be used effectively to engage local clinicians in health improvement or health-care quality initiatives. For example, an audit of statin prescribing to those people identified in a practice register as having coronary heart disease might be used to encourage greater rates of prescribing in women (which tend to be lower). Incentive systems may operate to encourage general practitioners to increase the amount of data collected, which can be used for audit and monitoring, as well as for one-to-one patient care during consultations. An example of an incentive system that has been used in England is the Quality and Outcomes Framework (QOF) [14].

Primary care data can provide a much better picture of morbidity within a population than hospital data. For example, data from the Global Burden of Disease study [15] indicate that the top five causes of death and disability in the UK are ischaemic heart disease, back pain, depressive disorders, headache disorders and chronic obstructive pulmonary disease (COPD). The management of all these conditions will mostly take place in primary care and only a very small proportion of people with back pain, depressive or headache disorders will ever be admitted to hospital.

How might you use primary care data to improve the quality of services and reduce inequalities? (See also Chapter 6.)

In the UK, the Royal College of General Practitioners runs a research and surveillance centre, which uses a network of practices across England and Wales [16]. This system collects data from participating practices and provides timely information about incidence of communicable and respiratory diseases such as influenza and asthma.

Accessing primary care data in England is complex. Data are collected from practices by NHS England (previously NHS Digital) and can be requested through the General Practice Extraction Service (GPES) [17]. An alternative approach is to access data that are collected by one of the clinical information system suppliers. These provide data collected by practices using that supplier's clinical system and are run on a commercial basis so data access can be expensive. Examples of this include the Clinical Practice Research Datalink (CPRD) [18] and The Health Improvement Network (THIN) [19]. Due to the way that clinical information systems have developed, there is some geographical clustering, and so results from analyses of these data may not always be generalisable across the population.

2.6.4 Specialist Disease Registers

It is possible to establish special data collection systems for some diseases. They provide richer sources of information than routine data, but are costly to establish and maintain. A good example of a disease register is that for cancer. Cancer registration is established in many countries including the UK, many European countries and the USA. In the UK, the Ministry of Health set up a system in 1923 through the Radium Commission to follow up patients treated with radium. This was the origin of the national cancer registration system [20], which collects details of age, sex, place of birth, occupation, site of primary tumour, type of tumour and date of initial diagnosis. Additional information about tumour pathology and markers and, increasingly, relevant genetic data are also collected. Information about incidence and survival are obtained, by tumour site, through linking the clinical data on individuals to the national death registration system. As with the other data sources, there are concerns about completeness of registration, accuracy of particulars and effectiveness of follow-up. However, cancer registration in the UK has a high level of data completeness and has proved an invaluable source of cancer morbidity and survival data. Increasingly, as more detailed pathological and genetic data are collected, registry data can be used to look at the effectiveness of different treatments and can also help researchers understand more about the contribution of genetics to the development and treatment of cancers.

More recently, the UK national cancer registration system has been extended to hold a separate register for rare diseases and congenital anomalies. In common with many other countries, the UK also has specialist disease registers which are run by clinicians, medical Royal Colleges or other interested groups working in the relevant field.

2.6.5 Data Linkage and Information Governance

Cancer registration is a good example of health data linkage [21]. This is the process by which two separate datasets can be linked together. Linkage is relatively easy if both datasets share a common identifier, but there are also more complex techniques which allow linkage of datasets without a shared unique identifier by matching several different variables.

Data linkage can hugely increase the utility of datasets and combined with modern analytical techniques, can generate new insights from data which have the potential to improve care and allow much more specific targeting of public health interventions. However, data linkage also increases privacy concerns and may make it possible to identify an individual within a linked dataset when it would not be possible to do so from the original unlinked datasets. The controls that are in place to protect privacy are collectively termed information governance (IG). Information governance is a complex area which, in the UK and many other countries, is governed by legislation. Full details of the legislative frameworks used in the UK can be found elsewhere [22].

The linkage of datasets requires considerable computing power. Large public health data systems may house billions of individual data items. Ensuring that these systems are storing data efficiently and safely, with appropriate access control, is a complex task requiring the specialist skills of data engineers and architects. These complex storage systems may be linked to a set of web pages (a 'front end') which allows users to access the data in the form of a dashboard or visualisation. In the UK, the 'Fingertips' platform is a good example of this kind of technology. Fingertips [23] links back to a large data store and can display a wide range of public health profiles or dashboards, along with sophisticated visualisations.

Explore the 'Fingertips' database. How might you use specific profiles for your local population to inform practice and recommendations?

2.7 Understanding Inequalities and the Wider Determinants of Health

As well as understanding morbidity and mortality within a population, public health practitioners need to understand the behaviours that influence health and the wider determinants of health. Relevant behaviours include things like whether an individual smokes and what the prevalence of smoking is in a population. Wider determinants of health, sometimes referred to as social determinants, include a wide range of factors, as outlined in the graphic by Dahlgren and Whitehead (1991) (see Figure 1.3). Understanding the patterns of wider determinants at a local level is crucial in supporting targeted public health interventions.

2.7.1 Routine Administrative Data

In the UK and many other countries, some of these data can be obtained from routine sources. For example:
- primary care data often include quite good information (e.g. about smoking status);
- local government holds data about housing, social care and local education services;
- tax authorities hold data on income and possibly welfare benefits; and
- police and highways authorities collect data on road traffic accidents.

However, unless these data can be linked or accessed at an individual level, they may not be useful in building an understanding of the health status across a population.

Many routine data sources will include information about protected characteristics such as gender and ethnicity. Such data are essential for exploring potential inequalities in health and outcomes between groups with different protected characteristics.

However, the recording of information about protected characteristics is variable as it relies heavily on individuals being willing to disclose information about themselves which they may not feel is relevant or necessary.

2.7.2 Surveys

Population surveys are an important source of data on both the wider determinants of health and the behaviours that influence health. Population surveys may be carried out at a national level, for example a regular census of the population, or they may be carried out at a more local level, for example across a local government area or the catchment of a health centre. In the UK, there are several national topic-specific surveys, for example the National Child Measurement Programme [24], the Active Lives Survey [25] and the National Diet and Nutrition Survey [26]. The National Child Measurement Programme aims to measure all children at specific ages within scope, but the limited sample sizes of the other two surveys that are mentioned mean that they do not provide very granular data. Although an essential tool for supplementing routine data sources, surveys are time-consuming and expensive. They are often subject to low response rates, unless a response is mandated such as in a census, and the data collected are usually self-reported.

2.7.3 Inequalities and Measuring Deprivation

Public health practitioners are interested in measuring inequalities with a view to being able to address them through appropriate interventions (see Chapter 14). Inequalities exist between sub-groups within the population. Sometimes these sub-groups are easy to define, for example data on gender are often collected as part of health datasets and so differences in morbidity or mortality between males and females can be identified easily. Other sub-groups may be harder to define, for example there are known differences in health outcomes between different ethnic groups; however, ethnicity is not straightforward to record, and many routine datasets have poor-quality data about ethnicity.

Inequalities are strongly associated with socioeconomic factors. Individual socioeconomic factors can usually be defined, but gaining an overall sense of socioeconomic deprivation requires the use of a composite measure in which measures of several individual factors are combined to produce a single measure of deprivation. Composite measures are complex and have limitations, but there are several composite measures of deprivation which have become widely known and used in the UK [27]:

- English Indices of Multiple Deprivation;
- Townsend score;
- Carstairs deprivation index; and
- Jarman score.

How could you compare inequalities for your local population with other similar 'statistical neighbours'?

The first of these, the Indices of Multiple Deprivation, are probably the most used in the UK, having first been developed in the 1970s. The Indices are made up of 39 indicators spread across seven domains and are calculated separately for England, Scotland, Wales and Northern Ireland, although not at a UK level:

- income;
- employment;
- health deprivation and disability;
- education, skills and training;
- crime;
- barriers to housing and services;
- living environment.

The Indices of Multiple Deprivation (IMD), Townsend score and the Carstairs deprivation index are relative measures of deprivation and result in a ranking of areas from least to most deprived. They can show how an area compares with other areas, but cannot be used to produce a time trend for a particular area. Townsend and Carstairs both use four indicators derived from the UK census and, like the Indices of Multiple Deprivation, have been used over the years to assist in allocating financial resources, although these days IMD tends to predominate.

Jarman scores were not developed as a measure of deprivation. They were created to measure GP workload and, therefore, help with resource allocation in primary care. They also used some census variables alongside information from GPs themselves. Over time, they started to be used as a proxy measure of deprivation. They are rarely used now, although they may still appear in the academic literature.

There are several limitations in all measures of deprivation. For example, the choice of variables is a particular issue – a good example of this being car ownership. Typically, car ownership is associated with living in a less deprived area; however, the absence of public transport in many deprived rural areas means that car ownership levels can be high, while in less deprived urban areas with good public transport car ownership has reduced in recent years. The utility of a specific variable may decrease over time. An example of this would be indicators of access to services such as post offices or banks. Closures of many of these local services as they move online alters how an access indicator would be interpreted now compared with a few years ago.

An alternative to using the standard measures of deprivation is to use geodemographic approaches to identify specific sub-groups within the population which may have similar characteristics. This is often done using commercial data sources, which combine routinely available data with geographical data and commercial data such as food sales and financial data.

2.8 Introduction to Predictive Approaches

The uses of information that have been covered so far are largely descriptive in nature. They use information which is either routinely available or specially collected for the purpose to describe a population, risk factors and behaviours in a population that influence health outcomes, and specific diseases, whether infectious or not.

Increasingly, health information is used to attempt to predict health outcomes. A simple example of this is where a population is 'segmented' using information about a range of population characteristics. Population segments can then be targeted for active case finding (e.g. for diabetes or hypertension) because it is known that a particular segment's characteristics are associated with a high prevalence of those conditions.

Much more sophisticated analytical techniques, often using machine learning algorithms, are being used to try and predict which individuals are at greatest risk of a particular outcome. This is often used in managing hospital services, but is also starting to be used in targeting prevention interventions - sometimes referred to as 'personalised prevention'. An example would be the use of smart devices that collect data about an individual's physical activity level then being used to deliver messages and interventions designed to change the device owner's behaviour.

2.9 Conclusions

The collation of the information described in this chapter to form succinct health profiles, which can be updated and utilised effectively, requires considerable skill - and effort. Observatories have been founded in some countries, and globally, to facilitate access to the data (such as the World Health Organization's Global Health Observatory, which brings together health data at a country level). In other countries, such as England, national public health organisations undertake much of this work on behalf of local systems. However, much of the data can only be found at small population levels and must be obtained through bespoke collection systems. Local interpretation is required of all data to enable appropriate public health action to be taken in the context of more anecdotal and qualitative information.

Public health practitioners must be familiar with the indicators that are established to monitor the health status of our communities. These indicators also help us to understand and evaluate the effects of current interventions and programmes. For some indicators, new research will be required to generate the information needed.

REFERENCES

1. UN Department of Economic and Social Affairs, Why population growth matters for sustainable development, United Nations, 2022. Available at: www.un.org/development/desa/pd/sites/www.un.org.development.desa.pd/files/undesa_pd_2022_policy_brief_population_growth.pdf

2. United Nations, Population. Available at: www.un.org/en/global-issues/population

3. D. Eayres, Commonly used public health statistics and their confidence intervals, Association of Public Health Observatories, March 2008, reprinted April 2010.

4. UN Institute of Migration, World Migration Report 2022, 2022. Available at: https://worldmigrationreport.iom.int/wmr-2022-interactive/

5. Office for National Statistics, Population and migration, 2022. Available at: www.ons.gov.uk/peoplepopulationandcommunity/populationandmigration

6. World Health Organization, International Statistical Classification of Diseases and Related Health Problems (ICD), 11th Revision, 2022. Available at: www.who.int/standards/classifications/classification-of-diseases

7. SNOMED International, 5-Step briefing (SNOMED CT), 2022. Available at: www.snomed.org/snomed-ct/five-step-briefing

8. Office for National Statistics, Life expectancies. Available at: www.ons.gov.uk/peoplepopulationandcommunity/birthsdeathsandmarriages/lifeexpectancies

9. World Health Organization, GHE: Life expectancy and Healthy life expectancy. Available at: www.who.int/data/gho/data/themes/topics/indicator-groups/indicator-group-details/GHO/life-expectancy-and-healthy-life-expectancy

10. E. MacKillop and S. Sheard, Quantifying life: Understanding the history of Quality-Adjusted Life-Years (QALYs), *Social Science & Medicine* **211**, 2018, 359–66.

11. M. Porta, *A Dictionary of Epidemiology*, 6th ed., Oxford, Oxford University Press, 2014.

12. NHS Digital, Hospital Episode Statistics (HES), 2022 [updated 6 June 2022]. Available at: https://digital.nhs.uk/data-and-information/data-tools-and-services/data-services/hospital-episode-statistics

13. Department of Health, *A Simple Guide to Payment by Results*, Leeds, Department of Health, 2012.

14. NHS England, Quality and Outcomes Framework (QOF) guidance for 2023/24. Available at: www.england.nhs.uk/gp/investment/gp-contract/quality-on-outcomes-framework-qof-changes/

15. Institute for Health Metrics and Evaluation, GBD Compare: United Kingdom. Available at: www.healthdata.org/united-kingdom

16. Royal College of General Practitioners, RCGP Research and Surveillance Centre (RSC). Available at: www.rcgp.org.uk/clinical-and-research/our-programmes/research-and-surveillance-centre

17. NHS Digital, General Practice Extraction Service (GPES). Available at: https://digital.nhs.uk/services/general-practice-extraction-service

18. Medicines & Healthcare products Regulatory Agency, Clinical Practice Research Datalink. Available at: https://cprd.com/

19. The Health Improvement Network, THIN. Available at: www.the-health-improvement-network.com/

20. NCRAS, The National Cancer Registration and Analysis Service [updated August 2022]. Available at: www.ncin.org.uk/home

21. A. Mayer and M. Stockdale, Developing standard tools for data linkage: February 2021. Available at: www.ons.gov.uk/methodology/methodologicalpublications/generalmethodology/onsworkingpaperseries/developingstandardtoolsfordatalinkagefebruary2021

22. NHS England, About information governance. Available at: www.england.nhs.uk/ig/about/

23. Office for Health Improvement & Disparities, Fingertips: Public health data. Available at: https://fingertips.phe.org.uk/

24. NHS Digital, National Child Measurement Programme, 2021 [updated 26 April 2021]. Available at: https://digital.nhs.uk/services/national-child-measurement-programme/

25. Sport England, Active Lives Online, 2022. Available at: https://activelives.sportengland.org/

26. Gov.uk, National Diet and Nutrition Survey, 2016 [updated 22 September 2021]. Available at: www.gov.uk/government/collections/national-diet-and-nutrition-survey

27. N. Dymond-Green, How can we calculate levels of deprivation or poverty in the UK? (part 1) [Blog], UK Data Service, 2020 [updated 24 June 2020]. Available at: https://blog.ukdataservice.ac.uk/deprived-or-live-in-poverty-1/

3

Epidemiology

Stephen Gillam and Mary Fortune

Key points

- Epidemiology concerns the study of the distribution and determinants of disease and health-related states.
- The uses of epidemiology include:
  - determination of the major health problems occurring in a community;
  - monitoring health and disease trends across populations;
  - making useful projections into the future and identifying emerging health problems;
  - describing the natural history of new conditions (e.g. who gets the disease, who dies from it and the outcome of the disease);
  - estimating clinical risks for individuals;
  - evaluating new health technologies (e.g. drugs or preventive programmes); and
  - investigating epidemics of unknown aetiology.

3.1 Introduction

At the core of epidemiology is the use of quantitative methods to study health, and how it may be improved, in populations. It can be defined as:

> the study of distribution and determinants of health related states and events in the population and the application of this science to control health problems. [1]

It is important to note that epidemiology concerns not only the study of diseases, but also of all health-related events - for example, we can study the epidemiology of breastfeeding or road traffic accidents. Rational health-promoting public policies require a sound understanding of causation. The epidemiological analysis of a disease or activity from a population perspective is vital in order to be able to organise and monitor effective preventive, curative and rehabilitative services. All health professionals and health-service managers need an awareness of the principles of epidemiology. They need to go beyond questions relating to individuals such as 'What should be done for this patient now?', to challenging fundamentals such as 'Why did *this* person get *this* disease at *this* time?', 'Is the occurrence of the disease increasing and, if so, why?' and 'What are the causes or risk factors for this disease?'

This chapter briefly considers the origins of epidemiology and then examines some of its key concepts, including:

- disease variation;
- the concept of a population;
- measures of disease frequency – rates;
- quantifying differences in risk;
- types of epidemiological study design; and
- how to interpret the results of epidemiological studies.

3.2 The History of Epidemiology

The origins of modern epidemiology can be traced back to the work of English reformers and French scientists in the first half of the nineteenth century. John Graunt laid the basis of health statistics and epidemiology with his analyses of the weekly bills of mortality in the seventeenth century. Using these data, Graunt described the patterns of mortality and fertility and seasonal variations charting the progress of epidemics, most famously in the plague years. In 1747, James Lind, a British naval surgeon, undertook a study testing his hypothesis of the cause of scurvy and the controlled clinical trial was born.

Building on the ideas of Graunt, William Farr institutionalised epidemiology in Victorian England. He developed a system of vital statistics that was to form the basis of disease classification and developed methods for studying the distribution and determinants of human diseases.

Twentieth-century epidemiologists have added to the body of knowledge on disease patterns and their causes in the population by meticulously studying large sections of the population with respect to particular conditions or risk factors. Examples of landmark studies are given later in the chapter.

3.3 Studying Disease Variation

3.3.1 Time, Place and Person

Epidemiologists describe and study health states and determinants in terms of 'time, place and person':

- How does the pattern of this disease vary over *time* in this population? A decline in disease is as interesting as a rise.

- How does the *place* in which the population lives affect the disease? International differences in disease patterns often reflect the different demographics of their populations.
- How do the *personal characteristics* of people in the population affect the disease's pattern? Disease is caused by interaction between the genome and the environment [2]. In large populations, genetic makeup is relatively stable, and so changes in disease frequency over short time periods are typically due to environmental factors. However, in individuals, genetic makeup is profoundly important in shaping risk of disease.

3.3.2 Quantifying and Understanding Disease Variation

Firstly, we must precisely define the population we are interested in and the exposure we wish to study. Next, we must choose how to quantify disease risk. If we are interested in a single population, we could give a measure of how *common* the disease is in the population or how common *new cases* of the disease are. If we are interested in comparing two populations, we could study the *absolute difference* or the *relative difference* in risk.

Next, we need to design a study which will not only measure the disease frequency within the population we have sampled, but also enable us to generalise our results to the wider population which we are truly interested in. We need to choose a study design which avoids *bias* (informally, measured outcomes within the study population which are not representative of the true outcomes in the general population) and be careful with interpretation. An association may be due to our having discovered a true causal factor for disease risk, or due to a *confounder* (a variable which is associated with both exposure and outcome).

Above all, we need to be aware of the role of random chance. Epidemiology focuses on population-level health. Applying the results of an epidemiological study to an individual patient is not straightforward. An individual may be at high risk of developing a disease, but that does not guarantee that they will be affected. Individuals with no apparent risk factors may still develop the disease. It is possible that, even if an exposure does not change disease risk, participants in the study who are exposed will, by random chance, develop the disease more often than those who are not exposed. In order to interpret an apparent difference in risk as meaningful in clinical practice, we must first ask ourselves: how likely is it that we would see a similar difference in risk by random chance, if there were truly no link between the exposure and the disease? These key concepts are all further explained below and illustrated with examples.

3.3.3 The Concept of a Population

Epidemiology and public health policy depend on the notion of a *population*. Traditionally, health systems have been designed around a population of people with health problems who contact the service seeking help – the 'tip' of the 'clinical iceberg' (see Figure 1.1). Public health specialists, however, have responsibility for the whole population or 'iceberg', including those who are at risk of health problems and those who have them at an early stage and are unknown to health services.

Even among the symptomatic, only some people seek formal health-care. People with symptomatic disease can be further subdivided into those who are symptomatic not seeking medical help, those who are symptomatic but self-treating, and those who are symptomatic but accessing informal care. Below the surface there are a large number who may have latent, pre-symptomatic, undiagnosed disease. However, not all people without symptoms can be described as in perfect health. Many people may have risk factors that make them more prone to various diseases: for example, smoking, sedentary lifestyle and obesity put people at increased risk of coronary heart disease (see Chapter 12).

In order to quantify disease variation, we first need to define clearly the population of interest. This might vary from an entire country to a small community. It may be restricted by the disease studied (e.g. those suffering from diabetes). When the population is defined, we can then consider how the pattern of disease varies. This will allow us to plan services based on the pattern of disease in the population as a whole and not just among users of the service. We can also deliver modified services to sub-groups of the population who differ in terms of their needs and are not making effective use of existing services (e.g. homeless, non-native-language-speaking). Finally, by using knowledge of population trends and health status, we can anticipate the need for future services (see Chapter 2).

Populations may be *stable* or *dynamic*. A stable population is known as a cohort (a group of people with common characteristics). The population is defined at the start of the follow-up period and gradually diminishes in size as its members cease to be at risk of becoming a case (e.g. they die). In contrast, a dynamic population is one in which there is turnover of membership while it is being observed. People enter and leave the population at different times.

3.3.4 Epidemiological Variables

Disease patterns are influenced by the interaction of factors (variables) at social, environmental and individual levels. Consideration of these factors aids in the depiction, analysis and interpretation of differences in disease patterns within and between populations. Age, sex, economic status, social class, occupation, country of residence or birth and racial or ethnic classifications may be used to show variations in health status. Most variables used in epidemiology are proxies for complex, underlying phenomena that either cannot be measured easily or are poorly understood. For example, we might measure obesity levels in a population as a marker for the risk of diabetes.

A good epidemiological variable should:
- have an impact on health in individuals and populations;
- be measurable;
- differentiate populations in their experience of disease and health;
- differentiate populations in some underlying characteristics relevant to health (e.g. income or behaviour);
- generate testable aetiological hypotheses; and
- help to: develop health policy; and/or plan and deliver health-care; and/or prevent and control disease.

Worked example: Applying criteria for a good epidemiological variable

Table 3.1 Age as a useful epidemiological variable

Criteria for a good epidemiological variable	Criteria in relation to the factor age
Impact on health in individuals and population	Age is a powerful influence on health; chronological age is related to the general health of the individual.
Be measurable accurately	In most populations age is measurable to the day, but in some it has to be guessed.
Differentiate populations in their experience of disease or health	Large differences by age are seen for most diseases or their determinants.
Generate testable aetiological hypotheses	It is hard to test hypotheses because there are so many underlying differences between populations of different ages.
Help in developing health policy, and/or help to plan and deliver health-care and/or help to prevent and control disease	Age differences in disease patterns could affect health policy and planning of services. Knowing the age structure of a population is critical to good planning. By understanding the age at which diseases start, preventive and control programmes can be targeted appropriately.

Once we have identified that a disease varies according to such factors, we can begin to consider how the factor exerts an effect. For example, it is well known that the occurrence of heart disease is more common in men than women. Some of the possible explanations for this include differences in lifestyle factors, occupations and levels of co-existing diseases.

Geographical differences in epidemiological variables can also provide important clues to the causes of disease.

 For each of these qualities, consider whether geographical location can be considered a useful epidemiological variable.

3.3.4.1 Measures of Disease Frequency – Single Population

One measure of disease frequency is a count of the number of cases of a disease occurring in a population. However, the number of cases alone is not particularly informative. Account must also be taken of the size of the population and the length of time over which its members were observed. This gives rise to a comparison between the number of cases in the population and the size of the population, often expressed as a rate.

It is important to understand the difference between a risk and a rate.

- A **risk**, in this context, is the probability of having the outcome of interest – we calculate the disease risk as the number of cases in our population of interest.
- A **rate**, in this context, measures the frequency of the outcome of interest – we calculate the disease rate as the number of new cases in our population of interest over a specified time period per total person time.

The numerator of a rate is the number of 'cases', but defining cases can be difficult. For some diseases (e.g. rabies) case definition is clear; for others (such as hypertension) the disease shows a spectrum of severity and arbitrary criteria must be imposed to distinguish diseased from non-diseased.

In calculating a pregnancy rate, what might be an appropriate denominator?

The denominator of a rate is the 'population at risk' and this too must be carefully defined. For example, the ideal denominator for a pregnancy rate is dependent on the culture of the population being measured. In some cases, it is married women in the specific age groups. However, in some cultures, the denominator would not be restricted to married women. This leaves us with a problem if pregnancy rates are compared across populations, as the denominators do not match.

3.3.4.2 Prevalence

A measure of the burden of disease in a population is the *prevalence*. This is the number of cases of disease in a population at a given time and it is frequently used in planning the allocation of health-service resources. Generally, we use the term prevalence to mean a *point prevalence*, which is defined as follows:

$$\text{Point prevalence} = \frac{\text{Number of diseased persons in a defined population at one point in time}}{\text{Number of persons in the defined population at the same moment in time}} \quad (3.1)$$

Point prevalence is a proportion and does not involve time. *Period prevalence* is the number of cases of disease during a specified time (e.g. a week, month or year). When the period is long, the denominator is usually the number of persons at the midpoint of the time period (e.g. the mid-year population).

$$\text{Period prevalence} = \frac{\text{Number of diseased persons in a defined population during a specified period in time}}{\text{Number of persons in the defined population over the same period of time}} \quad (3.2)$$

3.3.4.3 Incidence

When researching the aetiology of diseases, measures of disease *incidence* are of primary interest. Cases of incident disease in a defined period of time are those which first occur during that time. There are two ways of expressing disease incidence: risk (or cumulative incidence) and incidence rate, but in most situations these give very similar results.

Risk is defined as the number of cases that occur in a defined period of time as a proportion of the number of people in the population at the beginning of the period:

$$\text{Risk in defined period of time} = \frac{\text{Number of persons who become diseased (or die) during the period}}{\text{Number of persons in the population at the beginning of the period}} \quad (3.3)$$

Risk is the probability of harm. It describes the way that populations as a whole experience disease. However, it may also be thought of as the risk an individual has of developing the disease in the specified period of time. Risk may also be known as *cumulative incidence.*

Incidence rate is defined as the number of new cases (or deaths) occurring in a defined period of time in a defined population. The sum of the periods of time for each individual when they are disease-free but may develop the disease is the denominator and is known as the person–time at risk.

$$\text{Incidence rate} = \frac{\text{Number of persons who have become diseased}}{\text{Person–time at risk}} \quad (3.4)$$

Figure 3.1 shows two populations, A and B, which are observed for 10 years. Over time, members of the populations die. The length of time each person spends alive

Figure 3.1 Populations at risk of death.

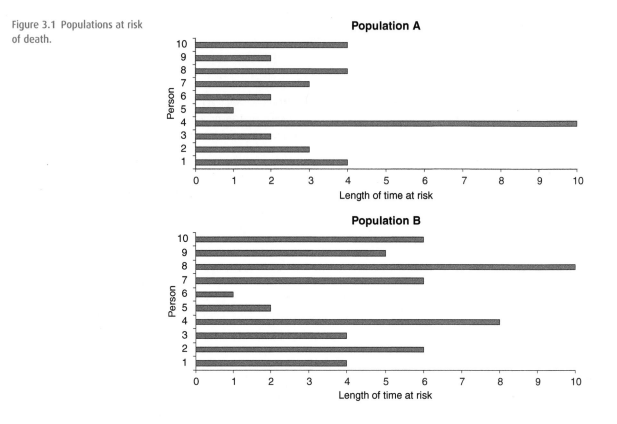

Figure 3.2 Incidence in dynamic populations.

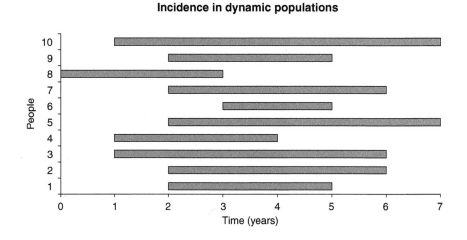

(and therefore at risk of death) is shown by the bars on the charts. Similar calculations can be done for dynamic populations. Figure 3.2 shows how incidence might look in a dynamic population.

Worked examples:

For population A:

- Person–time at risk = 10 people with 4 + 3 + 2 + 10 + 1 + 2 + 3 + 4 + 2 + 4 years at risk. Person–time at risk = 35 person years.
- Incidence rate at 10 years = 9 people who died/35 person years at risk = 0.257 people per year (number of cases is 9 as one person remains alive at the end of the period).

For population B:

- Person–time at risk = 10 people with 4 + 6 + 4 + 8 + 2 + 1 + 6 + 10 + 5 + 6 years at risk. Person–time at risk = 52 person years.
- Incidence rate = 9/52 = 0.173 people per year.
- Risk at 10 years = 9/10 = 0.9 people per year.

Calculate the risk and incidence for populations A and B.

Calculate the incidence in the dynamic population shown in Figure 3.2: person–time at risk at the end of year 7; incidence rate after 7 years; and the risk of the condition at the end of year 3.

Worked example:

a. Person–time at risk = 3 + 4 + 5 + 3 + 5 + 2 + 4 + 3 + 3 + 6 = 38 person years.
b. Incidence rate = 8/38 = 21.1% (two people remain at risk at the end of the period and are not counted in the numerator for incidence rate).
c. The total person years at the end of year 3 is (1 + 1 + 2 + 2 + 1 + 0 + 1 + 3 + 1 + 2 = 14) and person 8 died. Hence, the risk of the condition at the end of year 3 is 1/14, i.e. 7.14%.

Sometimes direct measurement of person–time at risk is not possible. This is true for mortality rates where we do not know when each individual became at risk (i.e. we do not know exact birth dates) or stopped being at risk (i.e. we do not know exact dates of death). Instead, as with estimates of period prevalence, an estimate of the person–time at risk is taken to be the population at the midpoint of the calendar period of interest × the length of the period (usually a year).

For example, the all-cause mortality rate for females in England and Wales for 2022 is defined as:

$$\text{Mortality rate per year} = \frac{\begin{array}{c}\text{Number of female deaths from all causes}\\ \text{in England and Wales in 2022}\end{array}}{\begin{array}{c}\text{Estimate of 2022 mid-year female population}\\ \text{of England and Wales}\end{array}} \qquad (3.5)$$

3.3.4.4 Relationship between Prevalence, Incidence and Duration of Disease

Figure 3.3 shows the prevalent population as the circle on the right and people entering this as incident cases from the non-diseased population on the left.

Figure 3.3 The relationship between prevalence and incidence.

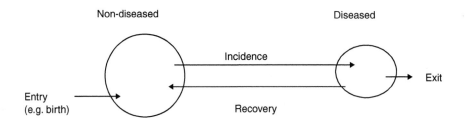

In a fixed population, prevalence rate is approximately equal to the incidence rate (the number of people entering the prevalent population in a defined period of time) multiplied by the duration of the disease (how long they stay there):

$$\text{Prevalence} = \text{Incidence rate} \times \text{Period of follow-up} \qquad (3.6)$$

For conditions with a long duration, prevalence is a good estimate of the burden of disease, but for conditions with a short duration, incidence is a better measure.

Worked example: Incidence and prevalence

10,000 miners were recruited to a study. At baseline, 50 were found to have lung cancer and were excluded from follow-up. The remainder underwent six-monthly reviews for 5 years. At the end of 5 years, nine miners had developed lung cancer.

a. What was the prevalence of lung cancer at baseline?
Prevalence at baseline = 50/10,000 = 0.5%.
b. What was the risk of developing lung cancer over 5 years?
Risk or cumulative incidence over 5 years = 9/9,950 = 0.905 per 1,000.
c. What is the approximate incidence rate of lung cancer among miners?
Incidence rate = 9/(9,950 × 5) = 0.181 per 1,000 person years.

d. Why is it only an approximation?
It is assumed that each person contributed a full 5 years of follow-up to the denominator and that a diagnosis of lung cancer is accurate, both at baseline and follow-up. However, it is likely that some either dropped out of the study or died of some other cause before the end of the 5 years.

3.3.4.5 Case Fatality and Survival Rates
The terms case fatality and survival rate are often used to compare the lethality of diseases. As they do not measure the rate per unit of time at risk at which death occurs, they are probabilities (forms of risk), not true rates. The case fatality rate is the ratio of deaths to cases, measuring the proportion of people with a disease (e.g. cancer) who die within a defined period of diagnosis. If we assume that all cases either die or survive, the case fatality rate is related to the survival rate from a disease:

$$\text{Probability (survival)} + \text{Probability (death)} = 1 \tag{3.7}$$

3.3.5 Quantifying Differences in Risk

Epidemiologists often compare rates of disease across populations. These may be populations with different risk factors, or populations who are being treated differently for a disease they already have.

The word 'risk' is a common one. However, in epidemiology, it has a specific meaning which can lead to confusion.

- Often, 'risk' has a negative connotation. This chapter uses risk of disease as its exemplar. However, some of the outcomes we might want to measure are positive outcomes (recovery from disease, improvement of symptoms).
- Often, 'risk' can be poorly defined. Consider 'the increased risk of COVID-19 for a patient with hypertension'. What does this mean? The probability that someone with hypertension will catch COVID-19? The possibility that someone with hypertension is likely to have worse outcomes if they catch COVID-19? How much more likely they are to have one of these outcomes than someone without hypertension?
- Sometimes the exposure being studied increases the risk of the outcome (the effect of smoke exposure on cancer occurrence) and sometimes it decreases the risk (the effect of adjuvant chemotherapy on cancer reoccurrence). Mathematically, Number Needed to Treat and Number Needed to Harm are computed in very similar ways. However, the clinical implications are very different.

Many of the concepts in the following section have more than one name. 'Relative Risk' and 'Risk Ratio' have identical meanings (and are both commonly abbreviated 'RR'). 'Attributable Risk', 'Risk Difference', 'Excess Risk' and 'Absolute Risk Reduction' have identical meanings.

3.3.5.1 Relative Risk

Relative risk tells us how much more at risk one population is than another. For example, we might want to compare how many children with meningitis die if they are treated using antibiotics alone with how many die if they are additionally given steroids. To begin, we must define the risk in both populations. There are two main ways of summarising this: as a proportion or as an odd.

For example, if 320 children developed meningitis during one year and 32 died, this can be expressed as a proportion: 32/320 (10%) – i.e. 32 children die for every 320 who get meningitis; or it can be expressed as the odds of dying: 32/288 – i.e. 32 children die for every 288 with meningitis who survive. Then, to compare the risk in two groups we can calculate the ratio between the risk measured in one group and the risk measured in the other group (i.e. divide the risk in one group by the risk in the other group).

The Relative Risk of death due to lung cancer among smokers is 15.34 compared to non-smokers. The same study found that the Relative Risk in smokers for coronary heart disease (CHD) was 1.45. What is your interpretation of these findings?

Worked example: Calculating relative risks of giving up smoking

In a trial of nicotine gum, a group of smokers were given gum and a control group were not. Out of 6,328 smokers who were given nicotine gum, 1,149 stopped smoking. Out of 8,380 smokers in the control group, 893 stopped. So the numbers who did not give up smoking is 6,328 – 1,149 = 5,179 and 8,380 – 893 = 7,487 respectively.

These figures can be shown on a 2 × 2 contingency table:

Table 3.2 A 2 × 2 table for calculating relative risks of giving up smoking

	Given nicotine gum	No nicotine gum
Gave up smoking	1,149	893
Did not give up	5,179	7,487
Total	**6,328**	**8,380**

The Relative Risk = risk of stopping smoking in nicotine-gum group/risk of stopping smoking in the control group = (1,149/6,328)/(893/8,380) = 1.70.

The Odds Ratio = odds of stopping smoking in the nicotine-gum group/odds of stopping smoking in the control group = (1,149/5,179)/(893/7,487) = 1.86.

This can be put into words:

- Someone who uses nicotine gum is 1.7 times more likely to give up smoking as someone who does not.
- The odds of someone stopping smoking if they use nicotine gum are 1.86 times greater than if they don't.

Note here that the word 'risk' has been applied to a desirable outcome (stopping smoking), rather than to a bad outcome. Relative risks and odds ratios can be used as a measure of the *strength of association* between a risk factor and an outcome (e.g. smoking and lung cancer) or a measure of the effectiveness of an intervention in causing an outcome (e.g. nicotine gum and stopping smoking).

When can Relative Risks and Odds Ratios be used? Relative Risks and Odds Ratios can both be calculated in cohort studies (described later in the section).

Relative Risks cannot be calculated in case-control studies, since in a case-control study, the investigators have artificially changed the prevalence by selecting the proportion of cases and controls to include. However, Odds Ratios can be calculated in case-control studies where we can derive the odds of exposure among cases (those with the condition of interest) and the odds of exposure in controls (those without the condition of interest).

In instances when the condition under study is rare, the Odds Ratio is approximately equal to the Relative Risk.

Worked example:

In the nicotine-gum example from earlier, the Relative Risk and the Odds Ratio are similar (1.70 and 1.86). Imagine that the prevalence of stopping smoking was much higher (Table 3.3):

Table 3.3 A 2 × 2 table for calculating relative risks for higher prevalence of smoking

	Given nicotine gum	No nicotine gum
Gave up smoking	3,000	2,000
Did not give up	3,328	6,380
Total	**6,328**	**8,380**

Calculating the Relative Risk and Odds Ratio now:

Relative Risk = (3,000/6,328)/(2,000/8,380) = 1.994
Odds Ratio = (3,000/3,328)/(2,000/6,380) = 2.87

The Relative Risk is now much smaller than the Odds Ratio. We cannot assume that an Odds Ratio quoted in a study for a very common outcome would be the same as a Relative Risk.

3.3.5.2 Absolute Risk Reduction

The *absolute risk reduction* (ARR) is the difference in the absolute risk (rates of adverse events) between study and control populations:

$$\text{Absolute risk reduction(ARR)} = \text{Risk in unexposed (control event rate, CER)}$$
$$- \text{Risk in exposed (experimental event rate, EER)}$$

$$(3.8)$$

The ARR is a measure of the absolute effect of exposure. It may be estimated in cohort studies, but not in case-control studies (see below).

In the case where the study population are at higher risk than the control population, we instead calculate the *absolute risk increase* (ARI), which is computed similarly:

$$\text{Absolute risk increase(ARI)} = \text{Risk in exposed(experimental event rate, EER)}$$
$$- \text{Risk in unexposed(control event rate, CER)}$$

$$(3.9)$$

In a clinical trial, the event rate in the control group is 40 per 100 patients, and the event rate in the treatment group is 30 per 100 patients. Calculate the Relative Risk and ARR.

3.3.5.3 Number Needed to Treat (NNT)

The *number needed to treat* is a summary measure of absolute risk that is helpful in making decisions over which interventions are effective. The NNT is the number of people who (on average) need to receive a treatment to produce one additional successful outcome. If, for example, NNT for a treatment is 10, the practitioner would have to give the treatment to ten patients to prevent one patient from having the adverse outcome over the defined period, and each patient who received the treatment would have a one in ten chance of being a beneficiary.

3.3.5.3.1 Calculation of NNT

If a disease has a death rate of 100% without treatment and treatment reduces that mortality rate to 50%, the ARR is (100/100 – 50/100) = 0.5. How many people would we need to treat to prevent one death? In this example, treating 100 patients with the otherwise fatal disease results in 50 survivors. This is equivalent to one out of every two treated, an NNT of 2.

Alternatively, the NNT to prevent one adverse outcome equals the inverse of the absolute risk reduction, i.e. NNT = 1/ARR.

> **Worked examples:**
>
> **Out of 6,328 smokers who were given nicotine gum, 1,149 stopped smoking.**
>   **Out of 8,380 smokers in the control group, 893 stopped smoking. What is the NNT?**
>   NNT = 1/ARR = 1/(1,149/6,328) – (893/8,380) = 1/(0.182 – 0.107) = 1/0.075 = 13.3. NNT is always rounded up and in this case it will be 14.
>   The ARR and the NNT give different information from Relative Risk and the Odds Ratio because they take into account the baseline frequency of the outcome.
>
> **A drug reduces the risk of dying from a heart attack by 40% (Relative Risk = 0.60). In terms of Relative Risk, this drug has the same 'clinical effectiveness' for everyone. Calculate the NNT if it is given to people with a 1 in 10 annual risk of dying from a heart attack and to people with a 1 in 100 risk.**
>   For a risk of 1/10:
>   The original risk is 1/10 (0.1) and with the drug $0.6 \times 1/10 = 0.06$
>   So the ARR is 0.1 – 0.06 = 0.04 and the NNT = 1/0.04 = 25
>
>   For a risk of 1/100:
>   The original risk is 1/100 (0.01) and with the drug $0.6 \times 1/100 = 0.006$
>   So the ARR is 0.01 – 0.006 = 0.004
>
>   And the NNT = 1/0.004 = 250
>
> So we can see that the NNT is much higher when the risk of the condition (incidence rate) is lower. If the drug causes serious side effects in 1 in 100 people, then we would probably not use it for people with a low risk, but it would still be an effective treatment for people with high baseline risk. So the NNT helps us estimate how likely the treatment is to help an individual patient.

3.3.5.3.2 Number Needed to Harm

When an exposure leads to an increased risk, then we calculate the Number Needed to Harm (NNH) – the number of people who (on average) need to be exposed in order to produce one more case of the outcome. It is calculated similarly to the NNT.

If a disease has a prevalence of 50% without the exposure and exposure increases that risk to 100%, the ARI is (100/100 – 50/100) = 0.5. How many people would need to be exposed to result in one more case of the disease? In this example, exposing 100 patients results in 50 additional cases. This is equivalent to one out of every two exposed, an NNH of 2.

Alternatively, the NNH to lead to one adverse outcome equals the inverse of the absolute risk increase, i.e. NNT = 1/ARI.

3.3.5.4 Relative vs Absolute Measures of Risks

Generally, Relative Risks are more useful for expressing a population and Absolute Risks are more useful when considering individuals.

If the risk of recurrence of a cancer goes from 5% down to 2.5% after treatment with a new drug, the Relative Risk reduction is 50% (2.5%/5% = 50%), but the Absolute Risk reduction is only 2.5% (5% - 2.5% = 2.5%). So, any one individual, who has a small risk to begin with, reduces their risk by a small absolute amount. However, across a population, this may be a significant risk reduction. Indeed, the NNT is 40 (100%/(5% - 2.5%) = 40): for every 40 patients we treat, we would expect to prevent a recurrence in one of them.

3.3.5.5 Measures of Population Impact

We also may wish to measure what proportion of death or disease can be attributed to specific causes.

For individuals, the Absolute Risk Increase (ARI) is also referred to as the *Attributable Risk* (AR), usually expressed as a percentage.

$$AR = \frac{(\text{Incidence in exposed} - \text{Incidence in unexposed}) \times 100}{\text{Incidence in exposed}} \tag{3.10}$$

This is the rate of disease occurrence or death ('risk') in a group that is exposed to a particular factor, which can be attributed to that factor. For example, in deciding whether or not to indulge in a dangerous sport such as rock climbing, the attributable risk of injury (i.e. the risk due solely to the rock climbing and not other causes) must be weighed against the pleasures of participation.

For populations, the *population attributable risk =*

attributable risk × prevalence of exposure to risk factor in population; or: (3.11)

Population attributable risk = Rate in population − Rate in unexposed

The population attributable risk tells us what proportion of a population's disease or death experience is due to a particular cause and can indicate the potential impact of control measures in a population (i.e. what proportion of disease would be eliminated in a population if its disease rate were reduced to that of unexposed persons). Population attributable risk is, therefore, particularly relevant to decisions in public health. The following exercises examine the risks attributable to smoking at a population level.

Worked example: A classic study of smoking and mortality [3, 4]

The British Doctors' Study

The British Doctors' Study was set up in 1951 to investigate the relationship between smoking habits and mortality. A total of 59,600 members of the medical profession in the UK were asked to fill in a simple questionnaire on smoking habits.

Complete replies were received from 34,440 men (about 69% of the male doctors alive when the questionnaire was sent). 17% of these were classified as non-smokers. In the first 20 years of follow-up (1951–71) a total of 10,000 deaths occurred, 441 of which were from lung cancer and 3191 from ischaemic heart disease (IHD); see Table 3.4.

Table 3.4 The British Doctors' Study [4]. Death rate for men by cause of death and cigarette smoking habit

	Death rate per 1,000	
Cause of death	Smokers	Non-smokers
Lung cancer	0.9	0.07
IHD	4.87	4.22

Table 3.5 Exercise on elativerisk and population attributable risk [4].

	Annual death rates per 100,000 from lung disease
Heavy smokers	224
Non-smokers	10
Total population	74

a. **Calculate relative risks (as Relative Risks) and attributable risk for the data in Table 3.4 relative to non-smokers.**
b. **(i)** Which disease is most strongly related to cigarette smoking?
   (ii) Which disease has the largest number of deaths statistically attributable to cigarette smoking?
      a. The Relative Risks are 12.86 (0.9/0.07) for lung cancer and 1.15 (4.87/4.22) for IHD. The attributable risk is 92% ([0.9 – 0.07] 10.9 × 100) for lung cancer and 13.3% ([4.87 – 4.22] 14.87 × 100) for CHD.
      b. (i) The data show that 92% of lung cancer is attributable to smoking and 13.3% of CHD. In CHD both Relative Risk and AR are not very high suggesting not less of the disease could be prevented, when compared to lung cancer.
      (ii) Ischaemic heart disease.

From Table 3.5, calculate the Relative Risk and population attributable risk of lung disease associated with smoking.
Relative Risk for heavy smokers 224/10 = 22.4
Compared to non-smokers
Population attributable risk 74 – 10 = 64 deaths per 100,000 person years

3.3.6 Summary

Table 3.6 summarises the concepts explained so far in the epidemiological description of disease (or risk factors) by time, place and person.

Table 3.6 Summary of concepts

Concept	Definition	Comment
Dynamic population	Population in which person–time experience can accumulate from a changing group of individuals	Ideal in cohort studies as everyone contributes to the denominator
Static population	Fixed population with no loss to follow-up	Difficult to achieve as people tend to drop out of studies
Period prevalence	The number of existing cases of an illness during a period or interval, divided by the average population	A problem may arise with calculating period prevalence rates because of the difficulty of defining the most appropriate denominator
Point prevalence	The prevalence of a condition in a population at a given point in time	Prevalence data provide an indication of the extent of a condition and may have implications for the provision of services needed in a community
Incidence	Number of new cases in a defined period of time	Used in cohort studies
Risk	Risk can be thought of as a probability of developing disease	Preventive measures try and address risk factors
Incidence rate	The proportion of new cases of the target disorder in the population at risk during a specified time interval. It is usual to define the disorder, the population and the time, and is reported as a rate	Can be calculated in cohort studies
Relative Risk	Incidence among exposed/incidence among unexposed	Important in aetiological enquiries
Risk ratio	Another term for relative risk	Important in aetiological enquiries
Odds Ratio	Ratio of odds of exposure in cases and controls	Used for studying associations
	In cohort studies, it is the odds of outcome in exposed and unexposed	Can be used in cohort studies
Absolute risk reduction	The absolute arithmetic difference in rates of unwanted outcomes between experimental and control participants in a trial, calculated as the control event rate (CER) minus the experimental event rate (EER)	Inverse of this provides number needed to treat (see below)
Number needed to treat (NNT)	The inverse of the absolute risk reduction or increase and the number of patients that need to be treated for one to benefit compared with a control NNT = 1/ARR	The ideal NNT is 1, where everyone has improved with treatment and no one has with control. Broadly, the higher the NNT, the less effective the intervention
Attributable fraction	The risk of disease occurrence or death ('risk') in a group that is exposed to a particular factor, which can be attributed to that factor attributable risk = (incidence in exposed − incidence in unexposed) × 100/incidence in exposed	This suggests the amount of disease that might be eliminated if the factor under study could be controlled or eliminated

Table 3.6 (*cont.*)

Concept	Definition	Comment
Population attributable risk or risk fraction	The difference between event rates in populations exposed or unexposed to a risk factor Population attributable risk = rate in population – rate in non-exposed Or Population attributable fraction = attributable risk × prevalence of exposure to risk factor in population	This provides an estimate of the amount by which the disease could be reduced in the population if the suspected factor is eliminated or modified

3.4 Types of Epidemiological Study

We now move on to consider how various epidemiological study designs help answer questions about health and health-care:

- **Description**. What is the extent of disease or risk factors in this population?
- **Prognosis**. How does this disease progress; what is its natural history?
- **Aetiology**. What are the causes of disease? Which risk factors are associated with disease?
- **Prevention/treatment**. How well does an intervention work to prevent or treat a condition?

Different types of study will help us answer the different questions above. Hennekens and Buring [1] classified epidemiological design strategies (see Box 3.2).

Box 3.2 Epidemiological study designs

Descriptive studies
    Population (correlation/ecological studies)
    Individual
        Case reports
        Case series
        Cross-sectional surveys
Analytical studies
    Observational studies
        Case-control studies
        Cohort studies
    Interventional studies
        Clinical trials

Descriptive studies help us to describe the health status of the population being studied, whereas *analytical* studies, which can be interventional or observational in nature, are employed to test hypotheses or establish aetiology. Interventional studies, in particular, are often used to study ways of treating or preventing a disease.

Epidemiological studies can be retrospective (i.e. study data are collected and analysed after the outcome being studied has occurred) or prospective (i.e. studies where participants who have not yet experienced the outcome of interest are monitored going forward). There are advantages and disadvantages to each. Retrospective studies can be cheaper and quicker to do, since existing data can be analysed. However, important data may not be available. Prospective studies can be tailored to answer a specific research question, but the burden of data collection is greater.

3.4.1 Descriptive Studies

These studies attempt to describe patterns of diseases within and between populations. They seek to answer the question 'What is the extent of disease or risk factors in this population?' They often use routinely collected data to identify relationships between the prevalence of disease and other variables such as time, place and personal characteristics. Data collection can take place at the level of the population or individual. A descriptive study does not seek to make generalisations to a wider population, nor does it seek to make inferences about causal effects.

3.4.1.1 Population Studies

In population studies, also called correlation or ecological studies, the unit of analysis is an aggregate of individuals. Information is collected on this group rather than on individual members. The statistical relationship between exposure and outcome is calculated using correlation coefficients.

For example, we could study childhood immunisation coverage at ward level using the Index of Multiple Deprivation (see Chapters 2 and 14 for information on IMD). Here, both deprivation (exposure) and immunisation coverage (outcome) are measured at ward level.

However, there are two problems with this approach. Firstly, the observed association may be due to confounding factors (see below). Secondly, observations made at population or aggregate levels may not be true at an individual level (the 'ecological fallacy'). Ecological studies generate hypotheses, but cannot test them.

3.4.1.2 Individual Studies

These are *case reports*, *case series* and *cross-sectional studies*. A case report describes the medical details of one case of disease, for instance in the post-marketing surveillance of licensed drugs when rare adverse outcomes not found in original studies may be seen. Case series (descriptions of several patients) can also be useful in generating hypotheses for further testing, for example when investigating out-breaks of communicable disease (see Chapter 10).

In cross-sectional studies, both exposure and outcome are measured at individual and population level at the same point in time. Classical examples are the health and lifestyle surveys undertaken in various populations. In the Health Survey for England, various health determinants and health-status indicators are measured in a sample of the English population (see Chapter 2). The major disadvantage of this design is that it cannot determine whether the outcome preceded the exposure or was due to the exposure, as both are measured simultaneously. Hence, this is not the study design best suited to testing hypotheses.

3.4.2 Analytical Studies

An analytical study aims to make an inference about the strength of an association between a suspected risk factor and a disease which can be generalised to a wider population.

Most analytical studies are about comparing two (or more) groups of participants: those who are exposed and those who are not exposed; those who were allocated the treatment and those who were allocated the placebo. However, it is not as straight-forward as simply directly comparing the outcomes. If we wish to perform a study which accurately analyses the effect of the proposed risk factor, we must also minimise interference from other variables, such as age and sex, which might have an independent effect on the development of disease. Such variables are called confounding variables (see below). We also must consider whether the results obtained do strongly support there being a significant effect of the risk factor, or whether apparent differences between the groups could have come about by chance.

Analytical studies can be grouped into *observational* studies and *interventional* studies.

Observational studies describe the distribution of diseases in populations and investigate possible aetiological factors to explain that distribution. The investigators have no control over who is or is not exposed to the factor under study. The most common observational study designs are *case-control* and *cohort* studies.

In interventional studies, the investigator decides who is exposed and who is not. They can only be performed when such allocation is both possible and ethical. The most common type of interventional study is the *randomised controlled trial*. There are many different types of clinical trial.

3.4.2.1 Observational Studies

3.4.2.1.1 *Case-Control Studies*

In case-control studies, people who have been identified as having the outcome (the *cases*) are compared with people who do not have the outcome (the *controls*) (Figure 3.4). The investigator looks back (retrospectively) to discover if in the past

Figure 3.4 A case-control study design.

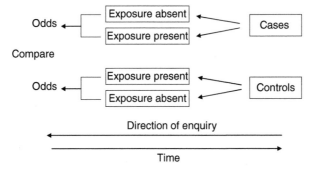

the cases had more or less exposure to the proposed risk factor than the controls. Should this be the case, then the investigator might conclude that there was, indeed, a relationship between exposure to the risk factor and development of disease (generally by calculating an Odds Ratio). It is important that the cases and the controls be as similar as possible (except for the presence of the disease) in order to reduce the effects of confounding variables.

A classic case-control study – oral contraceptives and pulmonary embolism [5]

In the late 1960s, Vessey and Doll interviewed women who had been admitted to hospital with venous thrombosis or pulmonary embolism without medical causes (cases). The controls were women who had been admitted to the same hospital with other diseases and who were matched for age, marital status and parity.

The investigators found that, out of 84 patients with deep-vein thrombosis or pulmonary embolism, 42 (50%) had used oral contraceptives during the month preceding the onset of their illness, while only 23 of the 168 controls (14%) had done so. From this, they concluded that the odds of those who had pulmonary embolism having used oral contraceptives were six times the odds of women who did not have the condition.

3.4.2.1.2 Cohort Studies

In cohort studies, a comparison is made between subjects allocated to groups on the basis of their *exposure* to the proposed risk factor. The aim is to compare the development of the disease in the exposed group with that in the unexposed group (see Figure 3.5). If the exposure occurred before the study started, then the allocation to groups is done at the beginning of the trial and the exposed group compared with a selected, unexposed, control group (e.g. a cohort study comparing rates of infection between two types of surgery). If, however, the exposure occurs during the study period, then allocation is done at the end of the study and those subjects who were not exposed

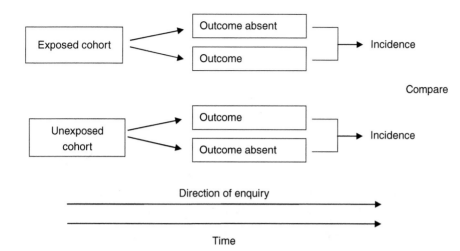

Figure 3.5 A cohort study design.

act as the controls for those who were (e.g. using a birth cohort, where participants are recruited at birth, to measure the impact of childhood adversity on adolescent mental health). Note that in a cohort study, as in all observational studies, the investigators have no control over which participants are exposed and which are not.

All subjects are followed up to record the development of the disease and, at the end of the study, the incidence of the disease in the exposed group is compared with the incidence in the unexposed group (usually calculated by a Relative Risk). Any difference between the two groups is likely to be due to the difference in their exposure to the risk factor, provided that the groups are similar in regard to possible confounding factors.

The evidence obtained from a cohort study is felt to be stronger than that from a case-control study due to the danger in the latter of introducing bias through inadequate selection of controls and the problems of reliable retrieval of historic information. Often, a case-control study is followed by a cohort study when more evidence of an association is needed. However, cohort studies tend to be more time-consuming and expensive to perform.

A classic cohort study – the Whitehall study [6]

The Whitehall studies of civil servants were set up in 1967 and included 18,000 men in the UK Civil Service. The first showed that men in the lowest employment grades were much more likely to die prematurely than men in the highest grades. The second Whitehall study that followed was set up to determine what underlies the social gradient in death and disease, and to include women. In 1985, all non-industrial civil servants aged between 35 and 55 in 20 departments in central

London were invited to a cardiovascular medical examination at their workplace. The authors recruited 10,308 civil servants. This study found an inverse relationship between socioeconomic position and the occurrence of coronary heart disease, diabetes and metabolic syndrome. A steep gradient in the incidence of coronary events with socioeconomic status was observed in the study, such that people of lowest socioeconomic status were between two and three times more likely than the wealthiest to suffer coronary events.

Many differences between the civil servants could influence health status. These include their income and socioeconomic status, access to and pattern of utilisation of health services, and lifestyle. For example, levels of smoking, obesity and physical activity could differ, leading to increased risk of diabetes and heart disease.

 Can you think of some of the possible reasons for the differences in health status observed among the civil servants?

3.4.2.2 Interventional Studies

In interventional (sometimes called experimental) studies, the investigators have control over who is and who is not exposed to the factor under investigation. Such intervention studies look at the effect of changing the exposure of the population to a factor. This is usually done by either removing a harmful factor or adding a beneficial or protective factor, and intervention studies provide information on prevention or treatment.

 What is the reference population?

The whole population (termed the reference population) cannot be practically studied, so two groups are chosen from the population to be representative. The reference group might be the whole population or those with a certain disease or condition. The desired intervention is administered to the intervention group, while a control (typically placebo or standard of care) is administered to the control group. This is normally only ethical if we have *equipoise* – when it is not known which of the exposures or treatments is more effective.

Both intervention and control groups are followed up and the development of disease in each group recorded (see Figure 3.6). A significant difference in disease incidence between the groups may indicate that this was the result of the intervention and that the factor added or removed has a real effect on the development of the disease.

 What do you understand by the term randomisation? What do investigators attempt to achieve by randomisation?

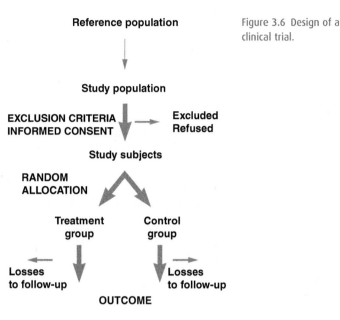

Figure 3.6 Design of a clinical trial.

The key benefit of being able to allocate interventions is that it ensures the two groups are similar except in terms of exposure to the intervention under study. This is typically achieved by ensuring that participants in the study have the same chance of being allocated to the intervention or control groups – a process called *randomisation*. A study where randomisation occurs between an intervention and a control group is called a *randomised controlled trial* (RCT). It is regarded as the best form of evidence of association as the randomisation process should ensure that, by random chance, the two groups should be equally balanced for any potential confounders, including those we may not be able to measure, or of which we are unaware.

What measure of association do you expect to be used in interventional studies? (Hint: Remember these are similar to cohort studies.)

Sometimes it is not possible to identify a control group and it may then be necessary to use the whole population before the intervention as a historical control against which the whole population after the intervention may be compared. These studies are often known as non-randomised trials, and can be considered as very similar to cohort studies, since they follow two groups of people over time to determine the outcome. However, these studies provide weaker evidence than randomised controlled trials since there is no way of ensuring that the two groups are balanced for confounders.

Why are interventional studies regarded as providing better evidence?

Worked example: A classic clinical trial – diabetes control [7]

The Diabetes Control and Complications Trial (DCCT) investigated whether intensive control of blood glucose in patients with insulin-dependent diabetes mellitus (IDDM) decreases long-term complications. Intensive control consisted of administration of insulin by external insulin pump or by three or more daily insulin injections and was guided by frequent blood-glucose monitoring. The control group received conventional therapy with one or two daily insulin injections. The researchers concluded that intensive therapy effectively delays the onset and slows the progression of diabetic retinopathy, nephropathy and neuropathy in patients with IDDM as the rate of neuropathy was around four times higher in the control group.

3.4.2.3 Summary

Table 3.7 summarises the main features of the different types of epidemiological study.

Table 3.7 Main features of the different types of epidemiological study

Design	Descriptive/ Observational/ Interventional	Retrospective/ Prospective	Aim	Specific comparison group/No such group
Case-series (clinical and population)	Descriptive	Retrospective in individuals	Describes diseases	No
Cross-sectional	Descriptive	Retrospective	Describes disease or risk factors in populations	Usually not
Case control	Observational	Retrospective	Examines association	Yes
Cohort (prospective and retrospective)	Observational	Prospective and retrospective	Examines associations of disease and/or outcomes with risk factors exposed to	Usually yes (though it may be integral to the study population)
Trial	Interventional	Prospective	Tests effectiveness of interventions to prevent or treat disease	Yes, with exceptions

3.5 Interpreting Results of Epidemiological Studies

Before we conclude that the results of studies are valid (true) and can be generalised to a wider population, we need to consider the factors that might fully or partly explain the observed results. Estimates of measures of associations such as Relative Risk and Odds Ratio may differ from their true value. This may be a result of random error or systematic error. Even if the estimates are close to the true values, we cannot imply anything about disease aetiology from the association; it is possible that there are many different causal factors working together to confer disease risk, or even that the true causal factors are merely correlated with the exposure we are studying.

3.5.1 Chance

The observed results of a study could be due to chance. The major cause of random error in epidemiological studies is *sampling error*, which is caused by the random nature of the sample. No sample will be truly representative of the population. By random chance, those in the sample might have worse outcomes than expected, or might have been exposed to some risk factor more than expected. Sampling error cannot be eliminated, but one of the aims of good study design is to reduce it to an acceptable level within the constraints imposed by available resources.

This random error might lead to us concluding that there is no association when there is one. This is called a *type II* or beta error (this can be thought of as a 'false negative' error). This type of error is harmful since it means we may not become aware of risk factors for disease, or we may reject effective treatments. Often, rather than talking about type II error directly, we talk about power, which is calculated as 1 - the probability of type II error.

Why might a type II error occur in a clinical trial?

Power is the probability we will detect an association, if there is a true association. A study must be designed with sufficient *power* to detect an association if one exists – if a study is clearly underpowered at the design stage, then undertaking it will be futile, and possibly unethical. Low power might be caused by the treatment having a small effect size, or there being a lot of variance in the outcome measure. Effects are harder to detect in smaller samples; a small sample size will reduce the power. Power is often increased by increasing the sample size in the study or by optimising the ratio of cases to controls.

Why might a type I error occur in a clinical trial?

Random error might also lead us to conclude that there is an association when in fact none exists. This is potentially more harmful as it may cause us to intervene in an ineffective way based on these results (e.g. to give an ineffective drug with potentially adverse effects). This is called a *type I* or alpha error. It can be thought of as a 'false positive' error.

In order to determine whether the results of the study are consistent with having come about due to sampling error and random chance, or whether the association between exposure and outcome appears to be significant, we must use statistical techniques. The two measures most commonly employed are the *p-value* and the *confidence interval* (CI). These are introduced briefly here, but readers are advised to refer to statistical texts to expand further their knowledge in this area [8, 9].

In epidemiological studies, the statistical framework typically used is null hypothesis testing. Here we have a null hypothesis, denoted H_0, the hypothesis that there is no association (i.e. the factor does not affect disease risk; the intervention does not have a treatment effect). We also have an alternative hypothesis, denoted H_1, the hypothesis that there is an association (i.e. the factor does affect disease risk; the intervention does have a treatment effect).

The p-value is the probability that the results observed in the study (or results even more extreme) would have occurred by random chance if the null hypothesis were true, and there was truly no association between exposure and the outcome. A p-value of 0.1 from a trial would indicate a 10% chance we would see data at least this extreme from a trial of a treatment with no effect. The smaller the p-value, the stronger the evidence that there is a meaningful association between exposure and outcome. If the p-value is sufficiently low, we say that the result is *statistically significant*.

Conventionally, we use a *significance threshold* of 0.05: if we obtain a p-value of 0.05 or below, we conclude that there is a statistically significant association between the exposure and the outcome. If there were truly no difference in outcome between those who are exposed and those who are not, we would expect to see a difference in our sample at least as extreme as the one we have seen here less than 5% of the time. If, however, we obtain a non-significant result (i.e. with the conventional threshold, a p-value of > 0.05), then we do not reject the null hypothesis that there is no association, and we conclude we have found no evidence of an association between exposure and outcome. However, this does not provide active evidence that there is an association.

With a significance threshold of 0.05, then about 5% of the time when the null hypothesis of no association is actually true, due to the effect of sampling error, we would still find an apparently statistically significant association in our data. If the potential harms of a type I error are high, or if we are performing many tests (e.g. testing many generic variants for disease association), it might be more appropriate to set a lower threshold – see Box 3.4.

Box 3.4 GWAS and the problem of multiple testing

Each time we perform a statistical test using a significance threshold of 0.05, when the null hypothesis is actually true there is a 5% chance that we make a false discovery, and incorrectly conclude that there is an association. False discoveries are unavoidable – there must always be a payoff between false positives and false negatives. (This is similar to the payoff between sensitivity and specificity in screening for disease. Any screening test will sometimes result in a false diagnosis; see Chapter 9.)

However, the more statistical tests we do, particularly in situations where the majority of the null hypotheses are true, the more likely we are to make at least one false discovery.

A common study design in genetic epidemiology is the Genome Wide Association Study (GWAS). Millions of genetic markers are analysed to determine whether they are associated with disease. The vast majority of them will not be associated with disease. However, 5% of these will have an associated p-value of < 0.05. If we were to report all of these as potentially disease-associated, they would drown out the true associations.

We can compensate for this by using a lower significance threshold for each test, in order to control the overall chance of making a type I error. In GWAS studies, the significance threshold usually chosen is 5×10^{-8}.

Even in a perfectly designed study, due to sampling error, we would still not expect our estimate of the measure of association to be precisely accurate. In order to quantify our uncertainty about the measurement, we calculate a *confidence interval* (CI). It is conventional to create confidence intervals at the 95% level – this means that if we were to repeatedly sample the population, 95% of the confidence intervals produced would contain the true value. The end points of the confidence interval are called confidence limits. These give the largest and smallest effects that are likely, given the observed data.

One useful feature of confidence intervals is that one can easily tell whether or not statistical significance has been reached, just as when using the p-value. If the confidence interval spans the value reflecting 'no effect' (e.g. the value 1 for a relative risk), this represents a difference that is not statistically significant. If the confidence interval does not enclose the value reflecting 'no effect', this represents a difference that is statistically significant.

3.5.2 Bias

Bias results when a systematic error causes a consistent discrepancy in measurement of exposures and outcomes. This results in inaccurate estimates. Two particularly common causes of bias in epidemiological studies are selection bias and information bias.

3.5.2.1 Selection Bias

Selection bias occurs when study participants differ systematically from the general population of interest. For instance, clinical trials typically recruit healthy young men, who may not be representative of the population who will go on to receive the intervention.

This is a major problem in case-control studies where it gives rise to non-comparability between cases and controls. It is found when cases (or controls) are chosen to be included in (or excluded from) a study by using criteria that are related to exposure to the risk factor under investigation.

> *Example*: In a case-control study of the aetiology of lung cancer, controls were selected from people who were suffering from non-malignant respiratory disease. Smoking is a cause of chronic bronchitis and thus the controls had a higher prevalence of smoking than the population from which the people with lung cancer was drawn. As a consequence, the strength of the association between smoking and lung cancer was underestimated. The controls should have been selected from the general population, which would have avoided this bias.

Much of the effort that goes into the design of good case-control studies is spent on the careful selection of controls in order to eliminate selection bias.

3.5.2.2 Information Bias

This involves study subjects being misclassified according to their disease status, their exposure status, or both. Differential misclassification occurs when errors in classification of disease status are dependent on exposure status or vice versa. For example, in a case-control study, a case's recall of his or her past 'exposure' to risk factors may differ from the recall of a control because the process of having the disease will have caused the person to think much more about possible exposures than is the case for the controls.

> *Example*: In a case-control study investigating the association between congenital defects in newborn babies and maternal exposure to X-rays, women with babies with congenital defects are more likely to recall their X-rays due to apparent association. The effect of this will be to over-estimate the strength of association, as the cases appear to have a higher exposure to the risk factor.

3.5.3 Confounding

This occurs when an estimate of the association between an exposure and a disease is confused because another exposure, linked to both, has not been taken into account. For a variable to be a confounder, it must be associated with the exposure under study and it must also be independently associated with disease risk in its own right (see Figure 3.7).

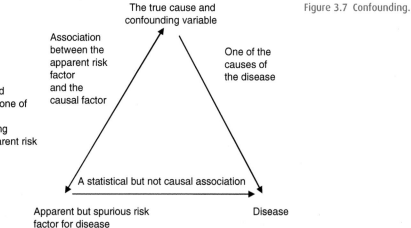

Figure 3.7 Confounding.

- The relationship can be considered as triangular

- The spurious confounded association results from one of the causes of disease (confounding factor) being associated with the apparent risk factor

Worked examples of confounding:

Example 1. Consider a study of the association between work in a particular occupation and the risk of lung cancer. A comparison of death rates due to lung cancer in the occupational group and in the general population may appear to show that the occupational group has an increased risk of lung cancer. However, it is possible this effect is caused by the confounding factor of age or the confounding factor of people in the occupational group having different smoking habits from people in the general population – if this is not taken into account, the inference is invalid. In practice, it is very difficult in this kind of study to control for the effect of socioeconomic factors.

Example 2. Age at menopause may confound estimates of the association between replacement oestrogens (taken for relief of menopausal symptoms) and breast-cancer risk. This is because an early age at menopause (the confounding factor) is associated with both a reduced risk of breast cancer (the outcome) and a greater use of replacement oestrogens (the exposure).

Confounding may be avoided by using an appropriate study design, such as a randomised controlled trial. If a specific confounder has been identified, the population under study can be made more specific. For instance, in Example 2, we could reduce the effect of age as a confounder by only studying women who had their menopause at a particular range of ages. However, it may also be controlled for in the analysis, provided that the confounding factors have been identified and information on them has been collected. The control of confounding at analysis is a widely used strategy, with much of the statistical methodology in epidemiology being concerned with this issue.

Use these questions to consider confounders for the following populations:

a. **People who drink alcohol have a raised risk of lung cancer.**

b. **People living in an affluent seaside resort have a higher mortality rate than the country as a whole.**

c. **African Americans are heavier users of crack cocaine than 'White' Americans.**

To consider the role of potential confounders, it is helpful to ask the following questions:

- What is the apparent association?
- What else might cause the outcome and could it also be related to the apparent cause?
- Therefore, what is the confounded factor and what is the confounding (causal) factor?
- How can we check whether the possible confounder is having an effect?

Worked examples: Confounding

Table 3.8 Confounding questions answered

The confounded association	One possible explanation	The confounded factor	The confounding (causal) factor	To check the assumption
a. People who drink alcohol have a raised risk of lung cancer	Alcohol drinking and smoking are behaviours which go together	Alcohol, which is a marker for, on average, smoking more cigarettes	Tobacco, which is associated with both alcohol and with the disease	See if the alcohol–lung cancer relationship holds in people not exposed to tobacco: if it does, tobacco is not a confounder
b. People living in an affluent seaside resort have a higher mortality rate than the country as a whole	A holiday town attracts the elderly, so has a comparatively old population	Living in a resort is a marker for being, on average, older	Age, which is associated with both living in a resort and with death	Look at each age group specifically, or use age standardisation to take into account age differences
c. African Americans are heavier users of crack cocaine than 'White' Americans	Poor people living in the American inner city are particularly likely to become dependent on illicit drugs	Belonging to the racial category 'African American'	Poverty and the pressures of inner-city living, including the easy availability of drugs	Use statistical techniques to adjust for the influence of a number of complex socioeconomic factors

As can be seen from the exercise above, we need to consider the potential confounders before we conclude that the association is causal. In case b, although we observe higher mortality in coastal towns, this is not due to the geographical area, but the different age structure between resort towns and other areas of the country. Resort towns tend to have a higher proportion of elderly as people tend to settle in these areas after retirement. Here, age is a potential confounder because it is a surrogate for age-related causal factors. There are various ways of tackling confounders, including advanced statistical techniques such as multivariate analysis.

3.5.4 Validity (Truth)

Once we have established that the results from the epidemiological studies are not due to chance or error (including confounding), we need to determine if our results are *valid* and if any association seen is causal. Validity is the extent to which a variable or intervention measures what it is supposed to measure, or accomplishes what it is supposed to accomplish.

In the context of epidemiological studies, validity has two components: internal and external validity. The *internal validity* of a study refers to the integrity of the experimental design and relates to inferences about the study population itself. The *external validity* of a study refers to the appropriateness by which its results can be applied to non-study participants. This will depend on how similar the study population and the population to which the results are extrapolated are. This is often termed the generalisability of a study.

When we are assured that the results of a study are valid, we can consider, where relevant, the issue of *causality*. Much of epidemiology seeks to determine aetiology; relate causes to the effects they produce. Epidemiological evidence by itself is rarely sufficient to establish causality, but it can provide powerful circumstantial evidence. We can be more certain of a causal relationship if our results come from a large, well-designed, randomised controlled trial, or from a meta-analysis of many such trials.

According to Hill, causality is more likely if the association can be shown [10] to be:
1. Strong (e.g. is statistically significant and has a large relative risk).
2. Dose-related (i.e. the greater the risk factor, the greater the effects).
3. In the right time sequence (cohort studies show that exposure precedes outcome).
4. Independent of recognised confounding factors.
5. Consistent between different studies. (We now look for systematic reviews and meta-analyses to increase our confidence in associations.)
6. Plausible. However, uncertainty about the biological mechanism should not automatically rule out causality. As medical science advances, our knowledge of the biological mechanisms will evolve in future years. In the 1980s, HIV/AIDS research was in its earliest stages. A relationship was discovered between the incidence of AIDS-like symptoms in homosexual men (the largest portion of the population displaying these symptoms at the time) and the use of alkyl nitrites,

more commonly called 'poppers'. As science stood at that time, the biological agent had not been identified and various mechanisms were put forward, including the 'poppers' hypothesis [11]. However, with the discovery of the causative agent, all these theories disappeared and a biological mechanism was established.

7. Reversible (removing the exposure should remove the risk). Two kinds of cause are sometimes distinguished. A necessary cause is one whose presence is required for the occurrence of the effect. A sufficient cause is one which can cause the effect alone. In practice, most causal factors are neither necessary nor sufficient, but contributory.

3.6 Conclusions

In this chapter, we have described the ways in which we measure the extent of health problems within and between populations and the scientific basis for conclusions we reach on disease causality, prevention and treatment. Without this knowledge, we cannot know where best to concentrate our efforts to have the greatest effect on population health. We recommend the accompanying book in this series, which provides a more detailed coverage of the field of epidemiology [12]. The next chapter continues this theme and looks at how we judge the strength of evidence on which we base health-care decisions.

FURTHER READING

H. T. O. Davies and I. K. Crombie, What are confidence intervals and p-values? *Hayward Communications* **3**(1), 2009, 1–8. Available at: www.bandolier.org.uk/painres/download/whatis/What_are_Conf_Inter.pdf.

J. Deeks, Swots corner: What is an odds ratio? *Bandolier* **25**, March 1996. Available at: www.bandolier.org.uk/band25/b25-6.html.

D. E. Lilienfeld and P. D. Stolley, *Foundations in Epidemiology*, New York, NY, Oxford University Press, 1994.

J. M. Last, *A Dictionary of Epidemiology*, 4th ed., New York, NY, Oxford University Press, 2001.

H. Motulsky, *Intuitive Biostatistics: A Nonmathematical Guide to Statistical Thinking*, 4th ed., Oxford, Oxford University Press, 2013.

D. Spiegelhalter, *The Art of Statistics: Learning from Data*, London, Pelican Books, 2019.

REFERENCES

1. C. Hennekens and J. Burling, *Epidemiology in Medicine*, Boston, MA, Little, Brown and Company, 1987.

2. Institute of Medicine (US) Committee on Assessing Interactions Among Social, Behavioral, and Genetic Factors in Health, *Genes, Behavior, and the Social Environment: Moving beyond the Nature/Nurture Debate*, Washington, DC, National Academic Press, 2006.

3. R. Doll and A. B. Hill, The mortality of doctors in relation to their smoking habits: A preliminary report, *British Medical Journal* **228**, 1954, 1451–5.

4. R. Doll and R. Peto, Mortality in relation to smoking: 20 years' observations on male British doctors, *British Medical Journal* **273**, 1976, 1525–36.

5. M. P. Vessey and R. Doll, Investigation of relation between use of oral contraceptives and thromboembolic disease, *British Medical Journal* 1968, **2**, 199–205.

6. J. E. Ferrie, P. Martikainen, M. J. Shipley and M. G. Marmot, Self-reported economic difficulties and coronary events in men: Evidence from the Whitehall II study, *International Journal of Epidemiology* **34**(3), 2005, 640–8.

7. The Diabetes Control and Complications Trial Research Group, The effect of intensive treatment of diabetes on the development and progression of long-term complications in insulin-dependent diabetes mellitus, *New England Journal of Medicine* **329**(14), 1993, 977–86.

8. D. G. Altman, *Practical Statistics for Medical Research*, London, Chapman & Hall/CRC, 1991.

9. B. R. Kirkwood and J. A. C. Sterne, *Essential Medical Statistics*, 2nd ed., Oxford, Blackwell Science, 2003.

10. A. B. Hill, The environment and disease: Association or causation? *Proceedings of the Royal Society of Medicine* **58**, 1965, 295–300. Available at: www.edwardtufte.com/tufte/hill.

11. J. P. Vandenbroucke and V. P. Pardoel, An autopsy of epidemiologic methods: The case of 'poppers' in the early epidemic of the acquired immunodeficiency syndrome (AIDS), *American Journal of Epidemiology* **129**(3), 1989, 455–7.

12. P. Webb, C. Bain and S. Pirozzo, *Essential Epidemiology. An Introduction for Students and Health Professionals*, Cambridge, Cambridge University Press, 2005.

4

Evidence-Based Health-Care
Padmanabhan Badrinath and Stephen Gillam

Key points

- Evidence-based practice integrates the individual practitioner's experience, patient preferences and the best available research information.
- Incorporating the best available research evidence in decision-making involves five steps: *asking* answerable questions; *accessing* the best information; *appraising* the information for validity and relevance; *applying* the information to care of patients and populations; and *evaluating* the impact for evidence of change and expected outcomes.
- Although practitioners need basic skills in finding evidence, a health librarian is an invaluable asset.
- There are specific checklists available to appraise research papers critically, and every practitioner should possess the skills to appraise the published literature.
- The COVID-19 pandemic has been a major test of evidence-based medicine demonstrating its limitations during a fast-moving global emergency.
- The major barriers to implementing evidence-based practice include the impression among practitioners that their professional freedom is being taken away, lack of access to appropriate training, and tools and resource constraints.
- Various incentives, including financial ones, can be used to encourage evidence-based practice.

4.1 Introduction

How much of what health and other professionals do is based soundly in science? Answers to the question 'is our practice evidence-based?' depend on what we mean by practice and what we mean by evidence. Some studies have estimated that less than 20% of all health-care interventions are underpinned by robust research [1]. This varies from discipline to discipline. For example, studies examining clinical decisions in the field of internal medicine found that most primary therapeutic clinical decisions are based on evidence from randomised controlled trials (RCTs) [2].

Sackett *et al.* defined evidence-based medicine (EBM) as:

> the conscientious, explicit, and judicious use of current best evidence in making decisions about the care of individual patients.

The practice of evidence-based medicine means 'integrating individual clinical expertise with the best available external clinical evidence from systematic research' [3]. The expansion of EBM has been a major influence on medical practice over the last 25 years. The demands of purchasers of health-care keen to optimise value for money have been one driver. A growing awareness among health professionals and their patients of medicine's potential to cause harm has been another. Since the early 1990s, EBM has steadily embraced other disciplines and public health is no exception. Public health practitioners with limited resources need to target these efficiently. Public health interventions are often costly and policy-makers need evidence to invest appropriately. One of the key competencies required for all public health professionals is the ability to form questions and retrieve evidence to advance population health and welfare.

In this chapter, we examine the nature of what is nowadays more broadly referred to as evidence-based health-care (EBHC) and discuss its limitations. It is worth noting that in the UK this field continues to expand, particularly into the arena of social care, which often goes hand in hand with the provision of health-care. Increasingly, the term 'evidence-based practice' (EBP) is used as a catch-all. While this chapter focuses on health-care, the principles of EBP we describe apply equally to other disciplines, including public health and policy [4].

4.2 Tools for Evidence-Based Practice

The tools needed to practise in an evidence-based way are common across disciplines. Doctors, public health practitioners, nurses and allied health and social care professionals all need the skills to ensure that the work they do, whether with individual clients or patients, or in the development of programmes and policies, is based on sound knowledge of what is likely to work.

Of the five essential steps in Box 4.1, the first is probably the most important.

Box 4.1 Five steps for evidence-based practice

1. convert information needs into answerable questions, i.e. by asking a focused question;
2. track down best available evidence;
3. appraise evidence critically;
4. change practice in the light of evidence; and
5. evaluate your performance.

4.2.1 Step 1: Asking a Focused Question

Before seeking the best evidence, you need to convert your information needs into a tightly focused question. For example, it is not enough to ask: 'Is alcohol-based gel more effective than soap and water in a hospital setting?' This must be converted into an answerable question: 'For persons entering a hospital, is hand rubbing with a waterless, alcohol-based solution as effective as standard hand washing with anti-septic soap for reducing hand contamination?' [5].

The PICO approach can be used as a framework to focus a question by considering the necessary elements. It contains four components (shown below with the alcohol-based gel question from above as an example):

- Patient or the population (those entering a hospital);
- Intervention (use of alcohol-based hand solution);
- Comparison intervention (use of antiseptic soap and water);
- Outcome (reduction in the contamination of hands).

Some practitioners add a fifth element to the question – time. It may be important to determine the time-frame; for example, when using an alcohol-based solution we may only be interested in contamination-free hands in the subsequent few hours, but when considering the effectiveness of cancer treatment we might want to know about mortality rates after 5 years.

 Form a focused clinical question using the PICO format to find the evidence for the effectiveness of smoking cessation interventions in adult smokers who have had a heart attack.

4.2.2 Step 2: Tracking down the Evidence

The second step in the practice of evidence-based practice is to track down the best evidence.

Health professionals in particular may all too easily assess outcomes in terms of surrogate pathological end points rather than commonplace changes in quality of life or the ability to perform routine activities (e.g. the hip operation was a success, but the patient still has limited mobility). Traditionally, clinicians making decisions about what works have attached much weight to personal experience or the views of respected colleagues. Over time, knowledge of up-to-date care diminishes [6, 7], so there is a constant need for the latest evidence and simple ways to access and use it. So, rather than rely on colleagues, simple Internet searches or textbooks, evidence-based health-care (EBHC) encourages the use of research evidence in a systematic way. Once a question has been formulated, the research base is then searched to find articles of relevance.

So, what evidence should be sought? What constitutes reliable evidence? Care needs to be taken in relying on published articles. Many reviews reflect the preju-dices of their authors and are anything but systematic. Even mainstream journals

Table 4.1 Levels of evidence (Scottish Intercollegiate Guidelines Network) [10]

1++ High-quality meta-analyses, systematic reviews of RCTs or RCTs with a very low risk of bias
1+ Well-conducted meta-analyses, systematic reviews or RCTs with a low risk of bias
1− Meta-analyses, systematic reviews or RCTs with a high risk of bias
2++ High-quality systematic reviews of case-control or cohort studies. High-quality case-control or cohort studies with a very low risk of confounding or bias and a high probability that the relationship is causal
2+ Well-conducted case-control or cohort studies with a low risk of confounding or bias and a moderate probability that the relationship is causal
2− Case-control or cohort studies with a high risk of confounding or bias and a significant risk that the relationship is not causal
3 Non-analytic studies (e.g. case reports, case series)
4 Expert opinion

have a propensity to accept papers yielding positive rather than negative findings, for example in assessing treatments, so-called 'publication bias' [8, 9]. Most books date rapidly, hence the prominence nowadays accorded to properly conducted systematic reviews at the top of the hierarchy of evidence. A widely used ranking of the strength of evidence is shown in Table 4.1 [10]. Another popular hierarchy of evidence is the one developed by the Centre for Evidence Based Medicine in 1998, which was revised in 2011 [11]. Most experts agree that the higher up the ranking, the more rigorous the study methodology is, and therefore the more chance of minimising bias.

Table 4.1 reminds us of the three main types of epidemiological study designs: descriptive, observational and interventional, which were considered in Chapter 3. When searching for evidence, we should look for the highest level suitable to our question. A question relating to the effectiveness of an intervention will most appropriately be answered by an RCT or a systematic review of RCTs. The RCT is the gold standard, as robust randomisation ensures that study and control groups differ only in terms of their exposure to the factor under study; the observed results are due only to the intervention and not to confounding variables.

However, in public health practice, with complex problems and situations, these types of studies are not always practical, or available. We can find answers to questions about the causes of a disease from case-control or cohort studies. However, questions beginning 'Why?' are often not answered by these kinds of study. What factors, after all, make a 'good nurse' or a 'good public health practitioner' and how easily are they measured? It is not possible to answer the questions 'Why do women refuse an offer of breast screening?' or 'Why do children take up smoking?' with any of the study types mentioned so far. Another example would be: 'What leads to inappropriate use of medicines in elderly inpatients?' In these cases, one looks for a qualitative study. Qualitative studies use methods such as interviews, diaries and direct observation to provide detailed information to describe the experiences of participants. Qualitative data are then analysed rigorously to lead to conclusions. Detailed coverage of qualitative methodology can be found in textbooks dedicated to this topic [12] and is beyond the scope of this chapter, but it is important to remember that not every question can be answered using the classical hierarchy above. Qualitative methods can generate a wealth of knowledge to contextualise many of the decisions health professionals must make.

What study type would be appropriate to answer the focused question: 'In smokers who have had a heart attack, does a smoking cessation intervention in comparison with usual care reduce mortality and improve quit rate?'

There are various sources of evidence. These include primary and secondary sources of literature. Primary sources are the thousands of original papers published every year in research journals. However, to deal with the vast amount of information available, more and more people now turn to secondary sources of evidence and the single most important source of systematic reviews remains the Cochrane Database (www.cochrane.org). The Cochrane Collaboration (named after Archie Cochrane, an early pioneer of EBM) is an international endeavour to summarise high-quality evidence in all fields of medical practice. It has slowly transformed many areas of clinical practice.

So, it is important to have basic skills in searching the literature, although the help of expert librarians may be needed. Research papers are catalogued in a variety of databases searchable on the Internet. For many medical or public health queries, the database Medline is a good starting place. Other databases are available for specialist queries such as those in the fields of social care, mental health and nursing (e.g. CINAHL or EMBASE). Using the PICO format here is helpful as it can be used to generate search terms with which to query the databases. Databases may have tools to support the user in this, such as the 'Clinical Queries' tool in PubMed, which is a US National Library of Medicine's service to search the bio-medical research literature [13].

List key words (using the PICO format) to search databases to answer the focused question: 'In smokers who have had a heart attack, does a smoking cessation intervention in comparison with usual care reduce mortality and improve quit rate?'

We can use our example question from earlier to demonstrate how a search might work. Our focused question was: 'In smokers who have had a heart attack, does a smoking cessation intervention in comparison with usual care reduce mortality and improve quit rate?'

In the search for evidence it should be remembered that not every piece of information which might help us answer our question may be published. Studies may be in progress which could inform our action; negative studies, which could help tell us what *not* to do, may not have made it as far as a publication; many pharmaceutical companies have unpublished information; conference reports might provide helpful information. As we move down the hierarchy, it becomes more difficult to find this kind of evidence (called 'grey' literature) from readily available sources, but some databases and repositories are available. This is a good time to seek the help of an expert librarian!

Review the standard checklists for RCTs, case-control studies, diagnostic studies, cohort studies, economic evaluations and qualitative studies and apply them to examples in your practice.

4.2.3 Step 3: Appraising the Evidence

To be able to determine whether we should act on the results of the studies found in the search, we must be able critically to appraise a range of study types. It is important to have an understanding of the basic epidemiological concepts outlined in Chapter 3, to be able to understand the results presented and to have a systematic approach to the appraisal. In brief, we are looking to determine whether we believe the results sufficiently to act on them and change our practice. In order to do this, we ask a series of questions about the study, which include:

- Did the research ask a clearly focused question and carry out the right sort of study to answer it?
- Were the study methods robust?
- Do the conclusions made match the results of the study?
- Can we use these results in our practice? This might include an assessment of whether the results are due to chance, 'big' enough to make a real difference and whether the same results are likely to occur in our own situation.

There are standard checklists available to support systematic appraisal of different types of study designs. We can use these to help determine how valid the findings of the study are, and whether the findings can be generalised to our own population.

Table 4.2 shows a checklist for appraising an RCT, the most appropriate primary design to generate evidence of effective interventions. This checklist is taken from the UK Critical Appraisal Skills Programme (CASP) in Oxford [14].

It is important to be able to analyse critically the results of all study types, but, as the volume of scientific literature increases, it is perhaps most important to be able to use systematic reviews effectively to guide practice. It has been estimated that a general physician needs to read for 119 hours a week to keep up to date; medical students are alleged to spend 1–2 hours reading clinical material per week – and that's more than the doctors who teach them [15]. Also, a single study of insufficient sample size or of otherwise poor quality may yield misleading results. The right

Table 4.2 The CASP critical appraisal tool for systematic reviews [14]

Are the results of the review valid?

1. Did the review address a clearly focused question? Yes / Can't tell / No

   Consider if the question is 'focused' in terms of:

   the population studied

   the intervention given or exposure

   the outcomes considered

2. Did the authors look for the right type of papers? Yes / Can't tell / No

   Consider if the included studies:

   address the review's question

   have an appropriate study design

Is it worth continuing?

Detailed questions

3. Do you think all the important, relevant studies were included? Yes / Can't tell / No

   Consider:

   which bibliographic databases were used

   if there was follow-up from reference lists

   if there was personal contact with experts

   if the reviewers searched for unpublished studies

   if the reviewers searched for non-English-language studies

4. Did the review's authors do enough to assess quality of the included studies? Yes / Can't tell / No

   Consider:

   if a rigorous strategy was used to determine which studies were identified

   Look for:

   a scoring system

   more than one assessor

5. If the results of the review have been combined, was it reasonable to do so? Yes / Can't tell / No

   Consider whether:

   the results of each study are clearly displayed

   the results were similar from study to study (look for tests of heterogeneity)

   the reasons for any variations in results are discussed

6. What are the overall results of the review?

   Consider:

   how the results are expressed (e.g. Odds Ratio, Relative Risk, etc.)

   how large this size of result is and how meaningful it is

   if you are clear about the bottom-line result of the review

7. How precise are the results?

   Consider:

   if confidence intervals were reported

8. Can the results be applied to the local population? Yes / Can't tell / No

   Consider whether:

   the population sample covered by the review could be different from your population and in ways that would produce
      different results

   whether your local setting differs much from that of the review

Table 4.2 (*cont.*)

9. Were all important outcomes considered?

   Consider whether there is other information you would have like to have seen

10. Are the benefits worth the harms and costs?

   Consider, even if this is not addressed by the review, what *you* think

Cumulative			Odds Ratio			Textbook Recommendations			
year	RCTs	Pts	0.5	1	2	Rout	Specif	Exp	NOT
1960	1	23							21
	2	65							5
1965	3	149						1	10
	4	316						1	2
1970	7	1793						2	8
	10	2544	P < 0.01						8
	11	2651					1		12
1975	15	3311					1	8	4
	17	3929					1	7	3
1980	22	5452	P < 0.001			5	2	2	1
	23	5767				15	8		1
	27	6125				6	1		
1985	33	6571							
	65	47185							
1990	70	48154	P < 0.00001						

Figure 4.1 Results of meta-analyses of thrombolysis for myocardial infarction (MI), according to when they could have been carried out, and the textbook recommendations at the time (Pts = patients): routine, in specified circumstances, as experimental treatment, or not recommended [16].

answer to a specific question is more likely to come from a systematic review. This is a review of all the literature on a particular topic, which has been methodically identified, appraised and presented. The statistical combination of all the results from included studies to provide a summary estimate or definitive result is called meta-analysis.

Antman *et al.*'s classic study of research into the effectiveness of thrombolysis demonstrates the importance of systematic review and meta-analysis for proponents of EBM [16]. The first study, showing that streptokinase reduced mortality following myocardial infarction, was published in 1960. The results of this meta-analysis are shown in Figure 4.1. While early RCTs showed a treatment effect (Odds Ratio below 1), the confidence intervals around these effect–size estimates were wide, showing imprecision, and went above 1, which indicates the possibility of no effect.

The power of meta-analysis is clearly demonstrated by the narrowing of these confidence intervals as the number of RCTs increased. From around 1970, the beneficial effect of thrombolysis seems clearly apparent, but some 30 years after the first RCT and nearly 20 years after meta-analysis might have decided the question, thrombolytics were still not being routinely recommended in clinical practice. Because reviews have not always used scientific methods, advice on some life-saving therapies has often been delayed. Other treatments have been recommended long after controlled trials have shown them to be harmful.

4.2.4 Step 4: Changing Practice in Light of Evidence

Actually following through on the results of your appraisal of new evidence – implementation – is the most difficult of the five steps. Some change can be self-initiated; other circumstances require change in those around you. The implementation of effective public health interventions often requires change in others, and public health practitioners often act as advocates for evidence-based practice, encouraging other professionals to act on results of an assessment of the evidence base. The management of people and an understanding of how they will react are invaluable. Chapter 7 covers the theoretical models of change in some detail and we can use evidence-based practice to determine how to implement change (see Box 4.2).

There is no magic bullet. Most interventions are effective under some circumstances; none is effective under all circumstances. A diagnostic analysis of the individual and the context must be performed before selecting a method for altering individual practitioner behaviour. Interventions based on assessment of potential barriers are more likely to be effective.

 Using the example of use of alcohol-based gel from Step 1, how would we assess whether practice has changed?

Box 4.2 Evidence of effectiveness of interventions to change professional behaviour [17]

There is good evidence to support:

> **Multifaceted interventions**. By targeting different barriers to change, these are more likely to be effective than single interventions.
> **Educational outreach**. This can change prescribing behaviour.
> **Reminder systems**. These are generally effective for a range of behaviours.

There are mixed effects in the following:

> **Audit and feedback**. These need to be used selectively.
> **Opinion leaders**. These need to be used selectively.

There is little evidence to support:

> **Passive dissemination of guidelines**. However, there is some evidence to support use of guidelines if tailored to local needs and associated with reminders.

4.2.5 Step 5: Evaluating the Effects of Changes in Practice

Commonly, this step will involve an evaluation or clinical audit (see Chapter 6). Depending on how frequently the intervention or activity under scrutiny is performed, a review of behaviour will be undertaken some months after instigation of the change. There are various ways of ascertaining whether practice has changed and further consideration of this role of evaluation is discussed in Chapter 6.

4.3 Limitations to EBHC

Evidence is only one influence on our practice. Education alone may not change deeply ingrained habits (e.g. patterns of prescribing). Knowledge does not necessarily change practice. This is true for practitioners and patients or the public. An example is the continued use by patients of complementary therapies such as homeopathy which professionals consider to be ineffective. Doctors are sceptical of their benefits and attempt to restrict their use on the basis of scientific evaluations. These are often of poor quality or show either evidence of no effect or no evidence of effectiveness [18]. The public continue to use them and research has shown that 26% of adults have taken a herbal medicine in the previous two years, possibly because they meet personal needs that conventional treatments do not [19].

Hence, we need to consider employing other incentives to change. Financial incentives are used to promote interventions known to be effective (e.g. target payments to increase immunisation uptake). In the NHS, the Quality and Outcomes Framework (QOF) payment system was introduced to improve the quality of clinical care and promote evidence-based practice [20]. Evidence suggests that financial incentives might improve provider performance in preventive interventions such as offering a stop smoking service [21]. Chapter 6 looks in more detail at quality improvement in health-care.

The most strident criticisms of EBHC have come from those physicians who resent intrusions into their clinical freedom. The use of evidence-based protocols has been demeaned [22] as 'cookbook medicine'. A more powerful philosophical argument is mounted by those arguing that a rigid fixation on RCTs risks ignoring important qualitative sources of evidence [23]. This argument may carry particular weight in the complex field of public health interventions.

In addition, there may be times when high-quality evidence from the upper echelons of the hierarchy simply does not exist. This should not prevent action! The lack of RCTs does not mean an intervention is ineffective, it means that there is no evidence that it is effective, a clear distinction. In these cases, one looks further down the hierarchy and uses the best level of evidence available. When no research evidence exists, there is nothing wrong with asking colleagues for their opinions; the practice of EBHC simply means we should at least carry out the search.

During the COVID-19 pandemic, there were reports of clinicians abandoning evidence and reaching for drugs because they sounded biologically plausible. Studies published during the early part of the pandemic often lacked control groups or enrolled too few people to draw firm conclusions. The COVID-19 crisis has exposed major weaknesses in the production and use of research-based evidence with many poor-quality studies with small numbers of patients. Efforts are underway to ensure that EBM still remains fit for purpose in a future pandemic or a health emergency [24, 25].

EBM has been described as a 'movement in crisis'. There have been concerns expressed regarding the viability and relevance of EBM as a noble goal in the practice of medicine [26]. Criticisms include the hijacking of the term by vested interests, the unmanageable volume of evidence, statistical significance trumping clinical significance, patient-centred care replaced by algorithms, and the inability of evidence-based guidelines to deal with multiple morbidities [27]. EBM has nevertheless been successful: producing a sophisticated hierarchy of evidence, promoting the need for systematic summaries of the best evidence to guide care and considering patient values in important clinical decisions.

4.4 Conclusions

The terms 'evidence-based medicine' and 'evidence-based health-care' were developed to encourage practitioners and patients to pay due respect – no more, no less – to current evidence in making decisions. Evidence should enhance health-care decision-making, not rigidly dictate it [28]. Public health practitioners need to consider their population's health and social care needs and what effective interventions are available to meet them. Finally, the practitioner must consider society's and individuals' preferences. The art of evidence-based practice lies in bringing all these considerations together.

REFERENCES

1. R. Smith, Where is the wisdom . . . ? *British Medical Journal* **303**(6806), 1991, 798–9.
2. G. Michaud, J. L. McGowan, R. van der Jagt *et al.*, Are therapeutic decisions supported by evidence from health care research? *Archives of Internal Medicine* **158**(15), 1998, 1665–8.
3. D. L. Sackett, W. M. Rosenberg, J. A. Gray *et al.*, Evidence based medicine: What it is and what it isn't, *British Medical Journal* **312**, 1996, 71–2.
4. J. Baron, A brief history of evidence-based policy, *Annals of the American Academy of Political & Social Science* **678**(1), 2017, 40–50.
5. A. DiCenso, G. Guyatt and D. Ciliska, *Evidence-Based Nursing: A Guide to Clinical Practice*, St. Louis, MO, Mosby, 2005.

6. N. K. Choudry, R. H. Fletcher and S. B. Soumerai, Systematic review: The relationship between clinical experience and quality of health care, *Annals of Internal Medicine* **142**(4), 2005, 260–73.

7. P. G. Ramsey, J. D. Carline, T. S. Inui *et al.*, Changes over time in the knowledge base of practicing internists, *Journal of the American Medical Association* **266**(8), 1991, 1103–7.

8. P. J. Easterbrook, J. A. Berlin, R. Gopalan and D. R. Matthews, Publication bias in clinical research, *The Lancet* **337**(8746), 1991, 867–72.

9. K. Dickersin, The existence of publication bias and risk factors for its occurrence, *Journal of the American Medical Association* **263**(10), 1990, 1385–9.

10. Scottish Intercollegiate Guidelines Network, SIGN 50: A guideline developer's handbook, Annex B. Edinburgh, SIGN. Available at: www.sign.ac.uk/assets/sign50_2011.pdf

11. OCEBM Levels of Evidence Working Group, The Oxford Levels of Evidence 2. Oxford Centre for Evidence-Based Medicine. Available at: www.cebm.ox.ac.uk/resources/levels-of-evidence/ocebm-levels-of-evidence

12. C. Pope and N. Mays (eds.), *Qualitative Research in Health Care*, 3rd ed., Oxford, Blackwell Publishing/BMJ Books, 2006.

13. PubMed, PubMed Clinical Queries. Available at: www.ncbi.nlm.nih.gov/pubmed/clinical

14. Critical Appraisal Skills Programme, CASP checklists. Available at: https://casp-uk.net/casp-tools-checklists/

15. D. L. Sackett, S. E. Strauss, W. S. Richardson *et al.*, *Evidence-Based Medicine: How to Practise and Teach EBM*, 2nd ed., Edinburgh, Churchill Livingstone, 2000.

16. E. M. Antman, J. Lau, B. Kupelnick *et al.*, A comparison of results of meta-analyses of randomized control trials and recommendations of clinical experts, *Journal of the American Medical Association* **268**(2), 1992, 240–8.

17. University of York, Centre for Reviews and Dissemination, Getting evidence into practice, *Effective Health Care Bulletin* **5**, 1999. Available at: www.york.ac.uk/media/crd/ehc51.pdf

18. E. Ernst, A systematic review of systematic reviews of homeopathy, *British Journal of Clinical Pharmacology* **54**(6), 2000, 577–82.

19. Medicines and Healthcare products Regulatory Agency (MHRA), Public perception of herbal medicines, Drug Safety Update, March 2009. Available at: www.mhra.gov.uk/Safetyinformation/DrugSafetyUpdate/CON088122

20. T. Doran, C. Fullwood, H. Gravelle *et al.*, Pay-for-performance programs in family practices in the United Kingdom, *New England Journal of Medicine* **355**(4), 2006, 375–84.

21. J. Roski, R. Jeddeloh, L. An *et al.*, The impact of financial incentives and a patient registry on preventive care quality: Increasing provider adherence to evidence-based smoking cessation practice guidelines, *Preventative Medicine* **36**(3), 2003, 291–9.

22. B. G. Charlton and A. Miles, The rise and fall of EBM, *Quarterly Journal of Medicine* **91**(5), 1998, 371–4.

23. J. Popay and G. Williams, Qualitative research and evidence-based healthcare, *Journal of the Royal Society of Medicine* **91**(Suppl. 35), 1998, 32–7.

24. H. Pearson, How COVID broke the evidence pipeline, *Nature*, 12 May 2021.

25. Editorial. Evidence-based medicine: How Covid can drive positive change, *Nature*, 12 May 2021.

26. T. Greenhalgh and N. Maskrey, Evidence based medicine: A movement in crisis? *British Medical Journal* **348**, 2014, g3725.

27. B. Djulbegovic and G. Guyatt, Progress in evidence-based medicine: A quarter century on, *The Lancet* **390**, 2017, 415–23.

28. S. E. Straus and F. A. McAlister, Evidence-based medicine: A commentary on common criticisms, *Canadian Medical Association Journal* **163**(7), 2000, 837–41.

5

Decision-Making and Priority Setting
Kirsteen Watson and Stephen Gillam

Key points

- In the UK, funding decisions are made at three main levels: nationally at the Department of Health; locally within commissioning organisations, and at the front line between clinicians and patients in hospitals and general practices.
- In order to make funding decisions, it is necessary to determine the priority status of different options and to make decisions between them.
- Priority setting should be a transparent process based on a clear set of criteria, for example:
  - Is there a need for the service?
  - Is there an intervention or service which is proven to be effective and which will meet this need?
  - Is the intervention acceptable and appropriate for the health-care system?
  - Is the service cost-effective?
- Priority setting needs to take place within a clear ethical framework.

5.1 Introduction

Health-care systems within most countries are resource-limited – budgets are finite and not every service one would like to provide can be funded. In publicly funded health systems, those responsible for procuring health-care need to be able to explain how taxpayers' money has been spent. Decisions are made at both an individual patient and a population level. At an individual level, the decision might be: should this patient get a prescription for a statin to lower her blood cholesterol and, if so, which statin should it be? At a population level, the decision might be: will a health and social care commissioning organisation purchase a heart-failure specialist nurse, an additional sexual health clinic or a new model of occupational therapy?

In the UK, funding decisions are made at various levels. Individual clinicians, managers within commissioning organisations and hospitals, local politicians using public health advice and expertise and civil servants in the Department of Health and Social Care all make decisions which affect what public health and treatment services are available to populations. Some decisions are more appropriately made by individuals at a local level, but the need for some specialised services for rare or complex conditions may be very low for small populations. For example, around ten liver transplants are needed for every million people and decisions over funding liver-transplant services are taken at larger population levels by specially configured service commissioning groups. In the UK, a national Specialised Services Commissioning Committee within NHS England decides on specialised services for rare conditions such as liver transplantation or for new drugs to treat cancer.

This chapter focuses on how such decisions are made and considers:

- a framework for priority setting;
- a discussion of what factors should be taken into account when comparing options;
- a consideration of basic health economic concepts; and
- an overview of ethical principles which influence decisions.

While this chapter primarily takes examples from health-care, the same principles can be applied to decision-making in other sectors relevant to the public's health, such as local government (e.g. social care, transport, leisure facilities).

5.2 A Framework for Setting Priorities

In order to plan services which are effective and can be adequately resourced, it is important to consider the need for each service within a clear public health framework. A series of questions need to be considered before a service is funded and these are shown in Figure 5.1.

5.2.1 Identifying the Proposed Service

This may sound easy, but it is frequently very difficult. Many services continue to be funded based on historical actions: the activity (say hip replacements) we saw last year is provided and funded again this year plus a little bit extra to account for population increasing and ageing. New interventions and service options are always potentially available, but very rarely are decisions made which lead to disinvestment in services rather than investment in new ones.

In reality, those funding and delivering health-care are making decisions within defined resource limits and choosing between different options.

5.2.2 Assessing Need

The assessment of needs is discussed in detail in Chapter 1. The use of needs assessment is crucial for determining which interventions for which health and

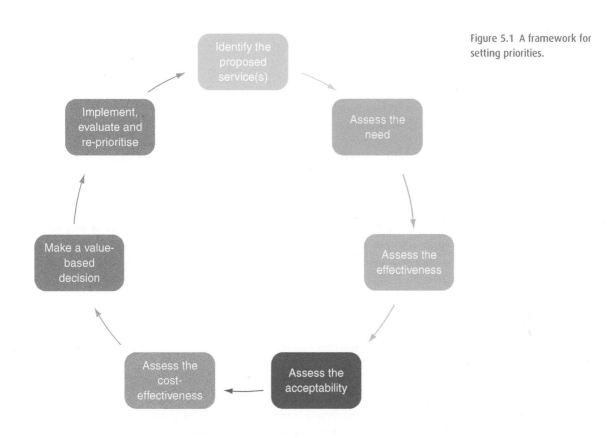

Figure 5.1 A framework for setting priorities.

health-care issues are likely to benefit the population most and so become priorities. Populations vary according to age, sex, ethnicity and many other determinants of health, and the need for health services will vary accordingly. The role of the public health specialist here is to ensure that services are targeted to those who most need them. One major way in which this is accomplished within the UK is via local authority-level collaboratively produced strategic needs assessments and health and well-being strategies, which identify core needs and priorities for the local population. These compile local-level epidemiological information with knowledge of local service delivery and therefore drive health and well-being service commissioning across a locality.

How might you apply this cycle to the commissioning of drug and alcohol services by a local authority, for example?

5.2.3 Assessing Evidence of Effectiveness

The concepts in this chapter are based on the moral judgement that if an intervention doesn't work, it shouldn't be provided by a publicly funded health-care system.

Repositories of evidence such as the Cochrane Library are valuable. Critical appraisal skills ensure the best possible assessment of the effectiveness of potential services or interventions (see Chapter 4).

However, evidence can be difficult to obtain. There are many interventions for which the quality and quantity of evidence are limited. Public health interventions often fall into this category as they may be multifaceted. Outcomes are only partly due to the intervention of interest (e.g. how much of a reduction in lung cancer mortality in men can be attributed to stop smoking services and how much could be due to treatment services or tobacco taxation?). Pragmatic solutions are often needed and the best available evidence is used to inform decisions.

The evidence base also changes over time and interventions previously thought to be effective may prove not to be in the light of further research. It can be difficult to reduce a service already in place and decisions such as these need careful implementation. For example, the evidence to support use of grommets in children with glue ear is limited. However, parents, and sometimes clinicians, need to be reassured that a useful service is not being withheld.

What methods could you use to ensure the views of the local population are taken into account when making decisions?

5.2.4 Assessing Acceptability

Services that are not acceptable to patients or the public will be less well used and potentially inefficient. When introducing new treatments, services or public health interventions, the views of patients and the public on what services are needed must be taken into consideration.

When introducing public health interventions which rely on people to change their behaviours, the people being targeted should be involved in the planning stages. Chapter 1 discusses some ways that patients, the public and local communities can be involved in health needs assessment. The same methodologies can be used to involve people in setting priorities.

5.2.5 Assessing Cost-Effectiveness

Costs must be factored into decision-making. However, money is not the only cost and saving lives is not the only benefit. Costs and benefits should be measured accurately and compared between different interventions and outcomes. For example, how do we determine whether £1 million spent on coronary care to improve cardiac outcomes is more useful than £1 million spent on cancer prevention?

Health economics applies traditional economic theory to consider problems in health-care. Economic evaluation helps decision-making by considering the outputs of competing interventions in relation to the resources they consume. Relevant outputs must be defined, costs measured and studies relating outputs to their costs undertaken.

5.2.5.1 Economic Evaluation

Economic evaluation can be defined as '... the comparative analysis of alternative courses of action in terms of both their costs and consequences' [1]. For a stop smoking service, for example, we would be comparing the costs (i.e. the resources consumed) and the consequences (outputs or benefits) of having this service against the costs and consequences of not having it.

Costs are generally divided into direct and indirect costs. Direct costs can be easily identified as the expenditure associated with the activity (e.g. the cost of 10 minutes of a general practitioner's time and the cost of a prescription). Indirect costs are more difficult to measure and might include items such as a share of the overheads (e.g. heating and lighting) for the building in which a service is provided. Opportunity costs should also be considered (see Box 5.1).

Consider an example. What might be some of the direct, indirect and opportunity costs of providing pneumococcal vaccines to an elderly population? How might this differ from the perspective of the health-care provider and the patient?

Options are rarely straightforward and the concept of *marginal or incremental* costs is helpful. This refers to the cost of (usually small) changes that can be made to an outcome or a service. Increasingly, health-care interventions make small, additional gains to health. Decisions are generally not whether to have a service or not, but whether to improve services in certain ways.

Thus, while we could compare, for example, a smoking cessation service with none, we are more likely to compare the current service (say, one nurse-led clinic per month) with an improved service (say, two clinics per month). In this case, we would compare the number of people who quit smoking from our original service with the

---

Box 5.1 Opportunity cost

An opportunity cost is 'the amount lost by *not* using the resource (labour, capital) in its best alternative use' (i.e. the benefit which could have been achieved if the money had been spent on the next best alternative).

For example, the financial cost of admitting an elderly patient with influenza and respiratory problems to a surgical ward (due to lack of beds) is relatively low (cost of bed, nursing, etc.). However, the opportunity cost of the admission may be much higher (e.g. cancelled operations due to a lack of beds for recovery, increased waiting lists, prolonged pain and disability for those unable to receive an operation).

Table 5.1 Types of economic evaluation

Type of evaluation	Costs measured in:	Benefits measured in:	Smoking cessation example:
Cost minimisation	Money	Not measured	Cost of one clinic compared to cost of two
Cost-benefit	Money	Money	Here you would need to value the benefits in terms of how much they were worth in financial terms – difficult to do
Cost-effectiveness	Money	Natural units – units relevant to the intervention	Costs per quitter
Cost utility	Money	Comparable units – often QALYs	Cost per QALY* gained for the quitters

* See Box 5.2.

number we predict for our improved service. We can then quote the benefits in terms of additional quitters per pound spent on the additional clinic. This is a marginal cost and tells us how much we could gain from our service improvement. An alternative is to focus on *programme budgets*, whereby expenditure can be broken down to identify funding for different types of disease areas and care, such as cancer, diabetes or mental health. Expenditure can be analysed against health outcomes to identify priorities, improve value for money and reduce health inequalities [2].

The process of comparing the costs and consequences of different treatments or services is called 'economic evaluation' and can be conducted in a variety of different ways according to what information is available to assess the consequences. Table 5.1 illustrates the different types of economic evaluation.

Cost minimisation does not count what is gained, but assumes the benefits of each option are the same. This type of analysis is often used, for example, in medicines management, when alternative drugs having the same clinical indication and effects are compared according to price and the cheapest prescribed. However, it is rarely the case that all consequences are equal.

Consider how you might persuade a health-care organisation that a more cost-effective but more expensive programme is a preferable investment.

In a *cost-benefit* analysis, both are measured in terms of monetary units, where a monetary value is placed on benefits such as cost savings, productivity or efficiency savings. Such analyses can be more transparent as they enable costs and effects to be compared using the same units. Often, monetary savings extend beyond direct savings in health to wider savings in the economy (such as productivity from employment), but it is difficult to quantify and compare these types of indirect savings from health-related interventions that might benefit society or individuals. One such workaround involves calculating a 'willingness to pay' – for example, how much an individual might be willing to pay for a product that monitors cholesterol levels to reduce their cardiovascular risk. One of the main limitations of cost-benefit analyses is the accuracy or ability to place an agreed monetary value on less tangible benefits, such as improvement in outcomes or well-being.

A *cost-effectiveness analysis* overcomes this challenge by comparing the outcomes in units of relevance for the intervention (e.g. lives saved or life years gained). In Table 5.1, the example is used of the number of people who quit after using a stop smoking service. However, this does not allow consideration of whether to invest in stop smoking services in preference to exercise classes or weight management, as the outcomes are not comparable.

This is where *cost-utility analyses* are useful as they measure all outcomes in terms of an index of benefit, which is comparable across different types of service. The quality-adjusted life year is the most commonly used index of benefit, used, for example, by the UK NICE technology appraisal programme [3]. This method allocates a quality of life value (between 1 (perfect health) and 0 (death)) and combines quantity and quality of life to derive the quality-adjusted life year (QALY). The process for this calculation is described in Box 5.2. Although the cost-utility method has the advantage that different interventions can be compared across a broad range of choices in resource allocation, a number of methodological problems remain, although this is also true of other approaches (see Box 5.3).

Box 5.2 How a QALY is constructed

A quality-adjusted life year (QALY) combines the quantity and quality of life. It is the arithmetic product of life expectancy and a measure of the quality of the remaining life years.

It takes 1 year of perfect-health life expectancy to be worth 1 and regards 1 year of less-than-perfect life expectancy as < 1.

Patients, the public and professionals are asked to judge the quality value (utility) for 1 year of life lived with the relevant condition and these values are then used multiplicatively with the number of years lived in this state to give the QALY.

For example, an intervention which results in a patient living for an additional 4 years rather than dying within 1 year, and where quality of life for both treated and untreated patients is 0.6, will generate:

4 years' extra life @ 0.6 QoL values = 2.4 less 1 year @ reduced quality = 0.6 generates 2.4−0.6 = 1.8 QALYs

QALYs can therefore provide an indication of the benefits gained from a variety of medical procedures in terms of quality of life and additional years for the patient.

Box 5.3 Disadvantages of QALYs

- It is argued that seeking to compare the incomparable (different treatments, different states) with crude tools is methodologically flawed and that their use oversimplifies complex health-care issues by reducing what should be a multifaceted assessment of options to simple quantitative values.
- QALYs are not based on an individual's assessment of value and the values determined by others may not reflect those of everyone.
- QALYs are controversial. They can be seen as 'ageist': reduced life expectancy results in lower QALY values, so interventions for elderly patients may compare poorly with those for young patients. Conversely, QALYs can be seen as 'insufficiently ageist' if one believes that the elderly have already had a 'fair innings' and the young are more deserving of treatment.
- QALYs may disadvantage those with disabilities or chronic conditions as their quality of life may be perceived by some as lower; interventions may yield fewer QALYs than for those in better 'background' health or fewer co-morbidities.
- QALYs may lack sensitivity within a disease area as not every subdivision within or level of complex conditions will have been valued and one value may be applied to subdivisions with varying health states (e.g. the quality of life with a condition like depression might vary considerably depending on the severity of the depression).

 How does a national organisation such as NICE utilise QALYs? Review their website and consider the pros and cons of this approach.

The most useful health economic analyses for public health tend to be *cost-utility* studies. Ideally, analyses should be carried out alongside the original effectiveness studies, but this adds to the cost of the study and is not always possible. It is important to understand from whose perspective the evaluation is being carried out as the costs and benefits will vary if considered from a health-care-provider perspective, as opposed to that of a patient or that of society. For example, in a study of nine alternative treatments for alcohol dependence, only three were found to be cost-effective when considered from the perspective of the patient who has to give time and money to attend the treatment [4]. However, while useful, the cost-utility model also does not reflect the complexities of measuring the impact of interventions on multiple outcomes.

5.2.6 Making Value-Based Decisions

There will always be competing needs to consider. Once we have assured ourselves that the proposed services are needed, effective, acceptable and cost-effective, we must still decide whether to fund them. This isn't as simple as asking 'Is there enough money to pay for this?' Frequently, funding one initiative means something else cannot be funded – there is an opportunity cost. Increasingly, there may be an additional requirement to ensure the overall expenditure on an intervention is cost-neutral or even cost-saving (i.e. that over time the ill health prevented saves the health system money). For example, identifying alcohol overuse in primary care and providing a brief intervention was estimated to be able to save the NHS in England £22 million per year in treatment costs from smoking-related admissions [5].

These kinds of judgements are ultimately also value-based. Options are weighed using ethical frameworks, implicitly or explicitly, to judge worth. Different ethical approaches upon which people base decisions, both in health-care and in daily life, are summarised in Table 5.2.

Table 5.2 Ethical approaches

Decisions are based on:	Explanation
The view that there is a right and a wrong	This approach is often seen in the popular press and media. Media headlines highlighting emotive issues around cancer treatments can make a dramatic impact on the public consciousness and influence the way in which decisions are made.
What powerful professionals think	There is a strong tradition, rapidly shifting now, of paternalism within health services. In a paternalistic system, decisions over treatment were pre-eminently the right of (mostly male) clinicians. There remain strong political preferences for or against imposing interventions on the population.
The greater good ('utilitarianism')	Public health decisions may use a 'utilitarian' framework, which aims to maximise the positive consequences for a population. This does not mean that everyone gets the same service, but that each receives health-care based on his or her need. This is equity rather than equality and attempts to bring the greatest good to the greatest number.
What we have always done	Health-care decisions about what services to fund are often made on the basis of what was bought last year. In these circumstances, services change very little and costs generally go up in line with inflation.
Standards or rights-based approach	We also tend to believe that everyone has the right to a minimum standard of service and many decisions are made based on guidance or targets set by experts (such as NICE). In England, interventions recommended in national NICE technology appraisals must be funded by each local health-care system.
Need in an emergency	Another way of making decisions is by applying the 'rule of rescue' [6]. Why do we mount a rescue for the survivors of a disaster when their chances of survival are slim? Why do we spend resources on critical care for patients where the effectiveness is limited? If we feel shocked by the circumstances of an individual and offer intervention based on this psychological imperative without thought for the opportunity costs, we are operating under the rule of rescue. For whole populations, this kind of decision-making may also take place in large-scale emergencies such as the COVID-19 pandemic, when funds are diverted to controlling an immediate threat.

Box 5.4 Beauchamp and Childress principles (and rules) of bio-medical ethics [7]

Beauchamp and Childress posit four major principles of bio-medical ethics and four minor rules:

Principles:

- **Respect for autonomy.** The right of an individual to make their own decisions about what to do. This important principle is implicit in the requirement for consent for procedures. It can be difficult to apply this principle to those who are unable to make informed decisions, such as minors or those with learning difficulties.
- **Non-maleficence.** Avoid harm. The need to avoid harm must frequently be weighed against the next principle when considering treatments with potential benefits and with some side effects.
- **Beneficence.** Do good. Too much beneficence can occasionally be paternalistic! For example, our need to prevent the harm caused by obesity might lead us to coerce overweight people into lifestyle changes.
- **Justice.** This principle reiterates the public health concept of equity in that a regard for fairness is important.

Rules:

- **Veracity.** The truth. It is difficult to make decisions based on falsehood, but the ability to be able to identify one common truth is debatable.
- **Privacy.** The right of patients to withhold information is seen to be important, but may hinder the diagnostic process.
- **Confidentiality.** This is of increasing importance in modern health-care and the need to handle patient-identifiable data sensibly is plain throughout many health-care systems.
- **Fidelity.** Trust. The relationship between clinician and patient requires trust; public health decisions which restrict treatments may jeopardise that trust.

 How would you apply the Beauchamp and Childress principles to decide whether it would be ethically justified to fund stop smoking services with specialist advisers to help individuals and groups quit through the use of motivational therapies and drugs?

Beauchamp and Childress' ethical framework [7] (see Box 5.4) is commonly used to guide clinical judgements. This can be adapted to form the basis of prioritisation decisions made in health-care settings. The principles may conflict with one another. For example, the decision to offer an expensive treatment to one patient from a limited budget permits them autonomy and enables the health carer to do good for that individual. However, the treatment may have side effects, which must be weighed against the benefits, and there may be insufficient funds left to treat others – thus unjustly restricting their right to treatment. Decisions around individual patient needs may conflict with the needs of populations and public health professionals are often involved in mediating over complex decisions.

A robust process not only serves the needs of patients and the public, but also enables organisations to assure their stakeholders that their decisions are fair and defend them, in a court of law, if necessary. An important element of decision-making is therefore not just 'distributive justice' or what resources are distributed to, but also 'procedural justice', the fairness of the processes that lead to the allocation of these resources. Making the values behind decision-making explicit is important. Daniels and Sabin offered an 'accountability for reasonableness' framework (AFR), which can be a useful model to consider and evaluate the fairness of priority-setting procedures [8]. It requires four conditions to be met:

- publicity – rationales for priority-setting decisions must be publicly accessible;
- relevance – these rationales must be considered to be relevant in this context, by 'fair-minded' people;
- appeals – there must be an avenue for appealing decisions; and
- enforcement – there must be some means of ensuring the first three conditions are met.

In the UK, NHS organisations are required to abide by a variety of laws as they make decisions which impact on patients, including those around equality and meeting the needs of patients, as well as remaining in financial balance. Priority-setting committees are frequently established by commissioning organisations, which utilise explicit frameworks to advise on the use of funds. The roles of such committees range from proposing rationing approaches for specific treatments (e.g. for IVF treatment) or setting clinical thresholds for certain treatments (e.g. varicose vein sclerotherapy), to the review of funding for 'exceptional cases' for individuals, in which the proposed treatment is not currently available.

What examples of decision-making frameworks have you seen in commissioning organisations? Many are available on their websites (e.g. exceptional funding review processes). Evaluate them from the perspective of distributive and procedural justice.

The notion of 'postcode' rationing, whereby different services – or different levels of service – are commissioned in different areas (or not), is a contentious aspect of priority setting. Many believe that geography should not determine to what care people have access. Yet there are significant inequalities across the country, some of which are attributable to the historic delivery of care and others would argue that prioritising by commissioners to 'rebalance local health economies is both inevitable and right' [9].

Beyond formal decision-making processes, it is useful to remember that various types of 'informal' or implicit ethical prioritisation decisions are made on a daily basis in health and social care [9]. 'Bedside' rationing ranges from seemingly ad hoc decisions made by individual clinicians or teams (such as which order inpatients are reviewed during a ward round, how long professionals spend with each patient and family), through to whether the availability of an intensive-care bed and treatment is allocated purely on medical need or other subconscious factors. It is important to be conscious of the potential biases, ethical values, frameworks or laws that influence our decision-making.

Globally, the ethics of rationing, as well as the ethical basis of restrictions of liberty and resources, came under significant challenge and scrutiny during the COVID-19 pandemic. For the first time in many countries, explicit discussions were taking place to decide how to use resources when a significant proportion of the population was affected by the virus, for example, how ventilators might be allocated to critically ill patients, how to triage admissions to emergency departments, how to deploy limited numbers of staff and how limited stocks of personal protective equipment might be allocated. Political decisions were made to restrict individual liberty and free movement for the sake of 'the greater good'. Ethical debates continue to balance the rights of individuals to go about their 'everyday' lives against the risk to extremely vulnerable individuals who might benefit from further mandatory restrictions, such as masks or social distancing. These debates and the introduction of legislation for the control of communicable diseases challenge public health specialists [10] and society at large, to deliver the best care and protection for the population.

 How might you define a set of criteria for access and use of critical care beds during a pandemic?

5.3 Conclusions

The aim of decision-making in public health is to provide a more robust decision than would be achieved through a less systematic approach, to ensure that resources are used cost-effectively, to enable improvement in the health of individuals and populations and to ensure decisions adhere to agreed ethical principles. Having made such decisions, the last stage of the framework proposes implementing the decision followed by evaluation and re-starting the cycle. A crucial element of prioritising and decision-making in health-care therefore involves quality, which is discussed in Chapter 6.

REFERENCES

1. M. F. Drummond, *Methods for the Economic Evaluation of Health Care Programmes*, Oxford, Oxford University Press, 1997.

2. Department of Health, Overview of Programme Budgeting Costing Methodology. 2011. Available at: https://assets.publishing.service.gov.uk/government/uploads/system/uploads/attachment_data/file/212911/Overview-of-the-Programme-Budgeting-Calculation-Methodology.pdf

3. National Institute for Clinical Excellence, Technology appraisal guidance. Available at: www.nice.org.uk/about/what-we-do/our-programmes/nice-guidance/nice-technology-appraisal-guidance

4. J. Dunlap, G. A. Zarkin, J. W. Bray *et al.*, Revisiting the cost-effectiveness of the COMBINE study for alcohol dependent patients: The patient perspective, *Medical Care* **48**(4), 2010, 306–13.

5. Public Health England, Guidance: Screening and brief advice for alcohol and tobacco use in inpatient settings, 2019. Available at: www.gov.uk/government/publications/preventing-ill-health-commissioning-for-quality-and-innovation/guidance-and-information-on-the-preventing-ill-health-cquin-and-wider-cquin-scheme#why-you-should-screen-and-give-brief-advice-for-alcohol-and-tobacco-use

6. A. R. Johnsen, Bentham in a box: Technology assessment and health care allocation, *Law, Medicine and Health Care* **14**(3–4), 1986, 172–4.

7. T. L. Beauchamp and J. F. Childress, *Principles of Biomedical Ethics*, 3rd ed., New York, NY, Oxford University Press, 1989.

8. N. Daniels, Accountability for reasonableness: Establishing a fair process for priority setting is easier than agreeing on principles, *British Medical Journal* **321**(7272), 2000, 1300–1.

9. R. Klein and J. Maybin, Thinking about rationing, King's Fund, 2012. Available at: www.kingsfund.org.uk/publications/thinking-about-rationing

10. World Health Organization, Ethics and COVID-19. Available at: www.who.int/teams/health-ethics-governance/diseases/covid-19

6

Improving Quality of Care

Nicholas Steel and Stephen Gillam

> ## Key points
>
> - Quality can be defined; it is multidimensional. The different dimensions of quality can be measured, but some (e.g. clinical effectiveness) are easier to measure than others (e.g. professionals' empathy for patients).
> - Problems with quality of care are widespread, with many people either not receiving effective health-care, or receiving care that is ineffective or harmful, and recurrent catastrophic failures at institutional level.
> - Approaches to improving quality have traditionally focused on regulation, education and clinical professionalism, including clinical audit.
> - Quality improvement involves the systematic and coordinated use of specific methods and tools to solve identified problems.
> - Quality improvement frameworks originating in industry (such as 'Plan-Do-Study-Act' and payment for performance) have been widely used with mixed results over the past 20 years.

6.1 Introduction

As we saw in earlier chapters in this book, effective health-care makes a large and increasing contribution to preventing disease and prolonging life, by reducing the population burden of disease. However, only the right kind of health-care delivered in the right way, at the right time, to the right person can improve health. Health-care interventions that are powerful enough to improve population health are also powerful enough to cause harm if incorrectly used. How can public health specialists know whether their interventions are having the desired effect? The last part of the planning cycle in Figure 1.4 concerns evaluation. Clinicians can monitor the impact of their treatments on an individual patient basis, but how do we examine the impact of a new service? This chapter looks at what we mean by quality of health-care and considers some frameworks for its evaluation.

6.2 What Is Quality and Can It Be Measured?

The science of quality measurement in health-care is still evolving, but it is generally accepted that elements of quality of health-care can be defined and measured. Quality has been defined as 'the degree to which health services for individuals and populations increase the likelihood of desired health outcomes and are consistent with current professional knowledge' [1]. 'Desired health outcomes' is a key phrase, as it deliberately does not specify who is doing the desiring. It implicitly accepts that different people will want different outcomes.

Some dimensions of quality, such as clinical effectiveness and its related outcomes of health status and mortality rates, are relatively straightforward to define and measure quantitatively. Other important but more subjective dimensions (such as patient-centred health-care) and attributes (such as respect and trust) are harder to measure. Yet measurement is an essential component of quality improvement. If we do not measure quality, we cannot know whether health services are achieving the level of population health benefit of which they are potentially capable. However, measures of quality need to be used carefully to avoid the risks of undermining professionalism and the doctor–patient relationship [2]. For example, zealous adherence to computerised treatment protocols may sometimes limit doctors' responsiveness to patients' priorities.

Desired health outcomes may be different for managers, patients and clinicians [3]. Managers may be rightly concerned with efficiency, and seek to maximise the population health gain through best use of an inevitably limited budget. Clinicians are usually more focused on effectiveness, and want the treatment that works best for each of their patients. Patients clearly want treatment that works and will not cause harm, and also place a high priority on how the treatment is delivered.

What aspects of care are important to you when you or your family use the health service?

Coulter has described the following health-care aspirations of patients [4]:
- fast access to reliable health advice;
- effective treatment delivered by trusted professionals;
- participation in decisions and respect for preferences;
- clear, comprehensible information and support for self-care;
- attention to physical and environmental needs;
- emotional support, empathy and respect;
- involvement of, and support for, family and carers; and
- continuity of care and smooth transitions.

A focus on health-care simply as a product rather than a service may undervalue the essential role of patients in the co-production of health, which Batalden describes as 'the interdependent work of users and professionals who are creating, designing, producing, delivering, assessing, and evaluating the relationships and actions that contribute to the health of individuals and populations' [5].

6.3 Dimensions of Quality and Their Evaluation

For the WHO, quality of care is 'the degree to which health services for individuals and populations increase the likelihood of desired health outcomes' [6] (see Box 6.1).

From a patient perspective, evaluation can be considered in terms of different dimensions of their care: access, assessment of preferences and goals, prevention, diagnosis, treatment and rehabilitation, and achievement of desired outcomes.

Evaluation has been defined as 'a process that attempts to determine as systematically and objectively as possible the relevance, effectiveness and impact of activities in the light of their objectives' [7]. A successful evaluation will tell us whether the intervention makes a difference, and whether the difference is worth the cost.

Where do we start when thinking about evaluation of a delivery system in the NHS? Avedis Donabedian, a guru in quality improvement circles, distinguished four elements (see Table 6.1): Structures, Processes, Outputs and Outcomes (SPOOs) [8].

Box 6.1 The World Health Organization proposes that health-care is rendered: [6]

- **effective** by providing evidence-based health-care services to those who need them;
- **safe** by avoiding harm to the people for whom the care is intended;
- **people-centred** by providing care that responds to individual preferences, needs and values, within health services that are organised around the needs of people;
- **timely** by reducing waiting times and sometimes harmful delays for both those who receive and those who give care;
- **equitable** by providing the same quality of care regardless of age, sex, gender, race, ethnicity, geographic location, religion, socioeconomic status, linguistic or political affiliation;
- **integrated** by providing care that is coordinated across levels and providers and makes available the full range of health services throughout the life course; and
- **efficient** by maximising the benefit of available resources and avoiding waste.

Table 6.1 Donabedian's model of examining health services and evaluating quality of care [8] and illustrated with an example

Element	Description	Example: Evaluation of the national screening programme for colorectal cancer
Structures	buildings, staff, equipment	The volume and costs of new equipment (colonoscopic, radiographic, histopathological), staff and buildings
Processes	all that is done to patients	The numbers of patients screened, coverage rates within a defined age range, numbers of true and false positives
Outputs	the immediate results of (medical) intervention	Number of cancers identified, operations performed
Outcomes	gains in health status, well-being or function	Complication rates, colorectal cancer incidence, prevalence and mortality rates

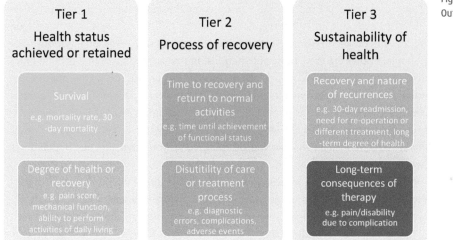

Figure 6.1 Porter's Hierarchy of Outcomes [9].

Use a structure, process, output, outcome model to consider what measures might be relevant to the evaluation of services; for example, immunisation programmes, a breast screening programme or a hip replacement pathway.

Michael Porter proposes a hierarchy for furthering considering outcome measures [9], which ensures outcomes are measured across the whole cycle or pathway of care (see Figure 6.1). For each dimension, success is measured by specific measures or metrics, and a decision is made on the timing and frequency for measurement. This is a helpful tool to consider what outcomes would reflect high quality, and to consider or choose appropriate metrics.

There are various examples globally of comprehensive outcomes measurement frameworks designed to share robust measures of health and well-being, and to enable comparison between geographical areas – for example, the UK Compendium of Population Health Indicators [10] or the Organisation for Economic Co-operation and Development's (OECD) 'Health Care Quality and Outcomes Indicators' [11]. Domestically, the UK government uses three national outcomes frameworks – one each for public health, adult social care and the NHS – which set out high-level areas for improvement, alongside supporting measures, to help track progress without overshadowing local priorities. A Quality and Outcomes Framework (QOF) is also used to remunerate general practices for providing good-quality care.

Use the SPOO framework and the hierarchy of outcomes to consider suitable outcomes and metrics to evaluate and monitor the quality of a variety of services; for example, a 'falls' pathway for those over 65 years, immunisation or screening service, or a cardiac rehabilitation programme.

The assessment of process as well as outcome measures is helpful for at least two reasons. Firstly, for many interventions it may be difficult to obtain robust data on health outcomes unless large numbers are scrutinised over long periods. For example, evaluating the quality of hypertension management within a general practice, you may be reliant on process measures (the proportion of the appropriate population with a current blood pressure measurement, treated and adequately controlled) as a proxy for good outcomes. The assumption here is that evidence from larger-scale studies showing that control of hypertension reduces subsequent death rates from heart disease will be reflected in your own practice population's health experience.

Secondly, one of the biggest problems in evaluating large-scale public health interventions is the effect of the many different factors influencing outcomes: background 'noise'. For example, assessing the impact of mass media campaigns against smoking might be complicated by the impact of laws to prevent smoking in public places, changes to what is taught in schools, increased taxation on cigarettes or background decline in the population prevalence of smoking. Similarly, it is difficult to measure the contribution of fruit and vegetable provision to, for example, reduction in colorectal cancer rates, due to the multifactorial nature of the determinants of bowel cancer. The complexity of the determinants of disease and of interventions designed to prevent them, the long time lag between some interventions and their expected effect (e.g. efforts to improve food labelling will not swiftly affect obesity levels) can all make it difficult to extrapolate the impact of specific interventions.

It must be remembered that readily available measures of quality are not necessarily the most important, and the most important elements of quality may not be easily measurable. For example, with their interest in equity of provision, public health specialists need to consider the accessibility of services particularly to disadvantaged groups.

Can you think of other factors that might complicate the evaluation of public health interventions?

6.4 Is There a Problem with Quality?

We have seen that health-care is a powerful tool for improving public health. Like all powerful tools, it can have adverse as well as positive effects. Problems with health-care fall into one of three broad categories, all of which are amenable to public health action:

- **Underuse**: effective health-care can be underused, so that people miss out on opportunities to benefit from it.
- **Overuse**: wasting resources by delivering care to those who do not need it, or where the potential for harm exceeds the benefit.
- **Misuse**: where patients suffer avoidable complications of surgery or medication – for example, a patient who suffers a rash after receiving penicillin as treatment for an infection, despite having a known allergy to penicillin.

We know that some effective health-care is underused. Many effective interventions are only received by half the people who should receive them [12]. There is also great variability in the quality of care experienced by different populations, by illness, age, sex, race, wealth, geographic location and insurance coverage. This problem of inequalities or disparities has been the focus of considerable policy attention, helped by Julian Tudor-Hart's devising of his famous 'inverse care law' 'as a weapon' over 30 years ago [13] (see also Chapter 14):

> The availability of good medical care tends to vary inversely with the need for it in the population served. This operates more completely where medical care is most exposed to market forces, and less so where such exposure is reduced. The market distribution of medical care is a primitive and historically outdated social form, and any return to it would further exaggerate the maldistribution of medical resources.

We also know that care can be overused. Wennberg first documented the wide variations in care received by similar populations. He showed that health-care is often driven by the availability of specialist services, rather than by the health needs of the population, with no detectable difference in health outcomes [14]. This variation in quantity of health-care with no apparent relationship to quality implies that some health-care is overused. The costs of such waste are substantial – upwards of $100 billion per year in the USA [15]. More importantly, too much medicine is a source of considerable harm [16].

What further examples can you identify of overuse, underuse and misuse within health-care?

Various entrenched factors drive overuse: commercial drivers and financial incentives, a medical culture that encourages excessive testing and treatment, lack of evidence on the effectiveness of new technologies or ignorance thereof. Multimorbidity and the accumulation of medical diagnoses is linked to the concept of over diagnosis: '... when people without symptoms are diagnosed with a disease that ultimately will not cause them symptoms or early death' [17].

About 850,000 'adverse events' occur in the NHS each year involving 10% of admissions. It is estimated that 3.6% of deaths in English hospitals are avoidable [18]. Adverse drug events have been shown to cause considerable morbidity, mortality, and cost in the UK and USA [19]. In an increasingly litigious environment, the numbers of written complaints about health-care are increasing. The NHS pays out over £2 billion each year to settle clinical negligence claims [20].

Reports into health-care scandals, such as the avoidable maternal and neonatal deaths at Shrewsbury and Telford Hospital over a period of nearly 20 years from 2000, repeatedly highlight the same problems: failure to learn and improve, underpinned by a failure to listen to patients; failures in leadership and systems; and staff bullying, often in a context of underfunding and inadequate staffing levels [21].

These widespread quality problems are not simply the result of individual clinicians making mistakes. Quality is a feature of health systems, and not simply of the health professionals in the system. Human beings will always make occasional mistakes, and experience from other industries has shown that dramatic quality improvement can occur when systems are designed that do not rely on humans avoiding mistakes. Some of the main approaches used to improve quality in health-care are described in the next section.

6.5 How Can Quality of Care for Populations Be Improved?

Many different approaches to improving the quality of health-care have been tried in the past, with varying levels of success. They can be broadly classified into the groups summarised in Table 6.2.

Table 6.2 Approaches to quality improvement in health-care

Type of approach	Examples
Regulation and standards	American Board of Medical Specialties in the USA
	General Medical Council in the UK
	UK National Screening Programmes and their quality assurance
Education and audit	Royal Colleges, professional organisations, Plan-Do-Study-Act
Market and financial	Payment for performance according to achievement of clinical indicators
System-level approaches	Lean; Six Sigma; implementation science (see below)

6.5.1 Regulation and Standards

A robust regulatory framework is important for assuring a basic standard of health-care, and regulation of medical professionals is a central component of quality improvement in nearly all countries. Historically, regulation has been primarily associated with the medical profession, but is increasingly used for non-medical health professionals. The three main purposes of professional regulation are:

- to set minimally acceptable standards of care;
- to provide accountability of professionals to patients and payers; and
- to improve quality of care by providing guidance about best practice [22].

In the UK, the General Medical Council regulates doctors. The UK Public Health Register is the regulator for public health specialists who come from backgrounds other than medicine. These regulators are currently adapting to environments where greater levels of public accountability are required. The UK Care Quality Commission assesses the performance of health-care organisations. In the USA, the American Board of Medical Specialties oversees certification of doctors. The requirements are a mixture of accredited training, cognitive examination, competency-based evaluation, and audit and clinical performance, and certification needs to be renewed every 6 to 10 years. Certification status has been shown to be associated with higher quality of care [22]. Accreditation of US hospitals for Medicare reimbursement takes place through the Joint Commission on Accreditation of Healthcare Organizations.

Standards of care can be set out in guidelines such as those published by the National Institute for Health and Clinical Excellence (NICE) and Scottish Intercollegiate Guidelines Network (SIGN) in the UK, and the US Preventive Services Task Force (USPSTF) in the USA.

A good example of the method by which standards of care are developed is the RAND/UCLA appropriateness method [23]. This was developed in response to the lack of randomised controlled clinical trial data on many interventions, and the problems with interpreting sometimes contradictory trial results for use in routine care. It combines research data with clinical expertise, and involves the following stages:

- identifying clinical area(s) of care for quality assessment;
- conducting a systematic review of care in the relevant clinical area(s);
- drafting quality indicators;
- presenting draft quality indicators and their evidence base to a clinical panel for a modified Delphi process. The Delphi process typically involves asking panel members to anonymously rate the draft indicators for validity, over two rounds with face-to-face discussion between rounds [24]; and
- approving a final set of indicators.

The quality standards produced by methods such as this can be used to assess the quality of care in a single clinic or a whole health system. An example of quality assessment on a very large scale is the payment of incentives to general practitioners

Table 6.3 Example clinical domains and indicators for UK general practitioners 2021–22 [25]

Clinical domain	No. of points (used to calculate financial incentives)	Example of indicator in each clinical domain
Hypertension	14	The percentage of patients aged 79 years or under with hypertension in whom the last blood pressure reading (measured in the preceding 12 months) is 140/90 mmHg or less
Asthma	20	The percentage of patients with asthma on the register, who have had an asthma review in the preceding 12 months
Depression	10	The percentage of patients aged 18 or over with a new diagnosis of depression in the preceding 1 April to 31 March, who have been reviewed not earlier than 10 days after and not later than 56 days after the date of diagnosis
Chronic kidney disease (CKD)	6	The contractor establishes and maintains a register of patients aged 18 or over with CKD with classification of categories G3a to G5
Diabetes	3	The percentage of patients with diabetes, on the register, with a diagnosis of nephropathy (clinical proteinuria) or micro-albuminuria who are currently treated with an ACEI (or ARBs)

in the UK on the basis of their performance against quality indicators. Table 6.3 gives examples of indicators from the 2021–22 revision of the British general practitioners' contract [25]. Income is determined by the total number of points obtained.

6.5.2 Education and Audit

The dominant approach for ensuring quality among health professionals has been education and audit. Education and audit are common requirements for regulation, but go beyond the requirements of regulation, in that they seek to go beyond a minimum standard and strive for excellence. Education has traditionally been professionally led, and is seen by many as an obligation of professional status. Professional organisations, such as the Royal Colleges in the UK, have been influential in setting high standards and encouraging audit.

The clinical audit cycle refers to the monitoring of performance against predefined standards (Figure 6.2). Measurement of one's performance against defined criteria can be demanding, but the real challenge is to make necessary adjustments and re-evaluate your performance – in other words, to complete the cycle.

 Consider an audit cycle you may have observed or where you could implement one in your practice. How would you define criteria and monitor performance?

Professionals have, of course, not had a monopoly on education. The evidence-based medicine movement and the Cochrane Collaboration have been very important in improving the quantity and quality of information on the effectiveness of health-care interventions (see Chapter 4). The Plan-Do-Study-Act (PDSA) cycle takes audit one stage further, and is widely used in health-care (see Figure 6.3). The PDSA cycle has four stages, designed to help with the development, testing and implementation of quality improvement plans. The stages are, firstly, to develop a plan and define the objective (plan). Secondly, to carry out the plan and collect data (do), then analyse the data and summarise what was learned (study). The final stage is to plan the next cycle with necessary modifications (act). For further information, see the Institute for Healthcare Improvement's website [26].

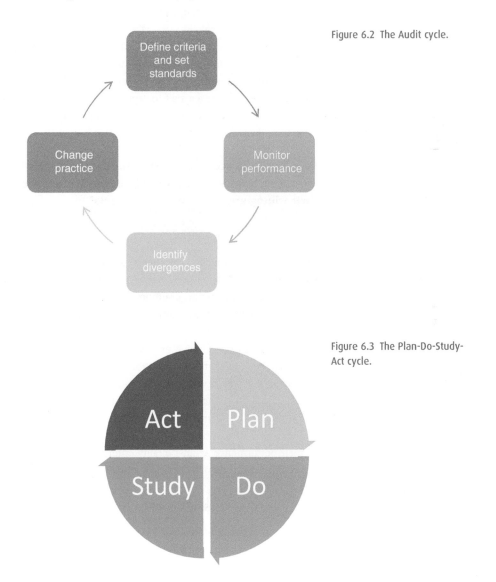

Figure 6.2 The Audit cycle.

Figure 6.3 The Plan-Do-Study-Act cycle.

The maintenance of a desired level of quality in a service and encouragement of continuous improvement – or quality assurance – requires attention to every stage of the process of delivery. The first rule of quality assurance based on experience in private production systems and public services across the world: when things go wrong and mistakes are made, the problem arises more often from faulty systems than from faulty individuals. In *An Organisation with a Memory*, the Department of Health laid down its approach to risk management in the NHS borrowing on experience in the airline industry [27]. It declared the need for:

- unified mechanisms for reporting and analysis when things go wrong;
- mechanisms for ensuring that, where lessons are identified, the necessary changes are put into practice;
- much wider appreciation of the value of the systems approach in preventing, analysing and learning from errors; and
- a more open culture in which errors or service failures can be discussed.

NHS England encourages staff to report incidents and 'near misses' without fear of personal reprimand. They should feel that, by sharing their experiences, others will be able to learn lessons and improve patient safety.

 In your experience, how 'open' is the culture of health-care? How does increasing litigation affect the way in which doctors practise medicine and their willingness to share adverse events?

6.5.3 Market and Financial

Market-based approaches have been most used in the USA, and rely on an informed consumer exercising choice. An example is the Consumer Assessment of Healthcare Providers and Systems programme. Public release of performance data alone has met with limited success in improving quality, perhaps due to lack of data to inform real choice, or perhaps because the data are not used by the public. However, data publication can be effective as part of a larger initiative. The publication of risk-adjusted mortality rates from coronary artery bypass grafting for hospitals and surgeons is nowadays widespread [28]. The data are used to inform quality improvement efforts and reduce operative mortality.

Payment for performance is a significant model internationally. Examples are the payment of a substantial portion of salary to British general practitioners according to their performance against quality criteria (see Table 6.3) and financial incentives to providers from the US Centers for Medicare and Medicaid Services.

6.5.4 System-Level Approaches

A common criticism of much of what health professionals do to try and improve the quality of their care is that it is piecemeal and poorly coordinated. Variable quality of care, particularly in the poorest, least healthy and least well-resourced parts of the country, has long been a fact of NHS life. In this section, we consider some widely used approaches at system level to improve quality: clinical governance, industrial models such as LEAN and Six Sigma, quality, service improvement and redesign (QSIR), and management of patient safety, including significant event audit.

6.5.4.1 Clinical Governance

The term 'clinical governance' (borrowing on notions of corporate governance from the private sector) refers to the framework through which NHS organisations and their staff are accountable for the quality of patient care. It covers the organisations, systems and processes for monitoring and improving services. The different components of clinical governance are listed in Box 6.2.

An element of clinical governance which has the potential to have a rapid impact on patient care is clinical audit, which is described in Section 6.5.2 above.

Box 6.2 Components of clinical governance

Processes for quality improvement	1. Patient and public involvement
	2. Risk management
	3. Clinical audit
	4. Clinical effectiveness programmes
	5. Staffing and staff management
Staff focus	6. Education, training and continuing personal and professional development
Information	7. Use of information to support clinical governance and health-care delivery

---

6.5.4.2 Industrial Models Such as Lean and Six Sigma

The business world has given us powerful examples of quality improvement initiatives that consider the whole system, and two that have been successfully adopted into health-care are Six Sigma, invented by Motorola, and Toyota's 'Lean' technique. The Lean technique entails assessing every process for its value to the patient, to cut waste and inefficiencies and improve patient care. The idea behind Six Sigma is simple: we should not accept the current common error rates of 50% in health-care, nor 10% or even 1%, but strive for near perfect error rates of less than 1 in 3.4 million [29]. Proponents of Six Sigma argue that these error rates are achievable in health-care, just as in manufacturing, and cite anaesthesia as an example of an area that has seen dramatic improvements in safety. Table 6.4 gives examples of the defect rates (which relate to a particular sigma level) in different industries.

Table 6.4 Sigma levels and defect rates in different industries [29]

Defects per million	Sigma level	Health-care examples	Other industry examples
3.4	6		Publishing: one misspelled word in all books in a small library
5.4		Deaths caused by anaesthesia during surgery	
230	5		Airline fatalities
6,210	4		Airline baggage handling Restaurant bills
10,000		1% of all hospitalised patients injured through negligence	
66,800	3		Publishing: 7.6 misspelled words per page in a book
210,000		21% of ambulatory antibiotics for colds	
	2	58% of patients with depression not diagnosed/treated adequately	
790,000	1	79% of heart attack survivors not given beta-blockers	

6.5.4.3 Significant Event Audit and Root Cause Analysis

Most health-care organisations will have a patient safety framework and management system. In the UK, the 'Patient Safety Incident Response Framework' (PSIRF) sets out the NHS's approach to developing and maintaining effective systems and processes for responding to patient safety incidents for the purpose of learning and improving patient safety.

Significant event audit (SEA) is a quality improvement and assurance process whereby 'individual cases in which there has been a significant occurrence (not necessarily involving an undesirable outcome for the patient) are analysed in a systematic and detailed way, to ascertain what can be learnt about the overall quality of care and to indicate changes that might lead to future improvements' [30]. This is used in clinical scenarios to evaluate every adverse event or potential adverse event to implement system-wide learning to prevent future incidents. It can be linked to root cause analysis (RCA), a systematic process to:

- gather and map information to determine what happened;
- identify problems with health-care delivery;
- identify contributory factors and root causes; and
- agree what needs to change and implement solutions.

Have you observed opportunities to improve the quality of care in your local service? How would you go about understanding the issue and implementing change?

6.5.4.4 Quality, Service Improvement and Redesign

NHS England has produced a comprehensive collection of proven quality, service improvement and redesign (QSIR) tools, theories and techniques [31]. This offers a vast range of different options for approaches to supporting 'grass-roots' change programmes within health and social care to identify and utilise opportunities to enhance quality. As is discussed further in Chapter 7, being aware of such tools and approaches, and their opportunities, strengths and limitations enables you to employ appropriate techniques in a variety of situations to analyse and improve quality.

6.6 Conclusions

We have seen that approaches to quality improvement can be grouped into four broad categories: regulation, education, market-based and system-level approaches. Whichever combination of these is used, the level in the health-care system at which quality improvement approaches are applied is important. Previously, most quality improvement took place in single clinics, in patients with single diseases. Multilevel approaches to change, that impact on individuals, groups or teams, the organisation as a whole, and the larger environment and system level, have greater chances of success [19].

Many different QSIR techniques have been successfully used in different parts of the NHS as well as other health-care systems, but examples of sustained scale-up and implementation of quality improvement are rare. Implementation science is starting to study the reasons for this [32]. A long-term phased approach that embraces complexity and uses social science to understand why people act in the way that they do in particular organisational and social contexts is likely to be needed for widespread implementation of successful initiatives. Excellent guides have been developed for health-care staff leading service change following the pandemic [33].

Furthermore, the risks of quality improvement should also be considered. Sometimes the most promising initiatives do not improve quality, and research and evaluation to assess the impact of quality improvement is essential [34]. Disparities in access to health-care are a problem in all countries, and any quality improvement programme may worsen disparities unless the improvement has proportionally greater benefit for the relatively disadvantaged population.

What are the opportunity costs of quality improvement? Do the benefits outweigh the costs?

The most important part of any quality improvement initiative is a group of committed people who consistently seek to make health-care better. The particular technique chosen is probably much less important than the dedication of the people involved. Chapter 7 looks further at how public health practitioners can employ leadership and management skills to wield influence and lead change.

REFERENCES

1. Institute of Medicine (IOM), *Committee on Health Care in America. Crossing the Quality Chasm: A New Health System for the 21st Century*, Washington, DC, National Academy Press, 2001.
2. D. Swinglehurst, N. Emmerich and S. Quilligan, Rethinking 'quality' in health care, *Journal of Health Services Research & Policy* **19**(2), 2014, 65–6.
3. N. Steel, Thresholds for taking antihypertensive drugs in different professional and lay groups: Questionnaire survey, *British Medical Journal* **320**(7247), 2000, 1446–7.
4. A. Coulter, What do patients and the public want from primary care? *British Medical Journal* **331**(7526), 2005, 1199–201.
5. P. Batalden, Getting more from health care: Quality improvement must acknowledge patient coproduction, *British Medical Journal* **362**, 2018, k3617.
6. World Health Organization, Quality of Care, Geneva, WHO, 14 October 2022. Available at: www.who.int/health-topics/quality-of-care
7. J. M. Last, *A Dictionary of Epidemiology*, 4th ed., Oxford, Oxford University Press, 2001.
8. A. Donabedian, *Explorations in Quality Assessment and Monitoring*, Vol. 1: *The Definition of Quality and Approaches to Its Assessment*, Ann Arbor, MI, Health Administration Press, 1980.
9. M. E. Porter, What is value in health care? *New England Journal of Medicine* **363**, 2010, 2477–81.
10. NHS Digital, About the Compendium of Population Health Indicators. Available at: https://digital.nhs.uk/data-and-information/publications/ci-hub/compendium-indicators
11. Organisation for Economic Co-operation and Development (OECD), Health Care Quality and Outcomes Indicators. Available at: www.oecd.org/health/
12. N. Steel, M. Bachmann, S. Maisey *et al.*, Self reported receipt of care consistent with 32 quality indicators: National population survey of adults aged 50 or more in England, *British Medical Journal* **337**, 2008, a957.
13. J. Tudor-Hart, Commentary: Three decades of the inverse care law [comment], *British Medical Journal* **320**(7226), 2000, 18–19.
14. J. E. Wennberg, Unwarranted variations in healthcare delivery: Implications for academic medical centres, *British Medical Journal* **325**(7370), 2002, 961–4.
15. W. Shrank, T. Rogstad and N. Parekh, Waste in the US health care system: Estimated costs and potential for savings, *Journal of the American Medical Association* **322**(15), 2019, 1501–9.
16. S. Brownlee and D. Korenstein, Better understanding the downsides of low value healthcare could reduce harm, *British Medical Journal* **372**, 2021, n117.

17. J. Treadwell and M. McCartney, Overdiagnosis and overtreatment: Generalists – it's time for a grassroots revolution, *British Journal of General Practice* **66**(644), 2016, 116–17.

18. H. Hogan, R. Zipfell, J. Neuburger *et al.*, Avoidability of hospital deaths and association with hospital-wide mortality ratios: Retrospective case record review and regression analysis, *British Medical Journal* **351**, 2015, h3239.

19. Committee on Quality of Health Care in America (IoM), *To Err Is Human: Building a Safer Health System*, Washington, DC, National Academy Press, 2000.

20. C. Dyer, NHS compensation scheme is 'not fit for purpose' and needs radical overhaul, say MPs, *British Medical Journal* **377**, 2022, o1085.

21. Independent review of maternity services at Shrewsbury and Telford Hospital NHS Trust, March 2022. Available at: www.ockendenmaternityreview.org.uk/

22. K. Sutherland and S. Leatherman, Does certification improve medical standards? *British Medical Journal* **333**(7565), 2006, 439–41.

23. R. H. Brook, M. R. Chassin, A. Fink *et al.*, A method for the detailed assessment of the appropriateness of medical technologies, *International Journal of Technology Assessment in Health Care* **2**(1), 1986, 53–63.

24. B. Graham, G. Regehr and J. G. Wright, Delphi as a method to establish consensus for diagnostic criteria, *Journal of Clinical Epidemiology* **56**(12), 2003, 1150–6.

25. NHS Employers and the General Practitioners Committee, Quality and Outcomes Framework guidance for GMS contract 2021/22. Delivering investment in general practice, London, NHS Employers, 2021.

26. Institute for Healthcare Improvement, Washington, DC. Available at: www.ihi.org/

27. Department of Health, *An Organisation with a Memory*, London, The Stationery Office, 2000.

28. B. Englum, P. Saha-Chaudhuri and D. Shahian, The impact of high-risk cases on hospitals' risk-adjusted coronary artery bypass grafting mortality rankings, *Annals of Thoracic Surgery* **99**(3), 2015, 856–62.

29. M. R. Chassin, Is health care ready for Six Sigma quality? *Milbank Quarterly* **76**(4), 1998, 565–91.

30. M. Pringle, C. P. Bradley, C. M. Carmichael *et al.*, Significant event auditing: A study of the feasibility and potential of case-based auditing in primary medical care, *Occasional Paper (Royal College of General Practitioners)* **70**, 1995, i–71.

31. NHS England, Quality, service improvement and service redesign tools (QSIR), 2022. Available at: www.england.nhs.uk/sustainableimprovement/qsir-programme/qsir-tools/

32. T. Greenhalgh and C. Papoutsi, Spreading and scaling up innovation and improvement, *British Medical Journal* **365**, 2019, l2068.

33. B. Jones, E. Kwong and W. Warburton, Quality improvement made simple: What everyone should know about health care quality improvement, London, The Health Foundation, April 2022. Available at: www.health.org.uk/publications/quality-improvement-made-simple

34. M. Dixon-Woods, How to improve health care improvement, *British Medical Journal* **367**, 2019, l5514.

7

Management, Leadership and Change

Kirsteen Watson and Jan Yates

Key points

- The delivery of improved population health outcomes requires a combination of expertise and influence, requiring the adoption and development of management and leadership skills for personal effectiveness and impact.
- Management and leadership are separate theoretical domains, but are often conflated. There are a large number of different theories and ideas and a critical analysis must be adopted to develop a personal toolkit that enhances one's leadership skills.
- Different styles of leadership and management are appropriate in different circumstances and an understanding of one's own preferences, strengths and areas for improvement are important in developing professional practice.
- Effective public health professionals work within a complex system of partners, agencies and organisations and must understand how to communicate and engage with individuals and teams effectively.
- Services and programmes are constantly evolving and public health professionals need to be able to lead and manage change effectively.

7.1 Introduction

Effective public health practice requires a combination of expertise and influence. The remainder of this textbook is devoted to the subject expertise required in public health: the skills to apply it to create solutions or improve outcomes are interwoven throughout with examples and suggestions. Yet gaining expertise in the subject matter is only one element of practice: the ability to influence outcomes, policy, services and the people who make decisions is crucial. To deploy your expertise to have an impact, you must hone leadership and management skills to persuade, encourage and empower others.

Leadership and management is an entire academic discipline in its own right, and the subject of a plethora of popular books, videos, websites, articles and courses. Even a potted history of key milestones in how leadership theories have developed, or current schools of thought requires a (large) textbook of its own! This chapter, therefore, aims to:

- offer a *brief* overview of different schools of thought in leadership;
- propose a simple framework of eight core domains for identifying skills and areas for professional development;
- introduce some popular theories for understanding others, which can enable you to work more effectively with individuals and influence within teams and organisations; and
- signpost to some key models of conceptualising change and how to lead or manage change.

7.2 Theories of Leadership and Management

Definitions in the literature tend to view 'leadership' as the act of encouraging others to pursue specific actions, with emphasis on inspiring others to follow you and to identify a course of action that will improve outcomes. 'Management', by contrast, usually refers to the consistent work of organising a team or programme of activity, overseeing performance and resources, and addressing any problems or challenges. Kotter offers a helpful distinction: 'leaders navigate change', while 'managers navigate complexity', and he notes that these are 'distinct but complementary functions' [1]. While this is somewhat oversimplistic (in reality, both functions involve change and complexity), it highlights how management is often perceived as overseeing the running of 'day-to-day' services and teams, whereas leadership often entails creating a vision for change and inspiring others to achieve this together.

Working in public health, you are likely to require management skills in working within or managing a team; coordinating and collaborating with others to create integrated systems or services; and working alongside different stakeholders and political groups to find a course of action which accommodates interests and agendas. Understanding how to manage and optimise such situations and interactions is crucial for personal effectiveness. Equally, much of public health practice involves striving for improvement, seeking the best use of public money and resources to deliver services and improve outcomes, and often requires significant leadership to bring about innovative or comprehensive solutions.

What do you think managers do? What managerial skills do you need?

7.2.1 The Evolution of Leadership and Management Theory

Leadership, like public health, can be considered both an art and a science, and involves assimilating and critically analysing various differing and interlinked models and ideas. It is challenging to conceptualise one overarching model of leadership – authors who have tried have created a complex 'mind map' of interlacing theories which can confuse rather than simplify the topic. Over the last century, enquiry into leadership and management and what they mean has evolved through various stages, and a basic summary of these phases in history is useful to understand where key theories arose.

Classical management theories evolved out of military theory and were developed as advanced societies industrialised. While they recognised the need to harmonise human aspects of the organisation, problems were essentially seen as technical. At the start of the twentieth century, Taylor proposed that work in factories could be better streamlined by considering how products were made using a 'scientific' method – this led to various practices to boost productivity [2]. Although considered to be limited and quite outdated, some elements of team-working and management in health services (and other sectors) today can be traced back to principles of scientific management – for example: defined roles and training; standardised procedures to maximise efficiency and minimise errors; supervision and the oversight of outcomes. Other process-focused theories of change and management have also been utilised for quality improvement interventions within health-care, such as the LEAN approach from the commercial sector [3] and business process mapping.

One of the most often-cited criticisms of the scientific approach is that it made individuals fit the requirements of the organisation, rather than taking into account the emotional and social needs of workers. Later theories, borrowing on behavioural psychology and sociology, suggest ways in which an organisation needs to adapt to meet the requirements of individuals. Psychology-based theories began to investigate what drives individuals and how best to motivate them to achieve desired outcomes at work.

More recent management theories tend to layer new (and sometimes contradictory) concepts and ideas on top of older counterparts rather than replace them. One strand of leadership theory distinguishes 'transactional' and 'transformational' approaches by different values, goals and the nature of follower–manager relations. Transactional leadership concentrates on exchanges between leaders and staff, offering rewards for meeting particular standards in performance. Transformational leadership highlights the importance of leaders demonstrating inspirational motivation and concentrates on relationships [4]. In reality, practice often encompasses elements of both – for example, performance management is still often used for service targets, yet many people find that engaging in relationships and working with staff can often result in deeper commitment and understanding of what is trying to be achieved and lead to better performance.

Other theories considered different styles of leadership that individuals might naturally adopt or can learn to employ, and these are considered in more detail later in the section on understanding yourself. Situational (sometimes called 'contingency') theory posits that leadership styles and approaches are adapted to suit the situational context. Hersey and Blanchard argued that there was no best way or style to lead, but that leaders must adapt their approach according to their followers [5]. John Adair coined the term 'action-centred leadership', which centres on the interplay between the leader, the team and also the task [6]. He proposes that each of these three domains must be considered and addressed to achieve the best course of action. 'Strategic leadership' has also been described as an approach which focuses primarily on 'the task', and highlights the importance of developing a strategic vision and developing a plan to lead a team to align behind specific goals.

More recent characterisations of effective leadership, especially within health and care settings, emphasise the importance of relationships. 'Compassionate leadership' involves a 'focus on relationships through careful listening to, understanding, empathising with and supporting other people, enabling those we lead to feel valued, respected and cared for, so they can reach their potential and do their best work' [7]. Proponents of 'authentic leadership' advocate specifically for the importance of self-awareness, modesty and humility, and empathic and ethics-based behaviour in a leader, alongside a focus on results [8]. A more collective view of leadership is that of 'systems leadership', which acknowledges and embraces the complexity of the systems in which we work and the roles that multiple groups or individuals play in improving the system [9].

The actual evidence-base for leadership theory is somewhat limited, and rarely falls within the usual types of evidence and research that many of us are comfortable with in public health practice. However, a pragmatic approach to identify theories, tools and ideas which may prove useful to your own practice and development, and critical analysis of their strengths and weaknesses in different situations, is an important aspect to enhance your own ability to influence others and improve outcomes in the systems in which you work. Adapting to an uncertain environment, and being willing to reflect on your experiences and performance, is important.

7.3 Developing a Toolkit of Leadership Skills and Approaches

For the modern public health professional, working in a complex environment, with interconnected forces and often across different organisations, it is therefore helpful to develop a toolkit of leadership skills and approaches to draw on in different situations. Figure 7.1 offers a simple framework of eight domains in which you can explore different theories and concepts and hone your own knowledge and skills.

- Understanding our own strengths and preferences as leaders can enable us to optimise our approach and skills in influencing others and deploying our knowledge and expertise most effectively.
- Having an understanding of what motivates individuals and how this interplay works within a team setting is extremely useful.

Figure 7.1 Watson & Yates:
Elements of leadership and
management for professional
development.
Source: Watson and Yates,
2023.

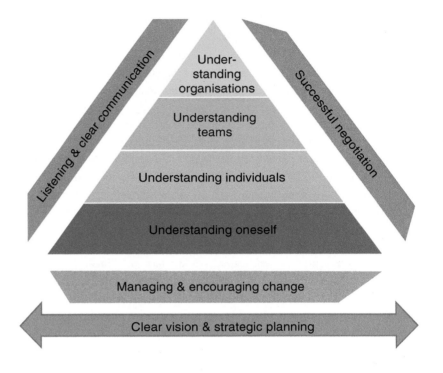

Figure 7.1 Watson & Yates: Elements of leadership and management for professional development. Source: Watson and Yates, 2023.

- Being aware of the culture, power and priorities of organisations and groups (our own and those with whom we work) is important to inform our actions and methods of communication and negotiation.
- In each of these situations, developing clear and persuasive communication is crucial, which requires careful and active listening at its core to understand the views of others.
- Listening and using 'emotional intelligence' to inform negotiations and interactions with others can significantly enhance our success.
- Developing a clear vision of what we wish to accomplish and a strategic plan for how to get there facilitates effective leadership, and understanding when and how to lead and manage change to improve outcomes can help us achieve our goals. Each of these areas is considered in more detail below.

The NHS Healthcare Leadership model and Medical Leadership Competency Framework and tools also describe some of the specific leadership skills outlined in Figure 1 (in the Introduction) in a more service-focused context [10, 11]. This is built on a concept of shared leadership and sets out the competencies doctors and other health-care professionals need to run health-care organisations and improve quality of care. Affiliated resources have also been developed which offer suggestions for how to gain workplace-based experience and achieve learning outcomes in each of the leadership domains described.

7.4 Understanding Yourself: Developing Your Leadership Style and Skills

Each of us, when asked to think of a 'great leader', can visualise a public figure or a personal mentor who inspires us, and often this person is characterised by a charismatic persona and engaging style that often we assume is an intrinsic part of their character. Early writers tended to suggest that leaders were born, not made, but no one has been able to agree on a particular set of characteristics required. Early 'trait' theories which defined such characteristics that a leader must inherently possess have mostly moved on nowadays, to instead recognise key skills that an effective leader can develop. Leadership and management skills can absolutely be taught and learned.

What qualities characterise the leaders you have encountered?

Leaders and managers wield power and must have the ability to influence others to achieve organisational aims. Therefore, how you carry out your managerial functions and the way you exercise power and authority – your management or leadership style – is central. It is worth remembering that being in a senior position will not automatically make you a good leader, and certainly not an influential one. Likewise, there are numerous examples of opportunities to influence situations or people when you do not have a formal position of power (see Box 7.1).

Box 7.1 Sources of power

Power based on the position of the individual

Positional power

Vested in individuals by virtue of the position they hold e.g. 'Team leader', Director

Resource power

Control over staff, funds or other resources

Power based on the individual

Expert power

Specialist expertise such as that of an NHS Consultant

Personal power

What an individual brings personally, such as style, charisma, skills

All of us have preferred leadership and management styles conditioned by personality and experience. Part of 'understanding yourself' requires a consideration of your preferred styles for learning, processing information, communication and negotiation, and interacting with others. Utilising opportunities such as peer or colleague feedback, anonymous '360' degree feedback tools and self-reflection, coaching or mentoring can help to develop and enhance this understanding [12]. The ability to practise and adapt your approach to different circumstances is a major determinant of effectiveness, just as communication skills require versatility according to circumstances.

In the 1940s, Kurt Lewin identified three styles of leadership that are often referred to today. Some people have a preference for 'authoritarian' behaviours and like to offer clear guidance; others prefer a more relaxed, *laissez-faire* or 'delegative' style; or a 'participate' or democratic approach. Daniel Goleman and colleagues expanded on this idea to present six leadership styles identified in a worldwide study of managers [13], in which they discovered that the best results seemed to come from those who utilised different styles effectively (see Figure 7.2).

So how do we determine what style is appropriate in what circumstance? The very attributes that might define a leader in one context may be inappropriate in other circumstances. Winston Churchill, for example, was famously rejected as Prime Minister by peacetime Britons. According to contingency theories of leadership, four variables have to be taken into account when analysing contingent circumstances. Unsurprisingly, the one over which you have most control is 'you'!

- the manager (or leader) – his or her personality and preferred style;
- the managed (or led) – the needs, attitudes and skills of her or his subordinates or colleagues;

Figure 7.2 Six leadership styles at a glance [13].

	Commanding	Visionary	Affiliative	Democratic	Pacesetting	Coaching
The leader's modus operandi	Demands immediate compliance	Mobilises people towards a vision	Creates harmony and builds emotional bonds	Forges consensus through participation	Sets high standards for performance	Develops people for the future
The style in a phrase	'Do what I tell you.'	'Come with me.'	'People come first.'	'What do you think?'	'Do as I do, now.'	'Try this.'
Underlying emotional intelligence competencies	Drive to achieve initiate, self-control	Self-confidence, empathy, change catalyst	Empathy building, relationships, communication	Collaboration, team leadership, communication	Conscientiousness, drive to achieve, initiative	Developing others, empathy, self-awareness
When the style works best	In a crisis, to kickstart a turnaround, or with problem employees	When changes require a new vision, or when a clear direction is needed	To heal rifts in a team or motivate people during stressful circumstances	To build buy-in or consensus, or to get input from valuable employees	To get quick results from a highly motivated and competent team	To help an employee improve performance or develop long-term strengths
Overall impact on climate	Negative	Most strongly positive	Positive	Positive	Negative	Positive

- the task – requirements and goals of the job to be done; and
- the context – the organisation and its values and prejudices.

A key personal element in effective leadership is that of 'emotional intelligence' [14]. This is the capacity for recognising our own feelings and those of others, motivating ourselves and managing emotions well in ourselves. This, too, is a skill which can be developed and enhanced, starting with exploring your own awareness and ability in this area. The next section aims to enhance your ability to interact with others, with a conceptual knowledge of what motivates others and influences their actions and responses.

Fundamental to all of this is effective listening and taking the time to try to understand the views and attitudes of your partners, stakeholders or audience. Scharmer describes four levels of, increasingly effective, listening, which offer a useful model for enhancing interactions with others [15] (see Box 7.2). Genuinely listening and taking on board the ideas, attitudes and feelings of others all inform your approach, your communication style and methods, your negotiation or discussion. As described further in Chapter 1, embedding the participation of key stakeholders, especially patients and the public, in public health programmes or activities is a crucial element of creating solutions and making shared decisions that are appropriate, sensitive and effective in local communities.

Finally, to bring your expertise to the metaphorical 'table' – be it in a public arena, in a multi-agency meeting, or even within your own team – you need to be able to communicate your assessment of the information available. Expertise is only useful if you can communicate it effectively and influence others to act on it. In public health, we rely on our communication skills daily: from chairing or contributing to a high-profile meeting; writing a succinct and persuasive briefing or report; giving a press interview or crafting a press release; to giving a verbal presentation or communicating effectively with a team via email and in meetings. A variety of communication tools and techniques ranging from Cicero's 'Five canons of rhetoric' in the time of

---

Box 7.2 Otto Scharmer's four different types of listening [15]

1. **Downloading** – 'what we know already' – listening by reconfirming old opinions and judgements.
2. **Factual listening** – 'Ooh, look at that' – paying attention to facts and to new or disconfirming data.
3. **Empathic listening** – 'oh yes, I know exactly how you feel' – appreciation of how the world appears through someone else's eyes, listening to a story of a living and evolving self.
4. **Generative listening** – 'I am connected to something larger than myself' – connecting to a future possible shift in identity and self; undergoing a subtle but profound change.

Ancient Greece to modern theories which consider elements of the 'source, message, channel and receiver' model [16] abound. Further detail is beyond the scope of this chapter, but all of these skills can be learned, practised and honed to enhance your ability to convey your expert opinion and urge action.

7.5 Understanding Individuals and What Motivates Them

As is evident in the examples throughout this book, the sphere of public health is a complex environment, which often involves working with numerous organisations and teams, to make decisions and to coordinate and integrate practice. Understanding how individuals, teams and organisations work is therefore crucial to maximise the motivation, performance and participation of staff, patients and the general public in public health practice – for example, encouraging an interdisciplinary team to work effectively together, share information, reduce duplication and create a joined-up experience for patients, carers and families. Managers everywhere are interested in how such concepts as job satisfaction, commitment, motivation and team dynamics may increase productivity, innovation and competitiveness.

Organisational psychologists identify three components of our attitudes to work:
- cognitive (what we believe, e.g. my boss treats me unfairly);
- affective (how we feel, e.g. I dislike my boss); and
- behavioural (what we are predisposed to do, e.g. I am going to look for another job).

Attitudes are important as they influence behaviour.

What motivates you at work, or in your personal life?

Various different theories of motivation exist, which can be broadly divided into 'content' theories which consider the needs and desires of individuals and how we can understand these and 'process' theories which look at how we can use this understanding to encourage, support and motivate individuals. An early and still widely quoted theory of job satisfaction was elaborated by Herzberg [17]. In his '2 factor' theory, 'hygiene' factors are those which individuals need to be satisfied in a job, but do not themselves lead to motivation (e.g. a good relationship with peers, working environment, status and security). 'Motivating' factors are related to the job itself and include recognition, advancement, responsibility and personal growth. The message for managers was that taking care of hygiene factors was a basic prerequisite; a focus on motivating factors could maximise job satisfaction.

The significance of positive reinforcement, setting goals and clarifying expectations is stressed in leadership-based theories. Job enrichment to give more control over content, planning and execution can help motivate employees. David McClelland considered the importance of matching people and job-related rewards, recognising three different sorts of personal need (Table 7.1 [18]).

Table 7.1 McClelland's motivational needs theory [18]

Need	Description
Need for achievement	The need to accomplish goals, excel and strive continually to do things better
Need for power	The need to influence and lead others, and be in control of one's environment
Need for affiliation	The desire for close and friendly interpersonal relationships

How much do you think you will need achievement, power and affiliation in your future work?

The work of psychologist Albert Bandura on 'self-efficacy' [19] can also be a useful lens through which to consider how to enhance a person's belief in their ability to achieve an outcome in a particular situation. Self-efficacy can be influenced by your own performance and successes and through 'vicariously' watching others' experiences and performances. Bandura also proposes that individuals gain confidence or self-belief through physiological feedback during situations which may be positive or negative; and that verbal persuasion and encouragement can be effective.

Another factor which may influence your job satisfaction is your expectations. Models such as Vroom's expectancy theory posit that the role of expected rewards can be very helpful in motivating individuals (e.g. career advancement, achieving personal goals, salary), so a mutual understanding and shared expectations with those you manage is important [20]. Adams' equity theory also highlights the importance of ensuring that individuals feel that the rewards they receive are fair and equitable, in comparison not only with what they put into their job, but also how this compares with what others offer and receive in return [21].

There are therefore opportunities for managers to create positive environments and working conditions to enhance performance and individual satisfaction. A final theory worth considering within this area is the impact of 'psychological safety' [22]. This refers to the ability to share your thoughts and feelings without fear of retribution or humiliation. The central tenet of this is that individuals should feel respected and accepted – and by encouraging a safe environment for any ideas or views, not only can we boost individual engagement and participation, but also foster a positive culture of innovation and learning from mistakes.

7.6 Organisational Behaviour and Motivation

It is also important to understand how people operate within the organisation in which they work. Organisational behaviour can be studied at three levels: in relation

Box 7.3 Handy's types of organisational culture

Power culture	Role culture
Power is held by a few and radiates out from the centre like a web. Few rules and bureaucracy mean that decisions can be swift.	Hierarchical bureaucracy where power derives from a person's position
Task culture	**Person culture**
Power derives from expertise and structures are often matrices with teams forming as necessary.	All individuals are equal and operate collaboratively to pursue the organisational goals.

to individuals, to teams and to organisational processes [23]. How organisations function is a combination of their culture and structures. Organisational culture has been described as a set of norms, beliefs, principles and ways of behaving that together give each organisation a distinctive character [24]. Culture and structure can be analysed. In a simple and early model, Charles Handy built on his own and earlier work to define types of organisations [25] (see Box 7.3). Johnson and Scholes designed a 'cultural web analysis' as a tool for understanding the current culture of an organisation and the desired culture, and any gaps between the two (see Figure 7.3) [26].

 In what type of organisation do you think you work? How does this influence your ability to do your job?
What factors affect the behaviour of staff and teams in your workplace?

7.6.1 Types of Team

We can see from this simple model of organisational culture that the type of teams which operate within an organisation may be determined by the type of organisation. However, all organisations may at some point form various types of team to carry out specific functions. Teams are often described as:

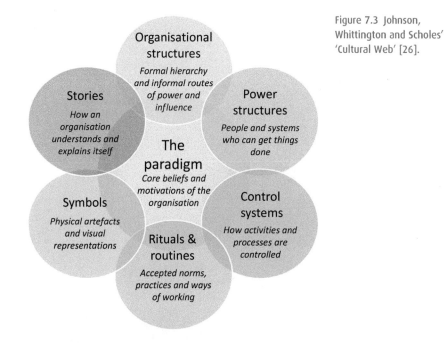

Figure 7.3 Johnson, Whittington and Scholes' 'Cultural Web' [26].

- **Vertical or functional**. Teams which carry out one function within an organisation, such as an infection control team within a hospital.
- **Horizontal or cross-functional**. Teams which are made up of members from across an organisation. These may be formed for specific projects, such as managing the introduction of a new service which might need operational, clinical and financial input, or can be long-standing teams such as an executive team running an organisation.
- **Self-directed**. Teams which do not have dedicated leadership or management. These may generate themselves within an organisation to achieve aims or they can be specifically designed to give employees a feeling of ownership.

Tuckman's model [27] (see Figure 7.4) offers an explanation of how teams develop over time and can be used to consider how individuals, including the leader, behave over time within those teams. Although the model is somewhat limited by the fact that it assumes all teams follow a linear process, which can be in reality much more complex, there are a variety of tools and approaches that can be useful to support the development of teams through these steps.

As a team leader, or a team member, how might you act at each of these stages to help move the team forward or encourage better team-working?

When creating a new team or trying to enhance the performance of an existing team, another useful model is that of Belbin's 'team roles' [28], where specific individuals can be identified who have the strengths or capability to perform specific

Figure 7.4 Bruce Tuckman's team-development model [27].

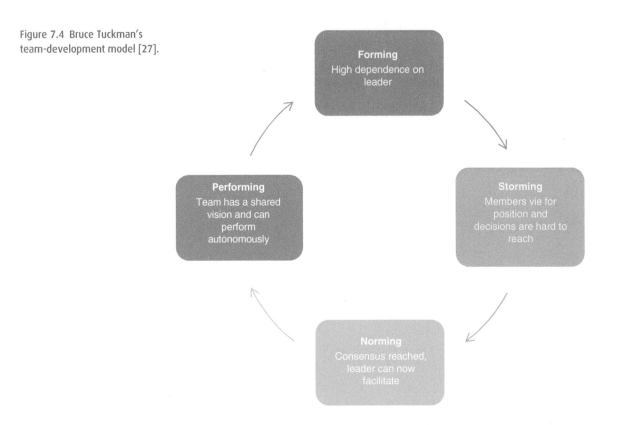

functions in the group (see Figure 7.5). This can be useful to help identify your own role within a group (which may change depending on the composition of the group) or to manage a team and ensure that each role is filled. Successful leaders often comment that one of their key skills is to be aware of their own limitations and weaknesses, and surround themselves by colleagues skilled in these areas.

7.6.2 Theories of Change

Change models in the literature fall into broadly two camps: theories which attempt to understand how change occurs, or what is needed to encourage individuals to change something; and theories which offer a framework or steps to follow to try and change a situation.

There are many management tools which can be used to analyse change and the forces which might support or hinder it. Lewin's force field analysis is a simple concept which essentially advocates analysing all of the positive or 'driving' forces to create a particular change, and all of the negative or 'resisting' forces to better understand how to foster or counter them [29]. A consideration of the strengths,

Team role	Description	Strengths	Allowable weaknesses
Resource Investigator	Uses their inquisitive nature to find ideas to bring back to the team.	Outgoing, enthusiastic. Explores opportunities and develops contacts.	Might be over-optimistic, and can lose interest once the initial enthusiasm has passed.
Teamworker	Helps the team to gel, using their versatility to identify the work required and complete it on behalf of the team.	Cooperative, perceptive and diplomatic. Listens and averts friction.	Can be indecisive in crunch situations and tends to avoid confrontation.
Coordinator	Needed to focus on the team's objectives, draw out team members and delegate work appropriately.	Mature, confident, identifies talent. Clarifies goals.	Can be seen as manipulative and might offload their own share of the work.
Plant	Tends to be highly creative and good at solving problems in unconventional ways.	Creative, imaginative, free-thinking, generates ideas and solves difficult problems.	Might ignore incidentals, and may be too preoccupied to communicate effectively.
Monitor Evaluator	Provides a logical eye, making impartial judgements where required and weighs up the team's options in a dispassionate way.	Sober, strategic and discerning. Sees all options and judges accurately.	Sometimes lacks the drive and ability to inspire others and can be overly critical.
Specialist	Brings in-depth knowledge of a key area to the team.	Single-minded, self-starting and dedicated. They provide specialist knowledge and skills.	Tends to contribute on a narrow front and can dwell on the technicalities.
Shaper	Provides the necessary drive to ensure that the team keeps moving and does not lose focus or momentum.	Challenging, dynamic, thrives on pressure. Has the drive and courage to overcome obstacles.	Can be prone to provocation, and may sometimes offend people's feelings.
Implementer	Needed to plan a workable strategy and carry it out as efficiently as possible.	Practical, reliable, efficient. Turns ideas into actions and organises work that needs to be done.	Can be a bit inflexible and slow to respond to new possibilities.
Completer Finisher	Most effectively used at the end of tasks to polish and scrutinise the work for errors, subjecting it to the highest standards of quality control.	Painstaking, conscientious, anxious. Searches out errors. Polishes and perfects.	Can be inclined to worry unduly, and reluctant to delegate.

weaknesses, opportunities and threats posed by a situation or opportunity ('SWOT analysis') is another often-used tool. A PESTLE analysis [30] can also be used to consider the context within which a specific change is occurring, in a more systematic way. The PESTLE acronym covers the influences on an organisation (Box 7.4).

Figure 7.5 R. M. Belbin's team roles [28].

Think about your own organisation or a health-care system. You could use the whole of the NHS.
Use the PESTLE model to analyse what is driving change in that system.

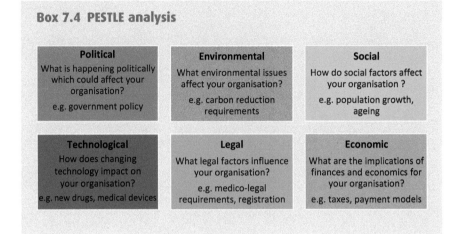

Box 7.4 PESTLE analysis

Political	**Environmental**	**Social**
What is happening politically which could affect your organisation?	What environmental issues affect your organisation?	How do social factors affect your organisation ?
e.g. government policy	e.g. carbon reduction requirements	e.g. population growth, ageing

Technological	**Legal**	**Economic**
How does changing technology impact on your organisation?	What legal factors influence your organisation?	What are the implications of finances and economics for your organisation?
e.g. new drugs, medical devices	e.g. medico-legal requirements, registration	e.g. taxes, payment models

Introducing a new service or changing an existing service in response to the kind of drivers identified by using a tool such as PESTLE is difficult. Many people will initially resist change even if the results are likely to benefit them. The process of change involves helping people within an organisation or a system to change the way they work and interact with others in the system. Leaders need to understand how people respond to change in order to plan it.

7.6.3 The Psychology of Change

Everett Rogers' classic model (Figure 7.6) of how people take up innovation is one model which can help us to understand different people's responses to change [31]. This was based on observations of how farmers took up hybrid seed corn in Iowa. The model describes the differential rate of uptake of an innovation, in order to target promotion of the product, and labels people according to their place on the uptake curve. This can be useful to devise communications or approaches to gain the support of different people or teams. For example, being aware of who in the team or the organisation is likely to be an 'early adopter' can enable you to involve them in trialling an idea and persuading others of its merits. Knowing likely opponents is also important because if they can be persuaded to support the change, they are likely to become important advocates. Rogers' original model described the 'late adopters' as 'laggards', but this seems a pejorative term when there may be good reasons not to take up the innovation. How soon after their introduction, for example, should nurses and doctors be prescribing new, usually more expensive, inhalers for asthma?

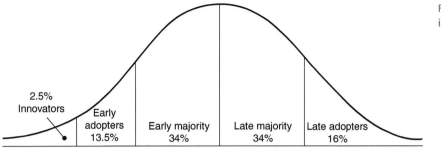

Figure 7.6 Roger's diffusion of innovation [31].

Individuals' 'change type' may depend on the particular change they are adopting. This depends on the perceived benefits, the perceived obstacles and the motivation to make the change. People are more likely to adopt an innovation:

- that provides a relative advantage compared to old ideas;
- that is compatible with the existing value system of the adopter;
- that is readily understood by the adopters (less complexity);
- that may be experienced on a limited basis (more trialability); and
- where the results of the innovation are more easily noticed by other potential adopters (observability).

As an illustration, pharmaceutical companies use this model in their approaches to general practitioners. The local sales representatives know from the information they have about GPs in their area whether a GP is an early adopter. Early adopters are often opinion leaders in a community. Early on in the process of promotion, they may target those GPs with personal visits, whereas they may send the late adopters an information leaflet only, as those GPs will not consider change until more than 80% of their colleagues have taken up the new product.

Anyone hoping to change people's behaviour is looking for the 'tipping point' [32]. This is the point or threshold at which an idea or behaviour takes off, moving from uncommon to common. You see it in many areas of life: new technologies like the uptake of mobile phones, fashion garments or footwear, books or television programmes. The change in behaviour is contagious like infectious disease epidemics: a social epidemic. Using the model of diffusion, the tipping point comes at the point between the early adopters and the early majority. It applies equally to changing behaviour of professionals and the public. This same technique can be used with staff going through a process of change. It is important to identify change types and opinion leaders.

7.6.4 Managing or Leading Change

There are some excellent free health-based resources available offering an overview of lots of different models and tools to achieve change [33]. Understanding people's psychological reaction to change is key to helping overcome their resistance. Bridges' 'transition' model offers applicable mechanisms for supporting individuals to

Figure 7.7 Kotter's eight-step
model for leading change [37].

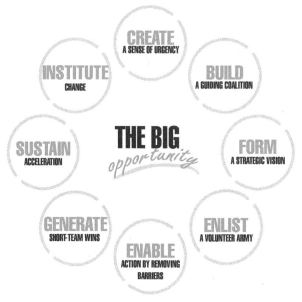

transition to adopt a new change to embrace 'new beginnings' [34]. Senge's 'commitment, enrolment and compliance' model has also been used in the NHS to facilitate quality improvement programmes, with a focus on engaging and gaining commitment from all stakeholders, identifying and addressing all barriers and resistance to adopting the change [35].

One of the most famous and influential 'macro' models is Kotter's '8 Steps for Leading Change', which provides a framework for moving through different elements of the change process (see Figure 7.7) [36].

How would you go about managing a new change or service that would require leadership and management to deliver?

Other similar models which offer a checklist or framework for overseeing a change process and emphasise different elements include, for example:

- '7 Rs of change management' – who Raised the change, Reason, Return required, Risks involved, who is Responsible, Resources required and Relationships.
- McKinsey's 7 Ss [38] – Structure, Strategy, Staff, Style, Systems, Shared Values and Skills.
- The ADKAR model [39] – Awareness, Desire, Knowledge, Ability and Reinforcement.

These strategic approaches can also be useful to consider in the 'task' element of leadership – how to devise a strategy to achieve a positive outcome and identify and plan for what needs to happen, when and how.

7.7 Developing a Vision and Strategic Plan

Strategy is at the heart of the change process and the development of a strategy offers a good example of how leadership and management skills can be applied in practice. Table 7.2 outlines the questions posed in strategy development and how some of the skills outlined in this chapter can be applied at each stage, in conjunction with the core public health skills described in this book.

Table 7.2 The leadership and management of strategy development

Examples of strategic questions	How do we achieve this?
How do we make the case for change?	• Assess local needs, taking account of national strategies, data and information, evidence and local feedback (see Chapter 1 on assessing need). • Define and account for the drivers for and against change (e.g. Lewin's force field analysis, PESTLE analysis).
What are we aiming to do?	• Clarify aims, objectives and desired outcomes – a leader/manager needs to bring the vision to life. Be creative: think laterally and use the ideas of others. • Define local standards and set targets.
How can we make change happen?	• Understand the principles of change management (e.g. Kotter's eight-step model) and plan to address the factors that might resist change. • Include a description of the steps and actions that are required, and an assessment of the resource implications of putting the new service into place, with clear financial plans. • Consider the organisational context and how teams and individuals need to operate in the new system.
How do we engage with partners and the public?	• Involve all stakeholders who are affected by the strategy, including commissioners, providers, managers, staff, patients and the public, and actively listen to their views, concerns and ideas. • Identify who will support and who will oppose it; develop an approach to building support and overcoming opposition. Consider who has the power in these relationships and how that affects the strategy development.
How do we know we have done what we wanted to do?	• Evaluate impact by demonstrating achievement against the standards and targets through monitoring routine data and special studies (see Chapter 6 for evaluating the impact of services). • Some form of progress report and/or debriefing meeting will enable people to see what they are achieving. The people as well as the task need evaluating, and the techniques of appraisal are important tasks for the leader of the team.
How do we make successful change become normal practice?	• The change in practice needs to be sustained to ensure that it becomes routine, as people tend to revert to their old ways of working. • This requires individuals to change the way they do things. Continuing education, appropriate management strategies, alterations to the work environment with a process of on-going monitoring/audit/feedback may all be required. • Consider what motivates people and how to use leadership and management skills to build a culture of psychological safety and continuous improvement.

7.8 Conclusions

The skills needed for leadership and management vary across an individual's career and must be assessed and developed over time. Based on individual values and strengths, the unique contribution we make and the purpose we have as a leader in this place at this time, each leader can begin to build a personal brand which informs their practice and development [40]. Leadership and management behaviours can be learned, but continuous improvement requires an open-minded approach to assessing our own skills level, an ability to seek and accept constructive feedback on our performance and a willingness to change. How can we lead and manage change if we are unwilling to lead, manage and change ourselves?

This chapter offers a basic framework for thinking about different skills to consider, and various professional frameworks and courses abound to offer the public health leader opportunities to broaden their skills 'toolbox' and practise modelling or implementing new skills or approaches.

REFERENCES

1. J. P. Kotter, What leaders really do, *Harvard Business Review* **79**(11), 2001, 85–97.
2. F. W. Taylor, *The Principles of Scientific Management*, New York, NY and London, Harper & Brothers, 1911.
3. J. P. Womack and D. T. Jones, *Lean Thinking: Banish Waste and Create Wealth in Your Corporation*, London, Simon & Schuster, 2003.
4. W. Bennis and B. Nanus, *Leaders*, New York, NY, Harper Collins, 1996.
5. P. Hersey and K. H. Blanchard, *Management of Organizational Behavior: Utilizing Human Resources*, Englewood Cliffs, NJ, Prentice-Hall, 1982.
6. J. Adair, *The Action-Centred Leader*, Franklin, TN, Spiro Press, 1988.
7. M. West and S. Bailey, What is compassionate leadership? The King's Fund, 2022. Available at: www.kingsfund.org.uk/publications/what-is-compassionate-leadership#:~:text=Compassionate%20leadership%20involves%20a%20focus,and%20do%20their%20best%20work
8. B. George, *Authentic Leadership: Rediscovering the Secrets to Creating Lasting Value Systems*, San Francisco, CA, Jossey-Bass, 2004.
9. NHS Confederation, The future of systems leadership, 2014. Available at: www.nhsconfed.org/publications/future-systems-leadership-scoping-project
10. NHS Leadership Academy, Healthcare Leadership Model, 2022. Available at: www.leadershipacademy.nhs.uk/resources/healthcare-leadership-model/
11. Academy of Medical Colleges and NHS Institute for Innovation and Improvement, Medical Leadership Competency Framework, 2010. Available at: www.leadershipacademy.nhs.uk/wp-content/uploads/2012/11/NHSLeadership-Leadership-Framework-Medical-Leadership-Competency-Framework-3rd-ed.pdf
12. NHS Leadership Academy, Healthcare Leadership model 360 feedback tool. Available at: www.leadershipacademy.nhs.uk/healthcare-leadership-model/360-degree-feedback-tool-2/

13. D. Goleman, Leadership that gets results, *Harvard Business Review* **78**(2), 2000, 78–90.

14. D. Goleman, *Emotional Intelligence*, London, Bloomsbury Publishing, 1996.

15. C. O. Scharmer, *The Essentials of Theory U: Core Principles and Applications*, Oakland, CA, Berrett-Koehler, 2018.

16. D. Berlo, *The Process of Communication: An Introduction to Theory and Practice*, New York, NY, Olt, Rinehart & Winston, 1960.

17. F. Herzberg, *Work and the Nature of Man*, Wenatchee, WA, World Publishing Company, 1966.

18. D. McClelland, *Human Motivation*, Englewood Cliffs, NJ, General Learning Press, 1973.

19. A. Bandura, Self-efficacy: Toward a unifying theory of behavioral change, *Psychological Review* **84**(2), 1977, 191–215.

20. V. H. Vroom and E. L. Deci, *Management and Motivation*, London, Penguin, 1983.

21. J. S. Adams and S. Freedman, Equity theory revisited: Comments and annotated bibliography, *Advances in Experimental Social Psychology* **9**, 1976, 43–90.

22. A. C. Edmondson, *The Fearless Organization: Creating Psychological Safety in the Workplace for Learning, Innovation, and Growth*, Hoboken, NJ, Wiley, 2018.

23. J. Greenberg and R. Baron, *Behaviour in Organisations: Understanding and Managing the Human Side of Work*, 2nd ed., Boston, MA, Allyn & Bacon, 1990.

24. A. Brown, *Organisational Culture*, London, Pitman Publishing, 1995.

25. C. B. Handy, *Understanding Organizations*, 3rd ed., Harmondsworth, Penguin Books, 1985.

26. G. Johnson, R. Whittington and K. Scholes, *Fundamentals of Strategy*, London, Pearson Education, 2012.

27. B. Tuckman, Developmental sequence in small groups, *Psychological Bulletin* **63**(6), 1965, 384–99.

28. R. M. Belbin, *Management Teams: Why They Succeed or Fail*, New York, NY and Abingdon, UK, Routledge, 2010. See also The Nine Belbin Team Roles. Available at: www.belbin.com/about/belbin-team-roles

29. K. Lewin, Defining the field at a given time, *Psychological Review* **50**(3), 1943, 292–310. Republished in *Resolving Social Conflicts & Field Theory in Social Science*, Washington, DC, American Psychological Association, 1997.

30. Chartered Institute of Personnel and Development (CIPD), PESTLE analysis factsheet, November 2010.

31. E. Rogers, *The Diffusion of Innovation*, 4th ed., New York, NY, Free Press, 1995.

32. M. Gladwell, *The Tipping Point: How Little Things Can Make a Big Difference*, London, Abacus, 2000.

33. J. Atkinson, E. Loftus and J. Jarvis, The art of change making, Leadership Centre, 2015. Available at: www.leadershipcentre.org.uk/wp-content/uploads/2016/02/The-Art-of-Change-Making.pdf

34. W. Bridges and S. Bridges, *Managing Transitions: Making the Most of Change*, Philadelphia, PA, Da Capo Lifelong Books, 2017.

35. P. Senge, *The Fifth Discipline: The Art and Practice of the Learning Organisation*, 2nd ed., London, Random House, 2006.

36. J. P. Kotter, *XLR8*, Boston, MA, Harvard Business Review Press, 2014.

37. Kotter, The 8 Steps for Leading Change. Available at: www.kotterinc.com/methodology/8-steps/

38. McKinsey & Company. Enduring ideas: The 7-S Framework. Available at: www.mckinsey .com/capabilities/strategy-and-corporate-finance/our-insights/enduring-ideas-the-7-s-framework
39. Prosci, The Prosci ADKAR Model. Available at: www.prosci.com/methodology/adkar
40. NIHR webinar, Your authentic leadership brand, 2021. Available at: www.youtube.com/ watch?v=wr5VS6jiQ38

8

Improving Population Health

Peter Bradley and Jan Yates

Key points

- Health and well-being are heavily influenced by social, economic, environmental and commercial factors, as well as individual genetics, lifestyle choices, and access to health-care and other services.
- Individuals, families and communities are central to any approach to promote health, but many different groups and sectors can promote health-enhancing environments, including governments, the public and charitable sector, the commercial sector and the media.
- In the twenty-first century, a sustained approach to promoting health should consider how to tackle inequality and disparity, mitigate the impact of climate change, promote political social stability, ensure digital literacy and use technology for the public good.
- Health promotion and tackling health inequality are, in part, political activities where choices are made about whose health is promoted and how this is achieved.
- Models used to inform health promotion activity tend to adopt a bio-medical focus, an individual focus, a societal focus or a combined perspective.
- Practitioners can promote health by working at many levels in the system: national, system, community, service, public and personal.
- Behaviour change is an essential component of health promotion and can be informed by behaviour sciences.

8.1 Introduction

As described in Chapter 2, life expectancy has increased in recent decades in many countries [1]. As a result of longer life spans, we are more likely to suffer from long-term conditions such as diabetes or dementia and more people end up having several conditions at the same time (see also Chapters 12 and 13). This, together with an ageing population and the increasing cost of health technology, puts considerable strain on our health and care services.

The causes of ill health and death are changing and, as we live longer, new preventable health problems emerge, bringing new challenges. Improving health (physical, mental or both) and promoting general well-being remain major priorities.

Just as important, the difference in health status between rich and poor continues to grow: on average, you are likely to experience 19 more healthy years if you grow up and live in a richer area, even within a relatively wealthy country such as the UK [2] (see Chapter 14). At a global level, the picture is even more complex (see Chapters 16 and 17). Although there is some evidence that life expectancy is beginning to plateau in developed countries such as the UK, the biggest potential to improve health still lies in addressing inequality between or within countries.

This chapter:

- summarises the models of health improvement that are prevalent today;
- introduces a combined conceptual model to describe the factors affecting health in modern times; and
- presents some case studies of interventions designed to improve health which offer important insight and learning.

8.2 Models of Health Improvement

Approaches to improving health reflect assumptions, values and beliefs about what can, and should, be done to improve health. Although the approaches are not mutually exclusive, the choice of approach may differentially benefit some sections of society. In broad terms, the approaches include:

1. a bio-medical model, where health improvement activities focus on reducing the risk of developing disease;
2. an individual-focused model, where emphasis is placed on supporting individual lifestyle choices; and
3. a model based on societal influences, where emphasis is placed on improving the conditions in society that might promote better health.

8.2.1 Model 1 – a Bio-Medical Focus

A bio-medical focus describes the progression of disease in the community and drives consideration of where along this pathway interventions might be made to reduce the development or progression of disease. Figure 8.1 shows the pathway through which a disease is seen to progress and where prevention can

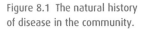

Distribution of health and disease in the community

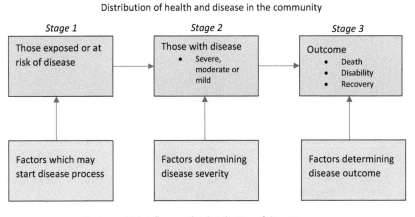

Figure 8.1 The natural history
of disease in the community.

Factors which influence the distribution of disease

be targeted as each stage. This perspective leads to a model of preventing disease which defines 'primary prevention' as actions to prevent the occurrence of disease, 'secondary prevention' as actions to detect and treat a disease before symptoms develop and 'tertiary prevention' as actions to limit disability once disease is established.

Apply the bio-medical model to a specific disease (e.g. vascular dementia) and consider the processes or factors that could be ameliorated at Stages 1, 2 and 3 to prevent them.

Often, we think of disease as being present or not, but for many conditions or risk factors such as high blood pressure, values fall along a spectrum. Decisions are made as to when to intervene – and also where and for whom. Thus, preventive treatment may be withheld from individuals whose risk for a disease is low (e.g. as determined by a threshold level of blood pressure) when the whole population may benefit from modifying this same risk factor.

This sort of decision is highlighted in epidemiologist Geoffrey Rose's description of two broad approaches to prevention (Figure 8.2). The high-risk strategy aims to protect those individuals at the high end of the risk distribution (generally a small proportion of the whole). The population strategy aims to reduce the underlying causes and is concerned with factors that affect risk across the whole population [3]. This is sometimes referred to as 'the prevention paradox', whereby the majority of cases of a disease actually come from a population at low or moderate risk, because of the volume of individuals in that risk category. Interventions that take a population approach intervene across the whole population regardless of their level of risk – for example, fluoridation of the water to

Figure 8.2 High-risk individual
and population-based
strategies for prevention.

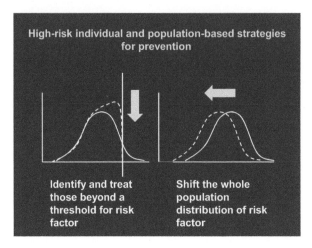

prevent dental caries in those with low fluoride in their diets, or strategies to encourage physical activity.

Can you describe further examples of a 'high-risk' prevention strategy and a 'population-level' strategy?

The bio-medical approach also raises questions about the cost and utility of preventive measures in the context of an expensive health-care system. Prevention should lead to more people living longer and having more years living in a healthy state and it is often held that 'prevention is cheaper than cure'. In other words, successful reduction of incidence rates of common diseases might, in theory, reduce health-care costs.

However, while prevention can be highly cost-effective, this is not enough to prevent costs rising in health services overall. Health-care costs are driven by other factors such as an ageing population, rising costs of medical technology and increasing numbers of people living with long-term conditions.

Nonetheless, prevention can be considerably more cost-effective than some traditional health services, even though they come with a significant expenditure across the whole population. Examples of interventions for which there is much evidence of their cost-effectiveness include smoking cessation services [4] and cervical screening [5].

Research the cost-effectiveness of other 'prevention' strategies in public health – for example, you might look at the evidence for supportive services for families with children aged 0–5 (see Chapter 11).

8.2.2 Model 2 – an Individual Focus

The bio-medical model focuses primarily on intervening with treatment, action or advice to prevent or reduce disease and its impact. Yet, in reality, making any sort of change often requires influencing individual (and group) attitudes and behaviour, which in turn shape health outcomes.

Health promotion is identified as 'the process of enabling people to exert control over and to improve their health' [6]. Health promotion is not something that should be done *on* or *to* people: it should be done *with* people either as individuals or as groups. The purpose of this activity is to strengthen the skills and capabilities of individuals to take action, and the capacity of groups or communities to act collectively *to exert control* over determinants of their health. Health promotion attempts to influence behaviour in many ways: from advertising campaigns – which aim to impart information – to 'nudge techniques' where the environment is subtly changed to make certain choices more attractive [7]. There are a variety of models used to consider whether an individual is ready to make a lifestyle change and to support them and these have their proponents and opponents.

Where have you observed behavioural techniques used to influence consumer behaviour, for example?

'Behaviour science' is the collective term for the discipline that studies cognitive, social, commercial and environmental factors that influence behaviours, such as health-related behaviour. Behavioural evidence can be used systematically to improve the design of policies and programmes. Behaviour science requires a multidisciplinary approach and generally focuses on the non-medical factors that influence health outcomes [7].

For example, local research on barriers to vaccination during the COVID-19 pandemic showed that some sections of the public considered vaccination centres too difficult to access (e.g. those with limited time). Vaccination was then encouraged by street messaging that informed passers-by that their vaccination centre was 'only ten minutes' walk away' and that walk-in appointments were available. Such an approach assumes that most people make most decisions unconsciously and non-rationally and are influenced by contextual cues [8], so their actions can be influenced by changing the way choices are presented to them.

Some people see these types of intervention as manipulative, restricting liberty and choice. To overcome this, new approaches that equip people with skills or tools to make better choices are now being used, referred to as 'boosting'. Rouyard and colleagues [9] explain the difference between 'nudging' and 'boosting' by considering interventions to reduce smoking rates. A nudge could consist of reducing the visibility of tobacco products in stores, whereas a boost strategy could consist of teaching smokers meditation techniques to overcome nicotine cravings.

It can be difficult to determine whether a behavioural science approach is best suited to meet health improvement objectives or whether regulation and legislation addressing the socioeconomic determinants of disease to promote health would be more appropriate. This potentially obscures a failure to address 'upstream' socioeconomic determinants of disease by continuing to focus on the downstream interventions focusing on individuals. In reality, these approaches are not mutually exclusive and a multifaceted approach is needed. For example, the challenging areas of tobacco and alcohol control require more than just encouragement to change individual behaviours. Michael Marmot's review of health equity in England 2010 and the further report after 10 years in 2020 [10] laid out much evidence for legislation, regulation, taxation and pricing policies of commodities such as alcohol and tobacco which could influence individual choices about whether and when to use them (see also Chapters 14 and 15).

Digital technology offers further opportunities to influence health behaviour. Health apps and wearable devices are increasingly available. These devices can directly provide users with health information, and data collected by an app or device can be used to monitor changes in health behaviour. Technology can also be used to support changes to the environment, such as 'smart' fridges that monitor nutritional intake and smart watches which monitor our sleep or daily physical activity. Artificial intelligence, using algorithms, can be used, for example, to provide health information through automated chat ('chatbot') services or to provide diagnostic interpretations from images taken as part of screening programmes. However, there are ethical implications and barriers in using these services. Not everyone has the skills to use digital technology. Digital services also generate data which raises questions about data security and use. The approaches adopted may not be easy to implement in real health-care situations and the use of algorithms can embed existing societal discrimination in practice [11].

8.2.3 Model 3 – a Societal Focus

Public health is by definition a political activity. There are always choices about who is helped and how they are helped and decisions about what to prioritise in developing the conditions to promote health (see also Chapter 7). Most governments will not be able to meet rising health-care demand if prevention activities are not available or strengthened.

If a programme promotes health overall, but widens inequality, can it be justified? For example, screening, vaccination, lifestyle services and health checks may improve health but, because uptake is lower in disadvantaged groups, they have the potential to widen inequalities.

This ethical dilemma is often ignored by governments, authorities and professionals in their efforts to emphasise the benefits of public health programmes [12]. However, those responsible for public health need to recognise this potential tension, reflect on their own and their organisations' values, and reflect on what they are trying to and what it is possible to achieve. Inequalities can be used to spur public health action with a socio-political focus on upstream determinants (e.g. housing, employment, green space, transport). They can also lead to inertia if tackling inequalities is seen as a problem that is too big to handle. It is therefore important to think in terms of the broad picture and work out how individuals and organisations can effect change in practice.

How might you address this ethical dilemma in terms of considering values and frameworks? For example, how would you argue for a programme to a commissioning body?

Box 8.1 uses the UK as an example of inequalities and social justice to suggest how a societal focus broadens the remit of health promotion.

> ## Box 8.1 Inequalities and social justice in the UK
>
> Some authors have suggested that tackling health inequalities is a question of social justice because deaths attributable to health inequalities are preventable. In the UK, it has been estimated that between 2011 and 2019, over 1 million people died earlier than they would have done if they had lived in more of the most affluent areas with the same age- and sex-specific death rates [13].
>
> To counter this, it is suggested that health promotion should focus on a wider range of policy areas, including:
>
> - giving every child the best start in life;
> - enabling all children, young people and adults to maximise their capabilities and have control over their lives;
> - creating fair employment and good work for all;
> - ensuring a healthy standard of living for all;
> - creating and developing sustainable places and communities; and
> - strengthening the role and impact of ill health prevention [14].

Although tackling inequalities in health is seen as a priority, there are many potential interpretations of what this means. Health inequalities can refer to inequalities in outcomes such as life expectancy; inequalities in access or uptake of services such as cancer screening services; or differential exposure to environments that impact on health, such as poor housing. Inequalities can be seen by age, gender, ethnicity or a range of other characteristics. See Chapter 14 for more information on health inequalities.

What societal factors might influence childhood asthma, for example? Or frailty in older people?

8.3 A Combined Model of Forces Driving Health

The models described above draw on assumptions about the determinants of health to inform ways to improve it.

Traditional models of health determinants such as Dahlgren and Whitehead's [15] account, in summary, for many of the major influences on health (see Figure 1.3). Although such models are helpful, they do not easily support conclusions about what is influencing health or lead to greater understanding on what action needs to be taken. Because of this, they can lead to a spurious sense of 'control' in the same way that medicine historically developed disease classifications, but did not have a range of effective treatments to offer patients.

In order to understand how to promote better health, it is important to recognise that health is rarely the sum of individual causes and effects: it is the result of complex interactions. Health is not just about using local health services or personal lifestyle choices. It is driven by wider social, economic and environmental conditions, all of which are mutually reinforcing and interlinked. Such conditions can have

Figure 8.3 A combined focus leads to an integrated model of health improvement. Pencheon and Bradley: Integrated health improvement model.

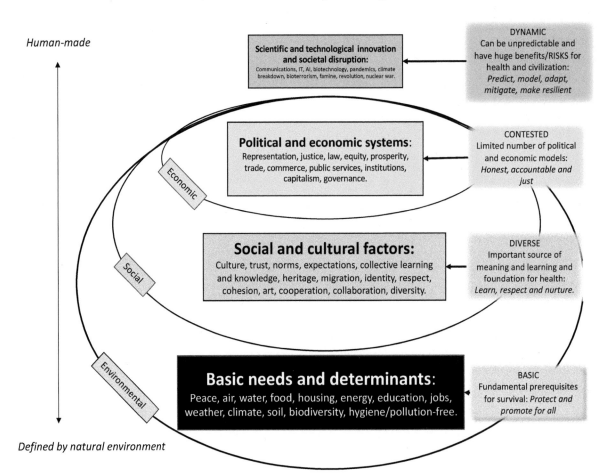

a long-term influence on health. This means that single actions often fail to yield better, long-lasting improvements in health. Traditional epidemiology, the study of the causes of disease, is therefore necessary but insufficient when trying to improve health trends over time and for large populations.

Figure 8.3 offers a new model for conceptualising these complex interactions or driving forces on health and well-being. This model recognises that politics and public health are inextricably linked and brings in ideas from fields that challenge traditional health improvement models, particularly acknowledging complexity and systems thinking.

- There are certain *basic needs and determinants* that are prerequisites of a good standard of health, whether we are talking about individuals or society as a whole. If we deem these to be ***basic***, they should be promoted and protected for all.
- The pattern of health across society is also shaped by specific *social and cultural factors* which determine, for example, who has access to specific protective or negative influences on health, lifestyle and behaviour. These factors are ***diverse*** and we should learn about them, and respect and nurture those that have a positive impact on health.
- These social and cultural factors determine the *political and economic systems* that drive even greater differences in health status between groups – for example, how wealth or benefits are allocated. As these factors are frequently ***contested***, society should be honest about these systems, accountable for choices made and seen as just by the population.
- Health can also be disrupted; by *scientific and technological innovation* or major societal events, such as the impact of social networks, artificial intelligence or war. These are highly ***dynamic*** and should be predicted and modelled so that populations can resiliently adapt and mitigate their impacts.

Implicit within this model is the concept of reducing inequalities in access to and benefit from all of these influences or factors. It is generally accepted that targeted action is needed to ensure that less powerful communities benefit from improvements in health, as they tend to live in less favourable economic and social conditions. To improve health, public health policy should aim to create the conditions in which health and fairness flourish over time. In addition, addressing inequality is not just about looking after the most dispossessed: it is about promoting a health-enhancing environment for everyone.

This model enables the framing of issues in health promotion to support conversations about causes and ways to tackle poor health and health inequities.

Boxes 8.2, 8.3 and 8.4 use the Pencheon and Bradley model in different ways to analyse three example issues of relevance in this decade. Box 8.2 looks at how commercial influences can harm or benefit health and considers what forces from the model are in play. Box 8.3 takes a case study from Mexico and uses the model to analyse what forces were driving the factors influencing the increasing burden of diabetes and how health improvement action was taken to counteract these forces. Box 8.4 uses the COVID-19 pandemic to explore how the forces had an impact on the generation of and response to a global public health issue.

Box 8.2 Analysis of the potential harms and benefits of commercial influences on health and health improvement

In 2005, the World Health Organization (WHO) Bangkok Charter for health promotion [16] recognised the importance of the commercial sector in influencing the public's health. The commercial determinants of health are defined by WHO as 'private sector activities that affect people's health positively or negatively' [17].

Using the health promotion model described above, some of the ways in which the commercial sector can benefit or harm health and its improvement can be analysed.

Impact	Does this have the potential to harm or benefit health/health improvement?		What Pencheon and Bradley model force is at play here?			
	Harm?	Benefit?	Dynamic societal and technological innovation and societal disruption	Contested impacts of political and economic systems	Diverse social and cultural factors	Basic needs and determinants
Developing products that are health enhancing (e.g. seat belts)		Yes	Yes			
Influencing governmental policy through donations or lobbying	Yes	Yes	Yes	Yes		
Sponsoring research which favours commercial interests	Yes	Yes	Yes	Yes		
Government banning advertising for unhealthy products such as tobacco		Yes	Yes	Yes		
Government disinvesting from companies that produce harmful products		Yes	Yes	Yes		
Government taxing unhealthy products such as sugary drinks		Yes	Yes	Yes		
Government assuring rights such as parental leave		Yes	Yes	Yes		

(cont.)

| Impact | Does this have the potential to harm or benefit health/health improvement? | | What Pencheon and Bradley model force is at play here? | | | |
	Harm?	Benefit?	Dynamic societal and technological innovation and societal disruption	Contested impacts of political and economic systems	Diverse social and cultural factors	Basic needs and determinants
Marketing of unhealthy products and consumer misinformation	Yes				Yes	
Source of income for communities		Yes			Yes	
Poor workplace health and safety practices	Yes					Yes
Discriminatory working environments and low wages	Yes					Yes
Pollution	Yes					Yes
Intensive farming and deforestation	Yes					Yes
Source of income and purpose for individuals		Yes				Yes
Providers of technology for health and social care		Yes				Yes
Promote health or social justice at work		Yes				Yes

As the model shows, these forces are interrelated and interventions must cover a complex range of issues to maximise the benefits and minimise the harms from the influences of the commercial sector on health.

Can you think of any other ways that the commercial sector can harm or benefit health and what force from the Pencheon and Bradley model would these demonstrate?

Box 8.3 A retrospective analysis of the approach in Mexico to obesity and diabetes

In Mexico in the early part of the twenty-first century, there was particular concern about rising rates of diabetes and obesity. Increased consumption of sugar-sweetened drinks and high-energy non-essential foods was associated with these worrying health trends.

What happened?

Availability of these products had been facilitated after Mexico signed the North American Free Trade Agreement in 1994.

Mexico's National Survey of Health and Nutrition [18] showed that between 2000 and 2006, deaths from diabetes doubled and was the leading cause of death, while childhood obesity rates rose by 40%.

In 2006, Mexico introduced a programme to tackle obesity which aimed to educate the public, encourage behaviour change and reduce advertising of unhealthy foods.

In 2014, a tax on sugar-sweetened drinks and high-energy non-essential foods was introduced.

Research suggests the introduction of the taxes was associated with a decline of 6% in the purchase of taxed beverages and of 5% in non-essential energy-dense foods in the first year [18, 19].

The drinks industry sponsored research to counteract conclusions on the impact of health improvement on behaviours and actively lobbied against the measures introduced to combat health harms [20].

This timeline of events can be analysed using the health improvement model proposed in this chapter.

Pencheon and Bradley model force	Example from this case study of influences on health	Health improvement action taken in this case
Dynamic societal and technological innovation and societal disruption	Prevalence of advertising acted as a disruptor and was enhanced by increased technology availability	Action taken to counteract advertising was political and cultural rather than technological or societally disruptive
Contested impacts of political and economic systems	Surveys and research were undertaken at a system level to understand the facts and by manufacturers to influence those systems	Action taken included regulation of advertising and taxation of high-sugar and high-energy foodstuffs
Diverse social and cultural factors	Cultural changes occurred, with behaviour changes related to availability of products and widespread advertising	Public education and behaviour techniques to encourage change were implemented
Basic needs and determinants	There appeared to be a link between access to cheap, high-energy consumables and prevalence of obesity and diabetes	Taxation reduced the availability of these products

Forces at all levels affect the impact of consumption of high-sugar and high-energy foodstuffs on health and therefore all levels must be considered when devising a method of intervention.

 Can you think of any way in which technological innovation could be used to imagine a health improvement intervention to counteract the advertising of high-sugar products?

Box 8.4 COVID-19 pandemic

Pencheon and Bradley model force	How this force affected the pandemic and the response to it
Dynamic societal and technological innovation and societal disruption	The risk of future pandemics is related to global farming practices [21] and environmental management and living with animals. Technology played a vital role to manage the pandemic (e.g. electronic certificates to give evidence of vaccination status, apps and electronic messaging to report test results and facilitate contact tracing).
Contested impacts of political and economic systems	Anti-vaccination sentiment developed partly because of a lack of trust in messaging from experts and authorities about vaccine safety [22] and the expedited safety checks and procedures.
Diverse social and cultural factors	Considerable misinformation was available about the dangers of vaccination. Digital exclusion was also an issue for those without Internet or mobile phone access.
Basic needs and determinants	Outcomes in the UK, including increased death rates, were worse for non-White British and poorer communities as a result of societal disparities (e.g. all-cause mortality rates for the entire period since the coronavirus pandemic began (24 January 2020 to 16 February 2022) were higher for males and females in the Bangladeshi ethnic group and males in the Black Caribbean and Pakistani ethnic groups compared with the White British ethnic group [23]).

How might you use this analysis to plan for a future infectious disease epidemic or pandemic? Refer also to Chapter 10.

Thus, for any health issue, each driving force in the model can be further explored conceptually to consider potential health impacts and potential health improvement interventions.

How might you use this combined framework model to create a health improvement strategy for tackling obesity in your local population?

Viewing health improvement through this wider lens demonstrates that for each driving force, interventions can be effected by many different groups and sectors, including governments, the public and charitable sector, the commercial sector and the media. Table 8.1 explores this further and provides an example checklist to use when analysing a health problem that is based around the Pencheon and Bradley model.

Table 8.1 Example checklist when analysing a Pencheon and Bradley model health problem

Force	Some examples of questions to ask when analysing a health problem – using tobacco use as an illustration
Dynamic societal and technological innovation and societal disruption	How are new technologies seen as relevant (e.g. vaping) and utilised or not in harm-reduction approaches to tobacco use?
	How do behaviours change in time of conflict and disaster and does this affect tobacco use or national policy?
	What health-care technologies are being developed to deal with the detrimental health effects of tobacco use?
	How do new data technologies affect advertising and targeting of advertising?
Contested impacts of political and economic systems	How do governments tax tobacco companies and respond to lobbying from both tobacco companies and charities opposing tobacco use?
	What legislation is put into place to restrict tobacco use and how is it enforced?
	How does the health-care-funding model of a country impact on the choices made around tobacco use in the population?
	How do companies manufacturing tobacco products affect the environment?
	How do companies manufacturing tobacco products affect the availability of work- and employment-related reward?
	What policies do governments put in place that counteract any of the harms of tobacco use (such as open spaces, physical activity)?
Diverse social and cultural factors	How do cultural norms affect takeup and stopping of tobacco use in certain sub-populations? This might be family or peer influences, or different tobacco products being seen as normal.
	How do the places people live affect the culture and the use of tobacco?
	How do economic policies affect levels of economic wealth and the consequent access to disposable income and behaviours of disadvantaged groups?
	What charities work in this sector and what influence do they have in communities?
Basic needs and determinants	What are individuals' inherent capacity for mental and physical health and well-being as smokers?
	How does the biology of nicotine dependence affect ceasing tobacco use?
	What health-care is provided to those who have tobacco-related ill health?

So what can practitioners working in public health do to influence and improve health?

Figure 8.4 shows some of the areas where practitioners can promote better health and some examples are given in Box 8.5.

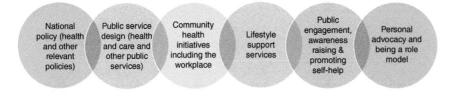

National policy (health and other relevant policies) | Public service design (health and care and other public services) | Community health initiatives including the workplace | Lifestyle support services | Public engagement, awareness raising & promoting self-help | Personal advocacy and being a role model

Figure 8.4 A hierarchy of health improvement intervention.

Box 8.5 Practical actions to improve health

Action	Who might do this	Examples
Act to ensure that national policy, whatever the topic area, is seen as an opportunity to improve health	Civil servants Lobbyists Professional groups (e.g. Medical Royal Colleges)	Road planning and its effects on community displacement and availability of green spaces
Be instrumental in designing better health and care services and promote health in other public services	Health and care commissioners Health-care managers and clinicians Public libraries providing health information	Clinical audit on inequalities in access to services Outreach services
Establish health-enhancing initiatives for communities or workplaces and design services that support healthier choices and lifestyles	Workplace health coordinators, human resources, occupational health Commercial companies Health and care commissioners	Healthy food choices in vending machines Water availability Health checks in the workplace Mental health champions
Raise public awareness of health issues and signpost individuals towards opportunities for self-help	Charities Health and social care workers School teachers and managers National and local media National and local government information campaigns	Social prescribing scheme promotion Information campaigns

(cont.)		
Action	Who might do this	Examples
Act as advocates for public health and adopt healthier, more sustainable lifestyles	Everyone	Minimise waste Eat healthily Undertake physical activity Moderate drinking of alcohol Cycle or walk more

 What actions could you or your organisation take to encourage physical activity, for example?

8.4 Conclusions

In conclusion, as life expectancy increases globally, health promotion challenges change. In addition to promoting health across the whole population, tackling health inequality is a central concern and involves political choices.

Health promotion can have a bio-medical, individual, societal or combined focus. The bio-medical focus emphasises the importance of disease prevention. Questions about the cost-effectiveness of prevention as opposed to the cost of health and care services are of particular importance. With the individual focus, the role of behaviour change is highlighted. Interventions to change behaviour can be informed by behaviour science, which studies the factors that influence behaviours.

With a societal focus, the importance of political choice is given weight, along with a recognition that commercial influences on health can be significant. Using the combined model, a range of factors are recognised: the choices of individuals and families; the existence of health, care, education and other services; food and water supply and the state of the local environment; the pattern of work and financial reward, together with wider influences such as climate change, political and social instability, inequality and disparity and use of technology and level of digital literacy.

Health can therefore be promoted in many different ways, including influencing national policy, driving system or service change, raising awareness of health issues, working directly with communities or by individuals acting as role models and advocates for health.

REFERENCES

1. World Health Organization, The Global Health Observatory. Available at: www.who.int/data/gho

2. Office for National Statistics, UK Census, 2021. Available at: www.ons.gov.uk/peoplepopulationandcommunity/healthandsocialcare/healthinequalities/bulletins/healthstatelifeexpectanciesbyindexofmultipledeprivationimd/2018to2020

3. G. Rose, *The Strategy of Preventive Medicine*, Oxford, Oxford University Press, 1992.

4. York Health Economics Consortium, *Cost-Effectiveness of Interventions for Smoking Cessation: Final Report*, York, University of York, 2007.

5. I. Bains, Y. H. Choi, K. Soldan and M. Jit, Clinical impact and cost-effectiveness of primary cytology versus human papillomavirus testing for cervical cancer screening in England, *International Journal of Gynecologic Cancer* **29**(4), 2019, 669–75.

6. World Health Organization, *Ottawa Charter for Health Promotion*, Geneva, WHO, 1986.

7. World Health Organization, Behavioural sciences for better health. Available at: www.who.int/initiatives/behavioural-sciences

8. C. Bonell, M. McKee, A. Fletcher *et al.*, Nudge smudge: UK government misrepresents 'nudge', *The Lancet* **377**(9784), 2011, 2158–9.

9. T. Rouyard, B. Engelen, A. Papanikitas and R. Nakamura, Boosting healthier choices, *British Medical Journal* **376**, 2022, e064225.

10. M. Marmot, J. Allen, T. Boyce *et al.*, Health Equity in England: The Marmot Review 10 Years on, London, Institute of Health Equity/The Health Foundation, 2020.

11. K. Igoe, Algorithmic bias in health care exacerbates social inequities – how to prevent it, 2021. Available at: www.hsph.harvard.edu/ecpe/how-to-prevent-algorithmic-bias-in-health-care/

12. E. M. Greenhalgh, M. M. Scollo and M. H. Winstanley, *Tobacco in Australia: Facts and Issues*, Melbourne, Cancer Council Victoria, 2023.

13. Institute of Health Equity, Contribution of inequalities in mortality to total numbers of deaths in England in the years 2009 to 2020, 2022. Available at: www.instituteofhealthequity.org/resources-reports/contribution-of-inequalities-in-mortality-to-total-numbers-of-deaths-in-england-in-the-years-2009-to-2020

14. M. Marmot, P. Goldblatt, J. Allen *et al.*, *Fair Society, Healthy Lives (The Marmot Review), Strategic Review of Health Inequalities in England Post 2020*, London, Institute for Health Equity, 2010.

15. G. Dahlgren and M. Whitehead, Policies and strategies to promote social equity in health, Institutet för Framtidsstudier, 2007.

16. World Health Organization, *Bangkok Charter for Health Promotion in a Globalised World*, Bangkok, WHO, 2005.

17. World Health Organization, Commercial determinants of health, 2023. Available at: www.who.int/news-room/fact-sheets/detail/commercial-determinants-of-health

18. National Institute of Public Health, *Mexico National Survey of Health and Nutrition Mid-Way 2016*, Mexico, Ministry of Health Mexico, 2016.

19. M. Arantxa Colchero, B. M. Popkin, J. A. Rivera and S. W. Ng, Beverage purchases from stores in Mexico under the excise tax on sugar sweetened beverages: Observational study, *British Medical Journal* **352**, 2016, h6704.

20. C. Batis, J. A. Rivera, B. M. Popkin and L. Smith Taillie, First-year evaluation of Mexico's tax on nonessential energy-dense foods: An observational study, *PLoS Medicine* **13**(7), 2016, e1002057.

21. Intergovernmental Science-Policy Platform on Biodiversity and Ecosystem Services, Workshop Report on Biodiversity and Pandemics of the Intergovernmental Platform on Biodiversity and Ecosystem Services, Bonn, Germany, IPBES, 2020.

22. N. F. Johnson, N. Velásquez and N. J. Restrepo, The online competition between pro- and anti-vaccination views, *Nature* **582**(7811), 2020, 230–3.

23. Office for National Statistics, Updating ethnic contrasts in deaths involving the coronavirus (COVID-19), England: 10 January 2022 to 16 February 2022. Available at: www.ons.gov.uk/peoplepopulationandcommunity/birthsdeathsandmarriages/deaths/articles/updatingethniccontrastsindeathsinvolvingthecoronaviruscovid19englandandwales/10january2022to16february2022

9

Screening

Sue Cohen and Jan Yates

Key points

- Screening is a tool to identify people at increased risk of a condition so that action can be taken to improve outcomes.
- Established criteria are used to judge when a screening programme should be introduced. These take account of the importance of the condition, the test, the treatment and the effectiveness of the programme as a whole.
- Screening tests are not 100% accurate: they will always identify false negatives and false positives.
- The performance of a screening test can be assessed using calculations of sensitivity, specificity and predictive values.
- Screening can incur harm and raises ethical questions. Health professionals and the public need to be aware of both the costs and the benefits to society and individuals from screening as a public health activity.
- For screening programmes to be effective, they must be organised with a screening pathway, have adequate resources, a quality assurance system and a strategy to address inequalities.
- Screening programmes must be regularly evaluated. It is important to be aware of potential sources of bias when assessing their effectiveness.

9.1 Introduction

The World Health Organization (WHO) defines the purpose of screening as:

'To identify people in an apparently healthy population who are at higher risk of a health problem or a condition, so that an early treatment or intervention can be offered. This, in turn, may lead to better health outcomes for some of the screened individuals' [1].

Screening is different from diagnosis in that it identifies those at increased risk rather than those having a disorder. By definition, screening looks for early signs in an asymptomatic individual (e.g. pre-cancerous changes in cervical cells, or unknown raised blood pressure in health check screening). Of particular importance from a clinical perspective, therefore, is that where diagnosis usually involves individuals presenting to health services to request help, screening invites those who may not otherwise be seeking care to participate and undergo tests, and further along the pathway, potential treatment. The term 'screening' is often used loosely to describe testing individuals for a condition opportunistically when they attend medical care or actively searching for cases of a disease. These examples would not be considered public health screening programmes, but may sometimes be described as 'screening'.

Screening that is carried out as part of an organised public health programme is termed 'population' or 'mass' screening when it is applied to a cohort of a population (such as all women between 50 and 70 years), or 'targeted' screening when it is only offered to a specific group of people who are considered to be at higher risk – for example, people with pre-existing conditions such as diabetes, or an exposure, such as smoking.

Screening is an important preventive public health activity. This chapter:

- provides examples of effective screening programmes;
- considers what criteria are needed to demonstrate the effectiveness of a programme;
- describes how screening tests can be used to guide action; and
- describes how screening programmes can be evaluated.

9.2 Should We Implement a New Screening Programme?

The concept of mass screening emerged during the early part of the twentieth century in part in the context of selecting recruits for the US army [2]. However, as its use was considered for medical settings, it became clear that the decision whether to implement a screening programme was not straightforward and in 1968 Wilson and Jungner, on behalf of the WHO, produced ten principles to guide policy-makers about whether to implement mass screening [3]. These principles remain relevant today and are fundamental to understanding whether a screening programme is an appropriate public health intervention. The principles have been adapted by many countries to produce national criteria for screening.

These principles evaluate the viability, effectiveness and appropriateness of a screening programme and can be split into four categories relating to: the condition; the test; the treatment; and the programme itself. In the UK, the National Screening Committee oversees the introduction of new screening programmes. It requires robust evidence for all the criteria for a new programme to be established.

Explore whether there are any screening programmes proposed which *haven't* been approved. Why? Do you agree?

Up-to-date schedules for the National Screening programmes for various countries can be found online. Below, examples of current UK screening programmes are used to illustrate key principles within these four key categories for assessing screening programmes.

9.2.1 The Condition

The condition screened for should be an important problem. A population-wide intervention such as screening will only be effective if it can prevent significant disease. For rare conditions without major health effects, screening would not be worthwhile.

Breast cancer is the most common cancer in women (around 25% of all cancer cases in women worldwide). Globally, in 2020, there were over 2 million new cases and it caused approximately 15% of all cancer deaths in women. Its incidence is higher in more-developed countries than less-developed ones. Colorectal cancer was the third most common cancer in 2020, causing 1.9 million new cases (around 10% of all cancer cases). Thus, both breast and colorectal cancer give rise to a high burden of disease [4].

In contrast, metabolic conditions in the newborn are extremely rare, for example phenylketonuria (PKU) occurs in approximately 1 in 10,000 newborns in the UK [5], yet there is a long tradition for screening for these conditions. The reason is that although rare, these conditions can be treated if identified early, but if untreated lead to a lifetime of disability with the associated cost to families and society, and they are therefore considered important public health problems.

The natural history of the condition sought should be adequately understood and there should be a recognisable latent or early symptomatic stage. To make gains in morbidity or mortality, it must be possible to identify an early stage of disease so that early intervention can prevent progression. For example, the aim of cervical cancer screening is to reduce the incidence of cervical cancer by detecting the presence of abnormal cells at a pre-cancerous stage and treating them to reduce the likelihood of these abnormalities progressing to cancer. Our understanding of the natural history of cervical cancer has improved in recent years and we know there is a clear causal path between infection with human papillomavirus (HPV) and changes in the cervical epithelium leading to cancer. This has led to a new screening test for cervical cancer by primary screening for HPV. Only if positive are abnormal cells looked for on cytology. This change has led to a more efficient and effective programme.

All practicable, cost-effective primary prevention measures should have been implemented. It is better to prevent the onset of disease rather than have to detect it early and then treat. Thus, screening programmes are more often established for conditions where preventive measures have not led to significant reductions in disease prevalence or incidence. An interesting case study is lung cancer, which is the commonest cause of cancer deaths worldwide, accounting for 18% of all cancer deaths in 2020. Many countries have invested in tobacco control measures as the most important cause of lung cancer. For example, the UK has seen a steady decline in smoking rates from about 25% in 1990 to about 14% in 2020 [6], but deaths from lung cancer remain the commonest cause of deaths from a cancer in the UK. For this reason, there has been interest in a targeted screening programme for heavy smokers using low-dose CT scans.

9.3 The Test

There should be a suitable test available which is simple, safe, precise and validated. As screening only identifies those at increased risk, it is necessary to have a test for the condition which maximises reassurance for those who do not need further investigation and rapidly refers as many appropriate people as possible for diagnosis and treatment. The population distribution of screening test values should be known and an agreed 'cut-off' value identified so that those people warranting further investigation can be identified.

 How might you determine an appropriate 'cut-off' value for a screening test?

The test or examination should be acceptable to both the public and to professionals. Screening programmes depend, for their effectiveness, on high proportions of the target population complying with screening offers. If the screening or diagnostic test is not acceptable, this will reduce the effectiveness of the programme, as many will not attend.

When screening for colorectal cancer (CRC) was started in the UK, there was a concern that asking people to collect faeces and send them into a laboratory for testing would be unacceptable, and the screening programme would be unsuccessful in reducing CRC mortality because of low uptake [7, 8]. This concern has receded over time as coverage in England for CRC was in the order of 65% by 2020.

It is important to remember that although the public as a whole may accept a particular test or diagnostic process, groups within a population may not accept the test or find it difficult to access it. This can lead to inequalities for certain groups. In CRC screening, some studies have shown inequalities in uptake across different ethnic groups, with all groups having significantly lower uptake than the White British group, except Asian Chinese [9, 10].

There should be an agreed policy on further diagnostic investigation. Those who receive a positive screen result must be informed of the choices available to them and access to diagnostic services should be available equitably for the whole screened population.

With reference to a specific screening programme, consider how inequalities might be exacerbated at each stage of the process.

Screening for CRC is often a two-stage process. Stool samples are tested for occult blood and if this is positive people are invited for a colonoscopy. If a country has limited endoscopy capacity, screening for CRC can add demand, leading to delays in diagnosis for both screened and symptomatic populations. Understanding the impact on diagnostic services is an important part of the planning before implementing a screening programme.

9.4 The Treatment

There should be an accepted and effective treatment for patients with recognised disease, facilities for treatment should be available and such treatment optimised by all health-care providers. Implementing a screening programme which raises hopes and uncovers demand for treatment services that do not exist or that do not have a firm evidence base would be unethical and an uneconomical use of resources. For example, a positive breast screening mammogram requires further investigation utilising hospital capacity, radiological, nursing, pathological and potentially surgical expertise, and the absence of or long waits for these adversely affects the effectiveness of the screening test.

There should be an agreed policy on whom to treat as patients, including management of borderline disease. Treatments may, however, be invasive and unpleasant and this must be explained clearly before screening is undertaken. In some screening programmes, the 'treatment' becomes more of an issue. For example, abdominal ultrasound of men aged 65 to detect and treat large abdominal aortic aneurysms has been shown to decrease aneurysm-related mortality by 42% [11]. However, the surgical aneurysm repair carries a 1–2% risk of dying within 30 days of surgery [12].

9.5 The Programme

There should be robust evidence that the screening programme is effective in reducing mortality or morbidity. Evidence from randomised controlled trials of screening programmes should be considered before initiating a screening programme.

There should be evidence that the programme is acceptable to the public and professionals such that individuals will be prepared to undertake the screening procedure and that the benefits outweigh the harms. All elements of the screening programme from invitations through to treatment should be acceptable and the outcomes of the programme in terms of morbidity and mortality should outweigh the physical and psychological harms caused by the test, diagnostic procedures and treatment.

Although both these principles seem straightforward, in practice they are hard to assess. The results of trials may not be easy to interpret. For example, should the outcome measure for a trial be a reduction of all-cause mortality or cancer-specific mortality? Can results of a trial be transposed from one country to another? How do you measure harms? How do you balance the psychological harms caused by anxiety in many against a reduction in mortality in a few? Making these judgements is complex and has led to considerable controversy over the years about whether certain screening programmes do more good than harm. We will look at this in more detail below.

The cost of early diagnosis and treatment should be economically balanced in relation to the total expenditure on health-care. Within a limited budget all health and health-care spend must be justified in terms of cost-effectiveness. Implementation of a screening programme must be demonstrated to be an efficient use of health-care funds in comparison to other interventions possible for specific conditions. For example, the WHO recommends that in low- and middle-income countries with poorly organised health services and late-stage presentation of breast cancer, investment should be in an early diagnosis programme rather than a breast screening programme [13, 14].

The programme must be adequately resourced. As well as all the staffing and other resource implications of the testing, diagnosis and treatment, screening programmes require significant money for management and monitoring, quality assurance and long-term evaluation. All of these resource implications must be determined before the programme is established.

9.6 Screening Can Lead to Harms as Well as Benefits

Screening can incur harms as well as benefits (see Figure 9.1). These can be harms to the individual in terms of physical and psychological well-being and the harm to a population from diverting resources from other needs into screening programmes that require significant resources.

No screening test is 100% accurate: it cannot pick up everyone at higher risk nor correctly identify everyone who does not have a condition. This means that screening tests may fail to detect a condition (or a higher risk of a condition) and offer false reassurance (false negative) or may identify healthy people as having a disease or at a higher risk (false positive). False positives can cause psychological harm, as well as expose people to unnecessary diagnostic investigations, which in themselves can cause harms (e.g. perforation from a colonoscopy).

An important feature of screening is that it can detect disease which would never have caused harm to the person in their lifetime (overdiagnosis); this is because screening can pick up very small lesions that would regress if left alone, or the lesions progress so slowly the person will die from something else. For the individual

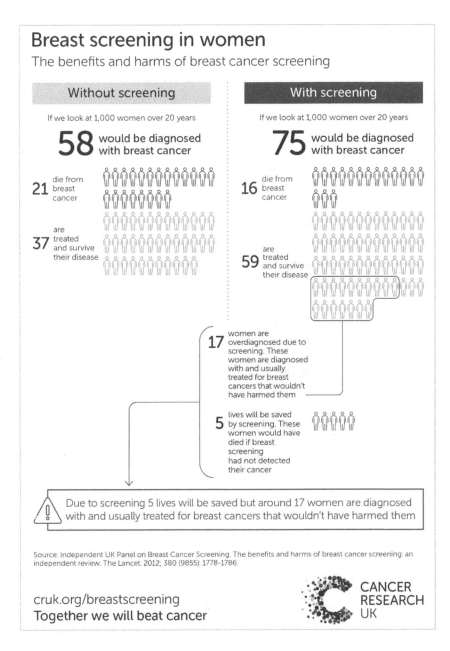

Figure 9.1 The benefits and harms of breast screening in women [15].

patient, it is not possible to distinguish those cancers that will harm from those that will not, so all patients are subjected to treatment. In the breast screening programme in the UK, it is estimated that screening saves about 1 life from breast cancer for every 200 women who are screened. However, about 3 in every 200 women screened every 3 years from the age of 50 up to their 71st birthday are diagnosed with a cancer that would never have been found without screening and would never have become life-threatening [16].

These women will be subject to treatment such as surgery and chemotherapy which can significantly impact on their lives (overtreatment). Some experts believe that this means the harm outweighs the benefit and that therefore we should not screen for breast cancer: others believe the lives saved justify the harms.

 List the pros and cons of a specific screening programme for an *individual* undergoing the screening test and the potential harms and benefits to them. How might you make this more acceptable to the public?

Screening programmes require significant human and material resources to set up and run effectively. They can generate a large number of referrals into diagnostic and treatment services and as such can place huge pressure on already stretched services. This can result in patients with symptoms having their assessments delayed and ultimately leading to poorer outcomes.

9.7 Ethics of Screening

The potential for harm for an individual, even though there may be benefits for the population leads to ethical debates about whether screening should be offered. Various ethical frameworks have been used to examine screening. Some use a 'utilitarian perspective' (see also Chapter 6) which says if benefits outweigh harms for a population then screening is justified; others say if it will cause significant harm to a single individual, screening is unethical. The WHO suggested a pragmatic use of values to support decision-making: respect for dignity and autonomy; non-maleficence and beneficence; justice and equity; and prudence and precaution [1]. As relatively high coverage is needed to produce health gains, there is a risk of pushing for high coverage rates and incentives to encourage screening, undermining participants' right to autonomy to make an informed decision. Therefore, effective health communication which explains the potential harms and benefits of screening and supports informed decision-making in the target population is an extremely important component of a screening programme. Communication methods should take account of disparities across populations and should be culturally appropriate and at an appropriate level of literacy and health literacy for all the population. Communicating risk is a challenging task, so current evidence in this area should be considered when devising material to inform populations about screening [17]. Leaflets, online resources and decision support aids all need careful testing to make sure they are accessible and appropriate.

9.8 Deciding Whether Screening Is the Right Course of Action

Thus, even with Wilson and Jungner's principles, deciding whether to start a screening programme is a complex and sometimes contested decision. In the UK and several other countries, committees have been set up to consider whether to start a programme (see Figure 9.2). The UK National Screening Committee (UK NSC) website [18] is a useful resource to illustrate how decisions about whether to continue, amend or establish a new screening programme are made, and it lists the conditions it has reviewed and considered and why a particular condition meets its criteria (or does not). In the UK, screening programmes cover the life course. There are antenatal programmes such as foetal anomaly screening, newborn programmes such as the blood spot programme which picks up nine conditions, including congenital hypothyroidism, cystic fibrosis and PKU, and newborn hearing programmes. The adult programmes include screening for cancers and conditions such as diabetic retinopathy and aortic aneurysms.

In recent years, the conditions that can be tested for have increased dramatically, as well as a growth in novel types of tests. Genetic and molecular testing and whole-body MRIs are readily available, often being sold directly to the public. These offer individuals the chance to find multiple diseases, including cancer and heart disease, as well as mapping their genetic profiles. Even though some of these tests may offer some potential of improving population health, most have not been subject to large-scale high-quality research studies, nor do they meet Wilson and Jungner's criteria, and in fact can pose risks to a population who may not understand the harms associated with screening. The challenge for many countries is to put in place regulatory frameworks that can respond to this burgeoning field while still implementing effective screening programmes [1].

9.9 Other Forms of 'Screening'

There are several other situations in which healthy individuals are tested that lie outside our definition of population screening. The underlying difference here is that this kind of testing relates to the need of the individual, rather than to reducing mortality or morbidity in populations (see Box 9.1).

Box 9.1 Not screening …

- pre-employment checks (e.g. sight tests for drivers);
- infection control (e.g. food handlers being cleared of an *E. coli* infection);
- to determine suitability for clinical interventions (e.g. pre-operative assessments);
- research studies; and
- fitness test prior to starting an exercise regime.

Figure 9.2 Process for deciding whether to implement a screening programme [1].

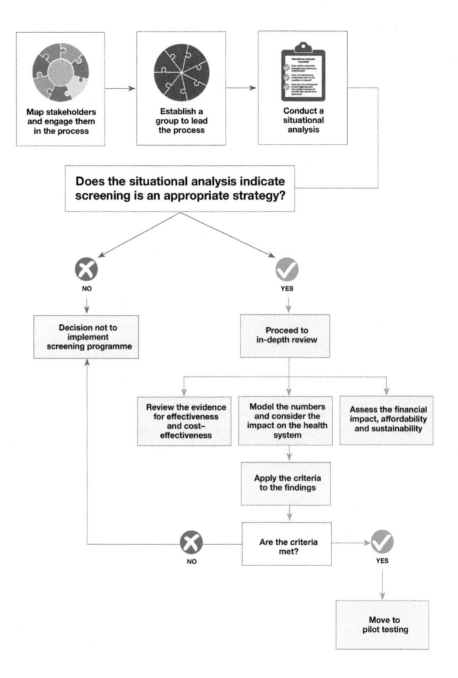

9.10 Screening Test Performance

Before implementing a screening programme, it is important to understand how the test will perform, using different measures of test performance.

9.10.1 Sensitivity and Specificity

No clinical or biochemical tests are 100% accurate and false positive and false negative values can be used to measure test performance.

Sensitivity is the proportion of those that truly have the condition (as measured by a gold standard test) who are correctly identified by the test. These are the true positives. Those that the test does not correctly identify with the condition are false negative results.

Specificity is the proportion of those who truly do not have the condition (as measured by the gold standard) who are correctly identified as not having the condition by the test. These are the true negatives. Those that the test incorrectly identifies with the condition, who is actually free of the condition, are false positive results.

A sensitive test keeps the false negative rate low, and a specific test keeps the false positive rate low. In the design of tests, it is usual that as tests are made more specific they become less sensitive and vice versa. A balance is needed and the calculated sensitivities and specificities are used to determine the best screening test for each condition. Figure 9.3 shows the impact on false negatives and positives of changing the threshold used to define a 'positive' screening outcome.

9.10.2 Calculating Sensitivity and Specificity

To calculate these measures, one needs to know the numbers screened, those found to have the condition with the test and the numbers then found to truly have the condition using the 'gold standard' test. Using these numbers, the number of true positives, true negatives, false negatives and false positives can be calculated and from this the sensitivity and specificity can be calculated.

The 2×2 in Table 9.1 illustrates this and the formulae used for the calculations.

In the example shown in Table 9.2, the test is very specific, but not very sensitive. This means that, at a population level, it is not very effective at picking up positive cases of the condition, but it is quite good at identifying people who do not have the condition. It is unlikely that a test with such a low sensitivity would be used as a widespread screening tool without further information being available for the clinician to inform decision-making following the test.

Figure 9.3 Defining the threshold
for screening [1].

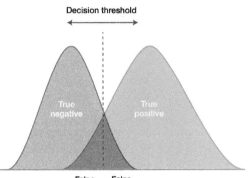

To increase the sensitivity, shift the threshold to the
left. However, this will increase the false positives
and reduce the specificity.

To increase the specificity, shift the threshold to
the right. However, this will increase the false
negatives and reduce the sensitivity.

Table 9.1 Generic 2 × 2 table showing the possible outcomes of a screening test and used to calculate its validity

		TRUE'		
		Positive	Negative	
TEST'	Positive	a	b	a + b
		True positive (TP)	False positive (FP)	
	Negative	c	d	c + d
		False negative (FN)	True negative (TN)	
		a + c	b + d	a + b + c + d
		All individuals with the condition	All individuals without the condition	
		Sensitivity	Specificity	
		TP/(TP+FN)	TN/(FP+TN)	
		a/(a+c)	d/(b+d)	

Table 9.2 Data for an imaginary screening test

		TRUE'	
		Positive	Negative
TEST'	Positive	6	6
	Negative	23	966

Use the formulae in Table 9.1 to calculate the sensitivity and specificity for the results of an imaginary screening test shown in Table 9.2 and explain what this means.

9.10.3 Predictive Values

The sensitivity and specificity of a test do not depend on the prevalence of the condition in question. However, the prevalence does affect our ability to predict if someone has a positive result whether they truly have the condition. Imagine a situation where a person is told they have a positive result for a very rare condition where the sensitivity and specificity of the test are quite high. What the person would want to know is what proportion of positive results are true positives. This is called the positive predicative value or PPV (true positives/true positives + false positives; note the difference in this measure to sensitivity). Because the condition is rare, most of the population will not have the condition, so even with a high specificity there will still be quite a lot of people with a false positive result. Similarly, because it is a rare condition, there will not be that many people who are true positives. So, if we take a proportion of true positives to all positives, the PPV will be quite low. If we repeat the calculation with the same test sensitivity and specificity, but now for a condition that is common, you can see that the number of people with true positives will increase and the number with false positives will decrease and so the PPV will increase.

Negative predictive value is a similar measure of true negatives as a proportion of all negatives.

PPV and NPV are very useful in understanding how the test will perform in each population, as demonstrated in Figure 9.4.

Thus, sensitivities and specificities are useful to convey how good a test is and determine what the best test is for any condition, and predictive values are useful as a measure of the usefulness of the test across populations.

The positive predictive value and the numbers of false positives vary according to the prevalence of the disease in each country (the sensitivity and specificity remain the same)

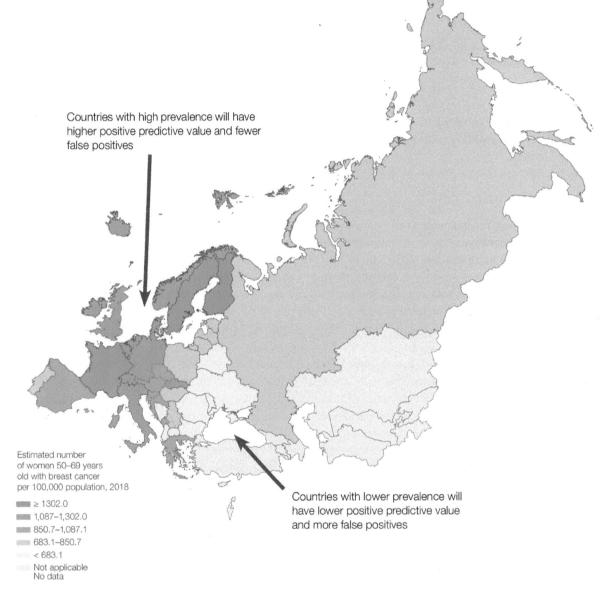

Countries with high prevalence will have higher positive predictive value and fewer false positives

Countries with lower prevalence will have lower positive predictive value and more false positives

Estimated number
of women 50–69 years
old with breast cancer
per 100,000 population, 2018

- ≥ 1302.0
- 1,087–1,302.0
- 850.7–1,087.1
- 683.1–850.7
- < 683.1
- Not applicable
  No data

In this case, the positive predictive value is the proportion of women with a positive mammogram who have breast cancer

Figure 9.4 The impact of prevalence on screening validity [1].

9.11 Implementing Screening Programmes

Criteria based on those of Wilson and Jungner are generally used to determine whether to put a screening programme in place, but they do not guarantee that a screening programme will work in practice.

In practice, an effective screening programme requires an agreed screening pathway, adequate resources, a quality assurance system and a strategy to address inequalities.

9.11.1 A Screening Pathway

This describes in detail how people who are screened are identified, invited, tested, referred, diagnosed and treated if needed. It includes explaining how people will receive information about screening and how to make sure there is informed consent; it defines cut-off points for referrals; what to do with equivocal results; and what should happen to people who are screen negative. It is used to develop IT systems to manage people's invitations and subsequent management; it can be used to calculate the impact of screening on diagnostic and treatment services; and it is useful in understanding weak points in a pathway where people may be lost and fail-safe systems may be needed. Mapping a pathway and understanding how it will work in practice is a fundamental step in implementing a new programme (Figure 9.5).

9.11.2 Adequate Resources

Screening programmes require lots of staff, equipment and IT, and can generate demand for more diagnostic and treatment services. A common reason for ineffective screening programmes is inadequate funding for part of the pathway, such as diagnostic and treatment services or information and communication materials.

9.11.3 A Quality Assurance System

All screening programmes require quality assurance systems. The core of the system are standards that set agreed parameters of process measures, such as uptake, coverage, detection rate and time to referral for diagnostic assessment (see Box 9.2).

It also includes protocols and guidelines that explain how to carry out all aspects of the screening pathway.

9.11.4 Addressing Inequalities

Recognising which population groups are likely to be subject to inequalities and implementing effective strategies to address this is a crucial part of making sure a screening programme will deliver its expected benefits. As previously described, the

Figure 9.5 Steps in a simplified
screening pathway [1].

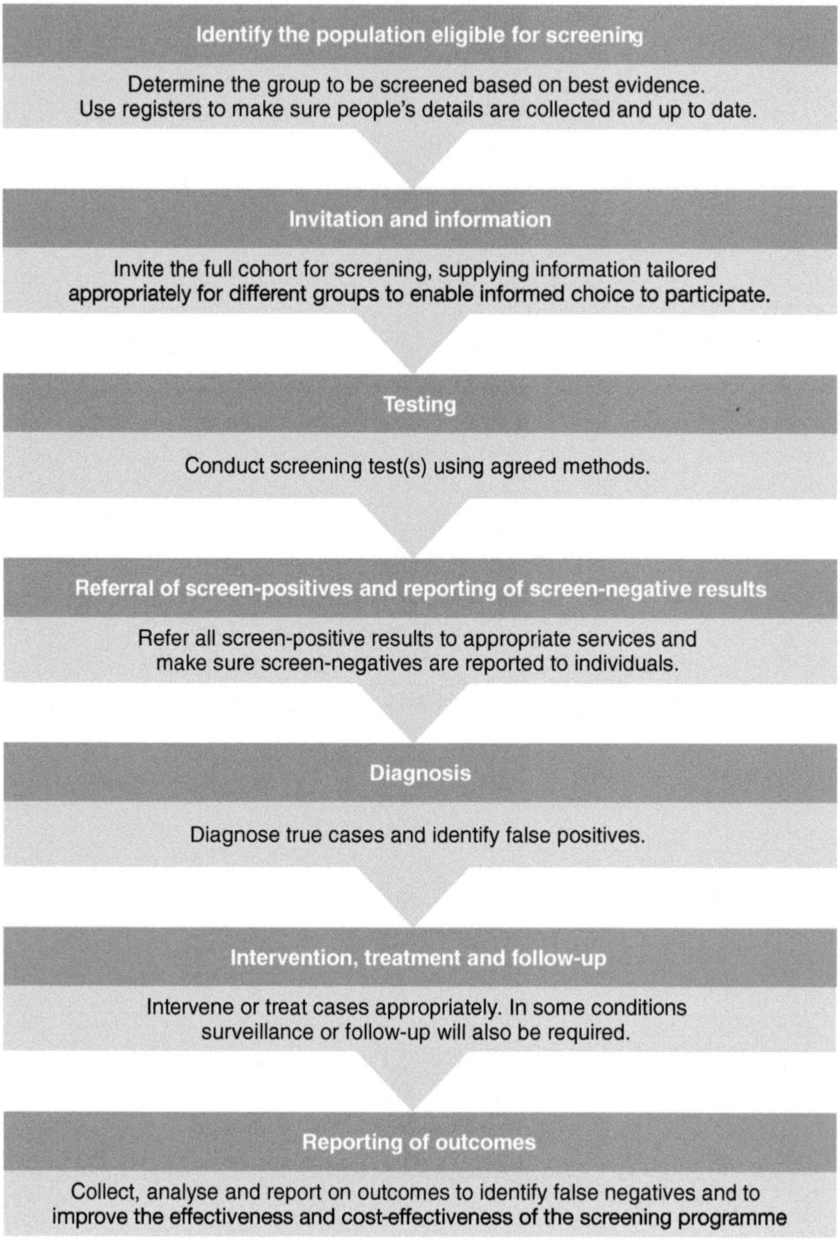

Identify the population eligible for screening

Determine the group to be screened based on best evidence.
Use registers to make sure people's details are collected and up to date.

Invitation and information

Invite the full cohort for screening, supplying information tailored
appropriately for different groups to enable informed choice to participate.

Testing

Conduct screening test(s) using agreed methods.

Referral of screen-positives and reporting of screen-negative results

Refer all screen-positive results to appropriate services and
make sure screen-negatives are reported to individuals.

Diagnosis

Diagnose true cases and identify false positives.

Intervention, treatment and follow-up

Intervene or treat cases appropriately. In some conditions
surveillance or follow-up will also be required.

Reporting of outcomes

Collect, analyse and report on outcomes to identify false negatives and to
improve the effectiveness and cost-effectiveness of the screening programme

Box 9.2 Monitoring screening programmes

Information which can be used to monitor the quality of a screening programme include:

- uptake (screened as a proportion of invited);
- coverage (screened as a proportion of eligible population);
- detection rate;
- number of referrals;
- number of test positives who are confirmed as true positives;
- number of true cases missed;
- number of cases effectively treated;
- clinical or laboratory expertise of those responsible for screening tests;
- the impact of the screening programme on other related services;
- the delays between different steps of the programme;
- the quality, accuracy and readability of the information provided to patients about the programme;
- coverage by different population groups to determine inequalities in access; and
- the training required to initiate the programme and maintain high standards.

challenge is to do this while maintaining an individual's autonomy to decide whether to participate in a programme. A successful and fair approach requires a dual focus on health literacy and ensuring informed consent, and at the same time addressing barriers to access through evidenced-based strategies.

9.12 Evaluation of Screening Programmes

To evaluate a screening programme, it is important to identify and analyse outcome measures that assess the programme's aims. This might be a reduction in mortality from a cancer screening programme or reduction in blindness due to diabetic retinopathy screening. However, it is not always straightforward to measure outcomes in screening programmes and it is also important to consider potential sources of bias that can occur.

9.12.1 Sources of Bias

9.12.1.1 Selection Bias

It is hoped that screening programmes attract all the intended population, but those who respond to invitations may be systematically different from the target population in some way. For example, deprived populations who may be at higher risk of cancers may have lower attendance rate for screening than the population as a whole. Because of this, it may appear that the screened population has a lower mortality rate from a cancer than an unscreened population, but this will be because the screened population is a healthier population rather than due to screening.

9.12.1.2 Lead Time Bias

Lead time bias occurs when detection by screening seems to increase disease-free survival, but only because disease has been detected earlier and not because screening is delaying death or disease. This is sometimes referred to as 'information bias' because the information about the disease has been detected earlier. Figure 9.6 shows how this works: person A and B develop disease, then die at the same time; however, it appears that A lives longer than B because she found out about her disease earlier through screening. This is one reason why it is important to evaluate a programme using mortality not using survival as an outcome and compare screened and unscreened populations. Where there is a lead time bias reduced improvements in mortality will be demonstrated.

Figure 9.6 Lead time bias.

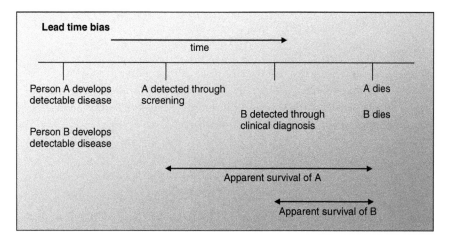

9.12.1.3 Length Time Bias

Length time bias occurs if the screening programme is better at picking up milder forms of the disease. Figure 9.7 shows how this occurs. Length time bias means that people who develop disease that progresses more quickly or is more likely to be fatal (person A) are less likely to be picked up by screening and their outcomes may not be included in evaluations of the programme. Thus, the programme looks to be more effective than it is. The programme evaluation must compare the type of disease

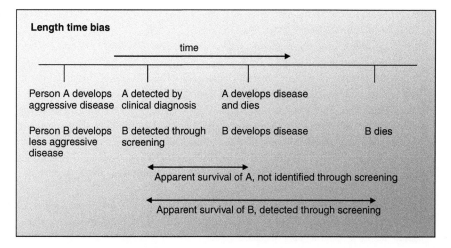

Figure 9.7 Length time bias.

which is picked up through screening with that picked up by routine diagnosis. Where length time bias occurs, the screening programme will systematically identify disease which has a better prognosis.

Can you identify an example of a particular screening programme which illustrates selection bias, lead time or length time bias?

9.13 Conclusions

Screening is an important public health intervention which has been demonstrated to have had a major impact on mortality for certain conditions. However, screening carries risks to individuals and is a good example of an area of public health where the needs of individuals and the needs of populations may conflict. Professionals working in screening, whether counselling individuals on screening choices or supporting screening at a population level, need to have a thorough understanding of the principles of screening and screening tests and need to be aware that their beliefs colour the way they communicate with people.

REFERENCES

1. WHO Regional Office for Europe, Screening programmes: A short guide, 2020. Available at: https://apps.who.int/iris/bitstream/handle/10665/330829/9789289054782-eng.pdf?sequence= 1&isAllowed=y

2. A. Morabia and F. F. Zhang, History of medical screening: From concepts to action, *Postgraduate Medical Journal* **80**(946), 2004, 463–9.

3. J. M. G. Wilson and G. Jungner, Principles and practice of screening for disease, Public Health Paper no. 34, Geneva, WHO, 1968.

4. International Agency for Research on Cancer, Cancer today, 2022. Available at: https://gco .iarc.fr/today/home

5. UK Health Security Agency, Newborn bloodspot screening: Programme overview, 2018. Available at: www.gov.uk/guidance/newborn-blood-spot-screening-programme-overview

6. Office for National Statistics, Drug use, alcohol and smoking: Smoking, drinking and drug taking in Great Britain and associated deaths and illnesses, 2020. Available at: www.ons.gov .uk/peoplepopulationandcommunity/healthandsocialcare/drugusealcoholandsmoking

7. C. von Wagner, A. Good, D. Wright *et al.*, Inequalities in colorectal cancer screening participation in the first round of the national screening programme in England, *British Journal of Cancer* **101**(Suppl. 2), 2009, S60–S63.

8. A. Chapple, S. Ziebland, P. Hewitson and A. McPherson, What affects the uptake of screening for bowel cancer using a faecal occult blood test (FOBt): A qualitative study, *Social Science & Medicine* **66**(12), 2008, 2425–35.

9. C. Campbell, A. Douglas, L. Williams *et al.*, Are there ethnic and religious variations in uptake of bowel cancer screening? A retrospective cohort study among 1.7 million people in Scotland, *British Medical Journal Open* **10**(10), 2020, 1–11.

10. A. Szczepura, C. Price and A. Gumber, Breast and bowel cancer screening uptake patterns over 15 years for UK south Asian ethnic minority populations, corrected for differences in socio-demographic characteristics, *BMC Public Health* **8**(1), 2008, 1–15.

11. H. A. Ashton, M. J. Buxton, N. E. Day *et al.*, The Multicentre Aneurysm Screening Study (MASS) into the effect of abdominal aortic aneurysm screening on mortality in men: A randomised controlled trial, *The Lancet* **360**(9345), 2002, 1531–9.

12. L. Meecham, J. Jacomelli, M. Davis *et al.*, Outcomes in men from the NHS abdominal aortic aneurysm screening programme with a large aneurysm referred for intervention, *European Journal of Vascular and Endovascular Surgery* **61**(2), 2021, 192–9.

13. World Health Orgnization, WHO position paper on mammography screening, Geneva, WHO, 2014.

14. R. Mandal and P. Basu, Cancer screening and early diagnosis in low and middle income countries: Current situation and future perspectives, *Bundesgesundheitsblatt Gesundheitsforschung Gesundheitsschutz* **61**(12), 2018, 1505–12.

15. Cancer Research UK, Overdiagnosis: when finding cancer can do more harm than good, 2018. Available at: https://news.cancerresearchuk.org/2018/03/06/overdiagnosis-when-finding-cancer-can-do-more-harm-than-good/

16. UK Health Security Agency, Breast screening: Helping women decide, 2013. Available at: www.gov.uk/government/publications/breast-screening-helping-women-decide

17. A. G. K. Edwards, G. Naik, H. Ahmed *et al.*, Personalised risk communication for informed decision making about taking screening tests, Cochrane Database of Systematic Reviews, 2013.

18. UK National Screening Committee. Available at: www.gov.uk/government/organisations/ uk-national-screening-committee

10

Health Protection and Communicable Disease Control

Beverley Griggs and Padmanabhan Badrinath

Key points

- The term 'health protection' covers threats to health (e.g. infectious diseases), environmental hazards (e.g. chemical releases) and radiological threats, natural hazards and terrorism.
- Health protection actions depend on the nature of the infecting organism (pathogen) or hazard, the transmission route and the response of the host to the hazard. Individuals can help to protect themselves by being aware of the nature of different risks, the methods by which individuals are exposed and any personal susceptibility.
- Vaccines are an effective way to protect whole populations against the serious health outcomes associated with some infectious diseases.
- Surveillance of infectious diseases is important to identify outbreaks, monitor levels of disease, plan control measures, monitor outcomes of control programmes and enable efficient targeting of resources.
- The public health effects of communicable disease are controlled through actions that affect hosts for the disease, transmission, susceptibility of the population, disease identification and disease treatment.
- Environmental health involves the reduction, investigation and control of potential health hazards, which arise from an environmental or man-made origin.
- Emergency planning and response is increasingly important as a mechanism to plan for and control the health effects of large-scale disasters and emergencies, including natural hazards and terrorist attacks.

10.1 Introduction

Health protection refers to threats to health such as infectious diseases, environmental threats, natural hazards and threats from terrorist acts. Health protection may also overlap with action tackling the determinants of health, especially legislative aspects such as workplace smoking bans or speed restrictions and even lifestyle choices and the health issues of ageing populations, such as increasing levels of chronic disease (which we now know may also be due to infections).

This chapter will outline the public health aspects of communicable disease control and touch on some of the other areas now included within health protection in the UK. Important health protection terms are included in the glossary.

10.2 Patterns of Communicable Disease

Based on the demographic transition, it was widely believed until recently that infectious diseases, especially childhood diseases, were a historic problem in developed countries. As a country develops, the burden of disease shifts from a primarily infectious one (such as diarrhoea and pneumonia) to non-communicable, such as long-term conditions and cancer. The eradication of smallpox, and the development of public health and medical interventions such as safe water supplies and vaccines appeared to signal their continuing decline. However, the WHO Global Burden of Disease project (2019) portrays a different picture. Globally, 23% of years of life lost are due to communicable diseases, but in low-income countries the figure is 45% compared to 4% in high-income countries. In sub-Saharan Africa, this years-of-life-lost burden is greater than that for non-communicable diseases and injuries combined [1]. While interventions to moderate the burden of infectious diseases have been shown to be cost-effective (e.g. a measles vaccination costs less than $1 per vaccination and less than $25 per quality-adjusted life year gained [2]), the resurgence of diseases once thought to be coming under control, such as tuberculosis (TB), illustrates an on-going failure to tackle basic causes as well as the natural ingenuity of causative micro-organisms. The lack of political and pharmaco-industrial will to develop low-cost remedies for 'unprofitable' diseases like leishmaniasis and TB also remains an obstacle.

New challenges continue to arise. Diseases once confined to certain parts of the globe now spread to other continents due to mass population movement and faster transportation systems. The COVID-19 pandemic, detection of polio virus in sewage systems in London and the USA, and outbreaks of Monkeypox in Western Europe are some examples of this phenomenon. The impact of COVID-19 in terms of morbidity, mortality, economic and social cost has been considerable and risk factors for death and chronic ill health in the form of 'long COVID' have graphically underlined the continued importance of health inequalities and poverty as determinants of ill health [3].

Health-care-associated infections (HCAI) are of increasing importance to health. *Clostridium difficile* is a major cause of nosocomial diarrhoea, having been recognised in the 1970s and identified as the causal organism in 1978 [4]. Different patterns of drug resistance continue to emerge and are linked in part to increasing use of antimicrobial or parasitic agents in medicine and animal husbandry; examples include carbapenem-resistant *Enterobacteriaceae*, extensively drug-resistant *Mycobacterium tuberculosis*, methicillin- or vancomycin-resistant *Staphylococcus aureus* (MRSA) and *Salmonella* species. Estimates of the global burden of bacterial antimicrobial resistance (AMR) suggest that this health problem is as significant as HIV or malaria (and possibly greater) [5]. Finally, more exotic threats to human health, such as variant Creutzfeldt-Jakob's Disease, avian and swine influenza, Ebola, Zika virus, SARS CoV-2, Monkeypox and a human case of *Brucella canis* in the UK, have further fuelled media interest in communicable disease.

To address the continued challenges associated with antimicrobial resistance, zoonotic infections and food security, there is an increasing focus being placed on implementing a 'One Health' approach. One Health advocates for a multi-sectoral response to developing policies and programmes which optimises the balance between the environment and animal and human health [6] (see also Chapter 17).

10.3 Controlling Communicable Diseases

In many ways, the public health challenges associated with infectious diseases are similar to those associated with other diseases:
- identify the burden of disease (identify the threat and quantify the risk);
- consider how to prevent or treat it; and
- take appropriate action (implement immediate and long-term, effective control measures to mitigate the risk).

However, there are some elements of dealing with infectious agents which set this field apart. Interactions between the cause (agent), host and environment are also important. For example, *Mycobacterium tuberculosis* is the direct cause of tuberculosis, but crowded housing and poor nutrition also increase the risk of infection. Causes of communicable disease have the ability to replicate. These agents are transmissible and can alter and evolve, as can the host's response to them. This host response is something we can use as a target for control when we utilise vaccines. Also, in contrast to much of public health, timescales in communicable disease control can be relatively short and there may be little time to initiate effective control measures. Thus, we often need to balance enforcement of control measures and education. The sporadic nature of outbreaks raises the importance of surveillance systems to spot problems early. Surveillance now also extends to monitoring sewage, which although initially intended for estimating antimicrobial resistance has proven to be very successful in supporting the public health management of the COVID-19 pandemic and in detecting once-eradicated pathogens such as the polio virus.

10.4 Controlling Transmission of Infectious Agents

Infection can be defined as the entry and multiplication of an infectious agent in the body of humans or animals. Control of infection relies on determining opportunities to interrupt transmission from reservoir to host. The organism causing the infection is termed an agent or pathogen and may be a protozoan (e.g. *Cryptosporidiosis*), a virus (e.g. polio, influenza), a bacterium (e.g. *Escherichia coli*) or a larger organism (e.g. worms, mites) – some of which may be vectors rather than the disease organism (a vector being any agent which transmits an infectious agent, e.g. mosquitoes transmitting malaria).

The means by which agents are transmitted from reservoir to host varies and determines what control methods are appropriate. In general, transmission is direct (e.g. touching or biting), indirect (e.g. via food or water) or airborne (e.g. via droplets carried in a sneeze).

So preventing transmission is easy in theory and there are a number of clear ways to do this, including:

- removing the agent (e.g. kill headlice, treat infections);
- controlling the reservoir (e.g. animal control of rabies, disinfection of potentially infected fomites);
- physically preventing transmission from the reservoir (e.g. barrier contraception);
- isolating or quarantining the infected host (e.g. in hospital-acquired infections); and
- preventing infection in a new host (e.g. vaccination).

Box 10.1 shows how individual control might work.

Box 10.1 Individual control of infections

Chlamydial infection

Chlamydia trachomatis causes one of the most common sexually transmitted infections in Europe, with the highest rates being seen in sexually active young people between 15 and 24 years of age [7]. Symptoms may be those of genital tract inflammation, but the majority of cases are asymptomatic. Untreated, chlamydial infection can lead to pelvic inflammatory disease, sub-fertility and poor reproductive outcomes in women. Individual control simply involves safe-sex practice and testing to enable cure before long-term effects are felt. Chlamydia screening appears to be relatively straightforward – it involves a simple and pain-free urine test, and treatment for those infected is a course of antibiotics. However, as a public health programme, *Chlamydia* screening is hard to implement across a young population who may not perceive infection as a risk.

Apply this framework to COVID-19 and consider the rationale for actions that were taken to reduce transmission during the pandemic.

However, difficulties arise when preventing transmission. One of these is where reservoirs of infection exist in animals (e.g. rabies, *Salmonella*) or the environment (e.g. *Cryptosporidium* and *Legionella*). Smallpox provided the World Health Organization's (WHO) greatest triumph, partly because humans are the only reservoir and an effective vaccine was available. Control is problematic where it depends on changing behaviours (e.g. controlling sexually transmitted infection relies on individual and cultural attitudes to behaviours such as condom use).

Organisms which have become resistant to some antimicrobial drugs are now being found in patients in both hospital and community settings. Organisms include *Enterobacteriaceae, Neisseria gonorrhoea, Staphylococcus aureus, Mycobacterium tuberculosis, Clostridium difficile* and certain strains of *E. coli*. While some organisms are naturally more resistant to antimicrobials (such as *M. tuberculosis*, which has thick cell walls), resistance can also occur through changes in an organism's genes or be introduced by transmission of resistance genes from other organisms. It is still possible to treat most drug-resistant infections, but the treatment options become limited and it is better to prevent the development of resistance. Resistance is particularly problematic in the care of hospital inpatients who are especially susceptible to infections. In general, solutions to the reduction of health-care-acquired infection (HCAI), including those due to drug-resistant organisms, are multifactorial and include: surveillance, clear infection control standards, maintaining clean hospital environments, strict antibiotic prescribing practices and isolation of infected patients. Again, control of resistance and use of antibiotics is challenging where it depends on attitudes and behaviours – for example, the perception of the population on whether they need antibiotics for certain infections, or whether they complete a full course of prescribed antibiotics.

What factors might you consider to reduce the transmission of *Clostridium difficile* in a ward setting?

Systems have to be in place to ensure that the control measures which prevent individuals transmitting or contracting infections are applied across large numbers of people. This type of control aims to reduce morbidity and mortality from these diseases in populations. While it would be ideal from a human point of view to *eradicate* infectious diseases (as we have with smallpox), pragmatism dictates that our control objectives cannot always be so ambitious. In some cases, we aim to *eliminate* infection from large geographical regions by preventing transmission, but accept that the organism still persists in our environment. We have achieved this to a large extent with *Salmonella enteritidis* in eggs through the vaccination of chicken flocks to eliminate the organism (British eggs from *Salmonella*-free flocks carry a 'Lion' mark and the US Food and Drug Administration have an Egg Safety Rule requiring producers to comply with control measures), and pasteurisation to eliminate milk as a vehicle for transmitting *M. tuberculosis* and *E. coli* O157. Lastly, we may accept that a disease cannot be eliminated or eradicated, but aim to *contain* it so that it does not present a significant public health problem. Winter outbreaks of influenza and more recently SARS CoV-2 are examples of where a disease is contained to minimise its impact on the population.

10.5 Protecting Populations through Vaccination

The term 'vaccination' derives from the historical origins of the process for inoculation with vaccinia virus against smallpox (first described by Edward Jenner in 1798). While immunisation is, strictly speaking, the protection (making immune) of an individual by the administration of a vaccine, the terms 'immunisation' and 'vaccination' tend now to be used synonymously by many people.

Vaccination is used to make large proportions of populations actively immune to bacterial or viral diseases such that the host is able to generate an active antibody immune response to combat an infectious agent. The agent administered (usually by injection) can be living but modified (e.g. yellow fever), a suspension of killed organisms (e.g. whooping cough (pertussis)) or an inactivated toxin (such as tetanus). The aim is to generate an immune response in those vaccinated, which will protect them from serious disease should they later be challenged with that organism. Killed organisms provide a limited immunity and may have to be given as a starter dose with boosters to provide optimal protection. Vaccines can also be given in pulses (repeated doses over time) to maximise immunity. Live, attenuated vaccines such as the oral polio vaccine provide better cover. These tend to be for viral infections. Sometimes a temporary, passive immunity can be generated with antibodies – for example, immunoglobulins against varicella are given to pregnant women who may have come into contact with chicken pox. In this case, the body does not produce its own antibodies, but depends on pre-produced antibodies.

Recent advances in messenger RNA (mRNA) technology have led to the development of vaccines which do not use live or attenuated virus, but instead enable our bodies to develop proteins which trigger the immune response when exposed to the infectious agent in question. The advantage of mRNA vaccines is that they can be created and produced more easily than our traditional live or attenuated vaccines, as seen with the rapid development and mass production of mRNA vaccines during the COVID-19 pandemic. This led to the swift production and approval of a bivalent vaccination for SARS CoV-2 which incorporated both the wild Wuhan and Omicron variants of the virus [8].

Immunisation may be general or targeted. General vaccination aims to eradicate, eliminate or contain infection similarly to other control methods. For example, mass measles vaccination resulted in a 78% drop in measles deaths between 2000 and 2008 worldwide. However, targeted vaccine programmes can sometimes be more

Box 10.2 Targeted vaccination – smallpox

When the incidence of smallpox was high, the dangers of vaccination (the vaccine causes death in approximately one in a million people) were vastly outweighed by the protection and reduction in mortality provided by the vaccine. As the occurrence of the disease declined, mass vaccination was not warranted, but when an outbreak occurred, all susceptible individuals in the defined area around the outbreak were vaccinated to contain the spread of disease (termed 'ring vaccination') [9]. The smallpox vaccine has also been used in controlling Monkeypox outbreaks through the targeted pre-exposure vaccination of at-risk groups (including health-care workers) and the post-exposure vaccination of close contacts.

effective than mass vaccination. Box 10.2 shows smallpox as an example. Influenza is another example of vaccination that is targeted at those most at risk and aims to contain infection.

No vaccine is 100% effective, as individuals mount different immune responses, which last varying amounts of time. However, it is not necessary for every person to be immune. *Herd immunity* is the degree to which a population is resistant to an infection as high general levels of immunity protect the non-immune. Herd immunity is an important concept in health protection and can be thought of as the immunity of a community. The basic reproductive rate (R_0) is the mean number of new cases generated by each case of a disease and can be imagined as the potential for growth of a disease epidemic. If $R_0 > 1$, a disease will continue to spread unless control measures are initiated. The R_0 of measles is 12–18, for example. However, if there is adequate herd immunity (i.e. enough people have been vaccinated and had a good response), the reproductive rate becomes less than one and the incidence of cases falls. This is why the coverage rate for vaccinations is considered important. If fewer people are vaccinated, the herd immunity drops and outbreaks of a disease occur. The proportion of a population which needs to be vaccinated to prevent sustained spread is given by $1 - 1/R_0$. Using measles as an example, the proportion of the population which needs to be vaccinated to provide herd immunity can be calculated as $1 - 1/18$ or 96%.

How might you explain, in lay terms, the term R_0 and what it means for controlling the spread of disease?

This is occurring in the UK with measles. Although the WHO recommended coverage above 95% [10], in the UK, coverage falls below 90%. Low uptake and incomplete coverage of vaccination in earlier years (partly due to low vaccine stocks and partly due to public apprehension around the MMR vaccine fuelled by negative media coverage) have resulted in an upswing in the number of measles outbreaks occurring in the UK.

How might you approach a conversation with an individual or family who are hesitant to receive a routine vaccination?

The population need for a vaccine is determined by consideration of the characteristics of the disease. Vaccines are then developed through clinical trials in much the same way as new drugs are. For example, a vaccine for *meningococcal group C* was introduced to the UK in 1999 because meningococcal disease, while quite rare (815 cases reported in England and Wales in 1998), is so devastating that a vaccine programme was considered cost-effective. The incidence has now fallen significantly to five cases in 2020/2021.

The aims of vaccination programmes vary depending on the disease and whether the control intended is harm reduction, eradication, elimination or containment. In general, vaccine coverage in the more-developed regions is higher. This means that more booster vaccinations may be given in less-developed countries in attempts to improve coverage. Not all infectious diseases have effective vaccines (e.g. Dengue fever) and not all countries need programmes for all the vaccines available. For example, BCG vaccination is currently given routinely in many countries where there is a high incidence of infection. However, in the UK (and some other countries), vaccination is targeted to those babies born in areas with a high incidence of infection (generally > 40 cases per 100,000 population), or those with a parent or grandparent from a high-incidence country. Thus, knowing the burden of diseases in various populations determines the vaccine policy developed. Hence, vaccination schedules differ by country depending on the local epidemiology of vaccine-preventable diseases (see Box 10.3).

Ensuring adequate vaccines for targeted diseases is a major industry and public health can provide useful advice to those developing and manufacturing vaccines through support for clinical vaccine trials, as well as supporting the delivery of vaccines to target audiences – for example, by managing the maintenance of a 'cold chain' (keeping the vaccine in a cold environment from production to administration) where necessary. This can be particularly problematic in developing countries. Public and professional attitudes to vaccination, as well as the complexity of decision-making when individual risk and community benefit are involved, mean

---

Box 10.3 Four features of a good immunisation schedule

1. epidemiological relevance;
2. immunological effectiveness;
3. operational feasibility; and
4. social acceptability.

that public health workers also have a role in educating the public and professionals about vaccination. At a national level, the management of programmes also includes vaccine funding and surveillance to monitor vaccination uptake and targets.

10.6 Identifying Threats, Planning and Monitoring Control Measures – Surveillance

The practice of surveillance – monitoring diseases through measuring morbidity and mortality – arose in the fourteenth and fifteenth centuries with the plague, or 'Black Death'. In this case, authorities wanted to be aware of ships with infected people aboard in order to prevent them coming ashore and infecting others. Surveillance can be defined as the on-going, systematic collection, collation and analysis of data and the prompt dissemination of the resulting information to those who need to know so that action can be taken.

Surveillance is used to identify individual cases of disease so that action can be taken to prevent spread (e.g. excluding food handlers from work if they contract food poisoning). This can also be used over time to detect changes in trend or distribution in order to initiate investigative or control measures. A microbiology laboratory, for example, might notice several cases of legionella infection and trigger an investigation into the possible source in order to prevent further cases. Trends in infection which are continuously monitored through surveillance systems can indicate changes in risk factors or that certain elements of a population are at increased risk (e.g. a rise in sexually transmitted infections in young women). This allows interventions to be targeted appropriately. Knowing the epidemiology of infectious diseases in close to real time through surveillance can help to evaluate current control measures such as vaccination programmes. A fall in incidence may allow control measures to be relaxed. For example, it is no longer necessary to vaccinate against smallpox. Lastly, and very importantly, surveillance allows new infections to be detected and hypotheses produced regarding their causes. Many countries have communicable disease surveillance programmes which carry out these functions.

Conversely, what are the challenges to an effective and comprehensive surveillance system?

Surveillance is, however, resource-intensive and it is important to make it as simple as possible to get the maximum amount of data reported (see Box 10.4). Reports generally come from individuals dealing with the diseases in question – clinicians and public health professionals or from information on laboratory diagnoses. The type and importance of the disease determines the type of surveillance. In some cases, reporting is mandatory; 'notifiable diseases' in the UK and the USA must be reported by doctors. It may, however, be preferable for surveillance to be voluntary and anonymous. Such is the case for HIV in the UK, which is monitored in

> ### Box 10.4 What makes a good surveillance system?
>
> **Clear objectives**. The system can then be evaluated to ensure that it is relevant to the needs of the population covered.
>
> **Clear case definitions**. Clear definitions are needed for the conditions under surveillance so that the same thing is counted accurately all the time. Data need to flow from clear sources to a clear collection point.
>
> **Easy reporting mechanisms**. These will maximise the number of cases reported and useful, timely feedback to reporters encourages participation and enables action.

annual surveys and where it is not possible to identify an individual patient from the data collected. In some infections, as with the HIV surveillance, it is not practical to collect details of every case. Representative samples can be taken and the true rates of disease extrapolated from them.

Surveillance of sewage systems both routinely and at large public events can also assist in monitoring the prevalence of infectious diseases. Use of whole genome sequencing in infectious disease surveillance has enhanced the ability to understand transmission dynamics and facilitates the monitoring of pathogens by genotype. This can have an important role in identifying clusters and outbreaks of infectious diseases and in using signals to support early investigation.

10.7 Containing Infection

10.7.1 Public Health Control Measures

Public health control measures have been used for many years to help break the chain of transmission for infectious diseases. Such measures are often implemented at the individual level or in defined areas to prevent secondary cases of infection or to contain clusters and minimise outbreaks.

The type of measures used may vary depending on the disease in question and the route of transmission, but may include isolation of cases, tracing, quarantining or testing of close contacts, administration of prophylaxis or vaccination for susceptible contacts, and the provision of hygiene and symptom advice to cases, contacts and affected settings. Much of this activity is undertaken by public health professionals and colleagues working in environmental health.

10.7.2 Containing Infection – Outbreak Investigation

When preventive measures fail (or when control was only ever going to contain the disease, not eradicate or eliminate infection), then control measures must be used retrospectively to contain the infection to as few people as possible. The management of an outbreak of a food-borne illness is a good example of how outbreaks are investigated and control measures implemented, although the methods used can be applied to any infectious disease.

How such an investigation might progress is described here and it highlights the stages and important points of such an investigation. In reality, the stages will not always occur in order. See Figure 10.1 and the example outbreak timeline in Box 10.5.

The COVID-19 pandemic saw the global escalation of public health control measures on an unprecedented scale. The response to the pandemic resulted in both individual controls (isolation, quarantine, etc.) and more widespread population-level measures, including travel restrictions, national lockdowns and mass vaccination programmes. Contact tracing and testing were scaled up in many countries to such an extent that rapid developments in technology and infrastructure were needed to support their implementation.

Behavioural science also contributed significantly to individual and population-level measures, such as social distancing, personal hygiene messaging, mask wearing and immunisation. It also played a role in tackling the vaccine hesitancy which emerged during the pandemic, in part in response to the attempt of many governments to introduce a vaccine mandate (a compulsory requirement for vaccination imposed on certain professional groups). Such attempts have not been uniformly successful and have therefore been abandoned by some countries.

Understanding the differential uptake of vaccination by different groups based on culture and beliefs is key for those working in behavioural science to help address vaccine hesitancy and improve uptake. This is of particular importance for infections such as COVID-19 which do not affect all sections of society equally, with those living in more deprived areas more likely to suffer from its impact and aftermath.

10.8 Environmental Public Health

Environmental hazards to health include chemicals released into the air, contaminated water sources or industrial accidents. The medical model of control applied to communicable disease control serves less well in these circumstances. Here, the environmental model (also called the pollutant linkage model and source-pathway-receptor model) is used. Methods to control the hazard are determined by identifying the source, the pathway and the receptor (Table 10.1).

The receptor need not be human – it may be animal or vegetable. Pathways can be air, water or ground. An example might be the release of a toxic chemical into the environment due to a road accident and a tanker spillage. The crashed tanker is the source. Pathways for this hazardous chemical to become a problem may be through the air if it is a fine powder or volatile liquid, through the ground if it leaks onto a

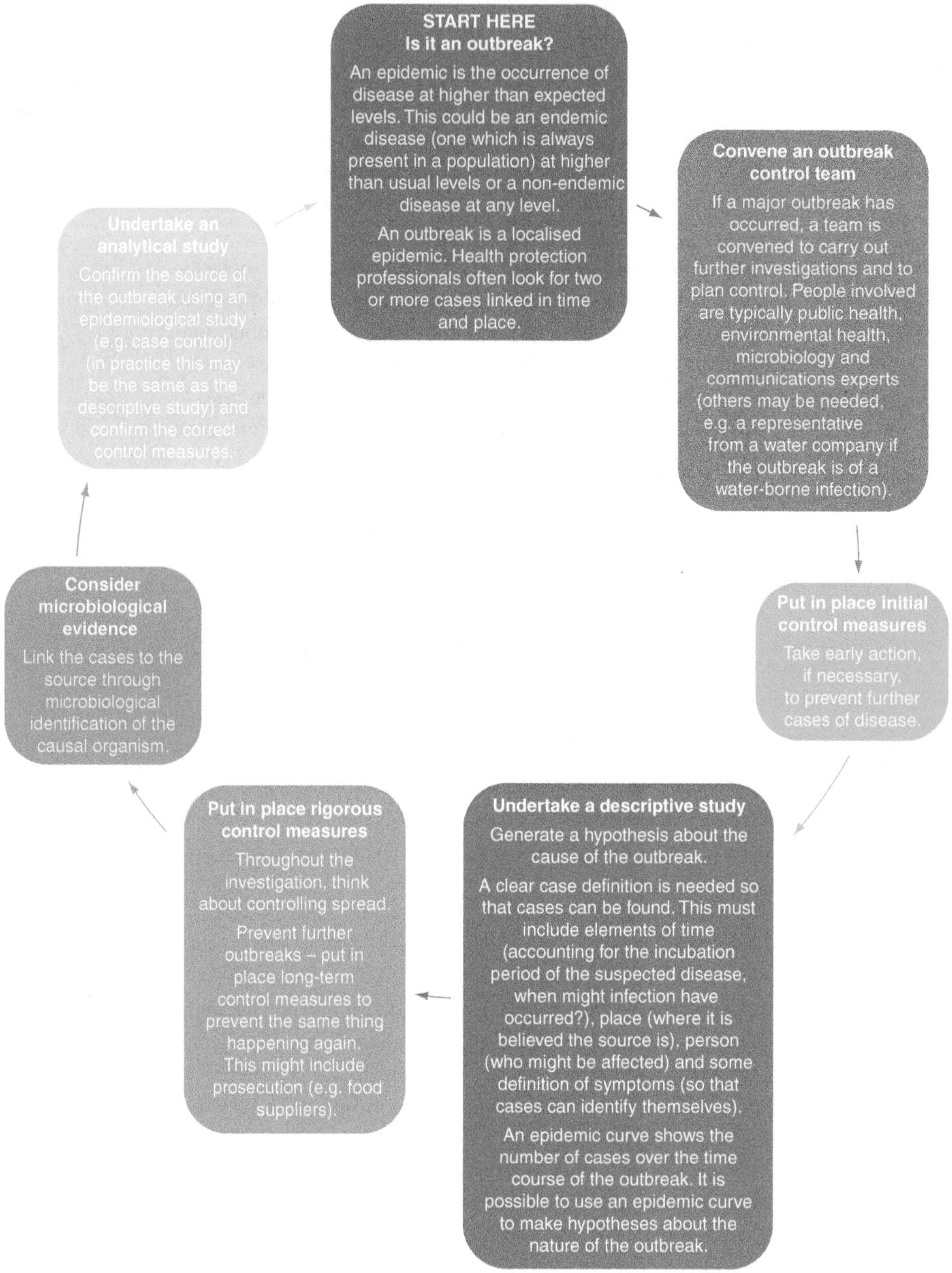

Figure 10.1 Outbreak investigation stages.

Box 10.5 Example outbreak timeline for a restaurant food poisoning episode

Sunday 2nd August – 17 people eat at the Golden Lion restaurant.

Tuesday 4th August to Thursday 6th August – several people report severe vomiting and diarrhoea.

Thursday 6th August – health protection specialists become aware, require the restaurant to close temporarily and form an outbreak control team to investigate. Environmental health and microbiology experts are included in the team.

Thursday 6th August – all current cases report having eaten at the same restaurant, so food remains from the relevant meal are taken for laboratory testing, stool samples are collected from those with diarrhoea.

Thursday 6th – local primary care clinicians are asked to identify any further cases and an epidemic curve is created over the next few days. This further suggests the single Sunday meal is the likely cause with the absence of further peaks suggesting no onward person-to-person transmission.

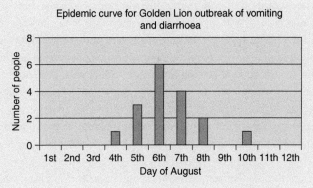

Saturday 8th August – the casual organism is identified as *E. coli* 0157, having been found in food remains and stool samples. All those who come into contact with a known case are investigated and advised as to control measures. In particular, food handlers, those caring for vulnerable people and those with poor personal hygiene are excluded from work or school until it is clear they are no longer carrying the organism.

Monday 9th – the restaurant staff have been re-trained, the premises fully cleaned and the restaurant is able to re-open.

porous surface such as fields, or through water if it enters a water course. From here, it may reach a variety of receptors – plant life through soil or water, and then animal life directly or via eating the plants. Animal life may also be affected directly from exposure to airborne matter. This model provides a methodology

Table 10.1 Examples of sources, pathways and receptors for some environmental hazards

Source	Pathway	Receptor
Chemical spillage from tanker crash	Air	Grazing cattle
	Ground	Humans
	Rivers	Allotment vegetables
Oil dump into the ocean	Ocean water	Wild fowl
		Fish
Factory fire, ash and smoke	Air	Humans
		Wild life
		Crops

for considering where the path from source to receptor can be interrupted or contamination prevented.

So we can think about containing an environmental hazard in a similar way to containing the hazards from communicable diseases – consider how the hazard transmits its effects to us and find ways to interrupt this. Some hazards such as air pollution cause a broad spectrum of harm to health and the environment and are challenging to address as they have multiple sources, both natural and manmade. However, the contribution of air pollution and other environmental hazards to climate change is recognised as a major threat, and is further described in Chapter 17.

In addition to this, there are many other complex areas of environmental health that a public health practitioner might be called on to contribute to, as described in Table 10.2.

It is important to note that some environmental hazards result from occupational sources and the effects of these and their modification are often dealt with by specialist occupational health practitioners. Some important areas of occupational health, in a range of countries including the UK, Australia and the USA, include the protection of the workforce from infectious diseases (e.g. hepatitis C in health-care workers), occupational cancers and mental disorders (e.g. work-related stress), physical injuries (e.g. related to poor workstation posture, physical trips and falls and lifting injuries) and chemical injuries (such as asbestosis and chemical burns).

In each case, the tools needed are those already highlighted in previous chapters, the effective use of epidemiological methods and risk assessment.

What public health action would be required to address any of the hazards in Table 10.2? What might you wish to consider?

Table 10.2 Environmental hazards

	Source	Pathway	Potential health effects
1	Nuclear waste spillage	Water, ground or air	Radiation poisoning
2	Gastro-intestinal disease organisms in flood water	Water, food	Intestinal infection/food poisoning
3	Radiation from radio masts	Air	Increase in leukaemia incidence
4	Earthquake	Ground	Physical injury from falling buildings
5	Volcanic ash	Air	Respiratory effects
6	Loud neighbours or new airport runway	Air	Psychological distress
7	Poor workstation posture	N/A	Repetitive strain injury
8	Terrorist chemical attack	Air or water	Toxic effects dependent on chemical used
9	Poor building design	N/A	Low physical activity levels and adverse health effects
10	Second-hand smoke in public places	Air	Increased lung cancer, coronary heart disease
11	Exposure to radon in the home	Air	Lung cancer

10.9 Preparing for Emergencies

Another specialist area within the field of health protection is disaster or emergency planning and response. There are a variety of interpretations of the words 'disaster' and 'emergency'. The UK Civil Contingencies Act of 2004 states that an emergency is an event or situation which threatens serious damage to human welfare; an event or situation which threatens serious damage to the environment; or war, or terrorism, which threatens serious damage to security. The UN Office for Disaster Risk Reduction (UNDRR) states that a disaster is 'a serious disruption of the functioning of a community or a society at any scale due to hazardous events interacting with conditions of exposure, vulnerability and capacity, leading to one or more of the following: human, material, economic and environmental losses and impacts' [11]. The UNDRR supports the implementation of the Sendai Framework for Disaster Risk Reduction 2015–2030, which lays out seven global targets to be achieved. This framework supports the other 2030 frameworks, including the Sustainable Development Goals and the Paris Agreement on Climate Change.

Responses to disasters and major incidents vary across nations. For example, since 2014, emergency services in the UK have worked under a framework known as the Joint Emergency Services Interoperability Principles (JESIP) [12], which seeks to ensure that response services work together coherently as a matter of routine.

Figure 10.2 shows the cycle of action which surrounds the planning for and response to disasters.

Beginning with preparedness, quantifying the scale of the risk to populations (Box 10.6) is important in prioritising planning and is dependent on the nature of the hazard and the vulnerability of communities.

Figure 10.2 Disaster cycle.

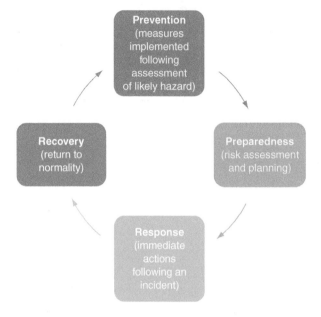

Box 10.6 Quantifying risk [13]

- Risk (probability of harmful consequences)
- Hazard (phenomenon which has the potential to cause harm)
- Vulnerability (capacity of a community to cope)

Risk = Hazard × Vulnerability

Sometimes the scale of the hazard is expressed as 'hazard × exposure' and the vulnerability of a community may be assessed as the balance between its various vulnerabilities and its capacities. An additional factor may be added: deficiencies in preparedness, which becomes a multiplier in the equation.

Three main types of emergency are planned for: those which creep up on us like a rising tide, those that hit with a 'big bang' and those which emerge completely out of the blue. In many countries, this planning process is highly organised within the top tier of national government such as the Cabinet Office in the UK, the Department of Homeland Security in the USA and the National Disaster Management Authority in India.

In the process of planning for disasters, the role of the health sector is to identify threats and deal with mass casualties and deaths, as well as, potentially, mass vaccination. With partners in local government, the emergency services and those in the armed forces, health-care organisations form the front line in responding to a wide range of incidents and have the primary responsibility for protecting health and maintaining health-care services during the emergency and restoring health afterwards. All agencies must also plan to maintain business continuity during times of disaster when the workforce may be significantly depleted due to illness, death or absenteeism. Box 10.7 illustrates how the health sector plans for a flu pandemic – a disaster for planning purposes as it could kill large numbers of people. In the 2009

Box 10.7 Disaster planning for a flu pandemic

We can use the disaster cycle to illustrate elements of how public health workers plan for and respond to an emergency such as a flu pandemic.

Prevention

Minimisation of opportunities for a highly pathogenic strain of animal influenza to acquire the ability to transmit to humans (e.g. slaughter or vaccination of bird flocks to prevent H5N1 transmission to humans).

Preparedness

Business continuity planning to deal with illness and absenteeism in the health-care sector:

- stockpiling of antiviral drugs and plans for distributing them;
- media awareness campaigns;
- worldwide surveillance of circulating virus strains.

Response

Rapid, coordinated development of case definitions and diagnostic tools:

- rapid development of treatment guidelines, vaccines, etc.;
- identification of at-risk staff and implementation of increased safety measures;
- isolation and treatment of cases;
- development of supply chains for antiviral drugs and vaccines;
- staff sharing to enable learning and cover of necessary functions;
- development of alternative access for maintaining urgent and intensive care when some centres may be closed due to mass infection;
- management *en masse* of infected casualties.

Recovery

Additional services to manage increased waiting lists due to cancelled procedures:

- cover arrangements for any staff who have worked overtime;
- provision of counselling for staff.

H1N1 pandemic, fewer infections and deaths were experienced than were planned for, but many of the measures planned for were instigated during the pandemic wave to reduce the anticipated impact.

 Which partners and local agencies would be involved in this type of disaster planning? Investigate your own local response teams and protocols.

10.6 Conclusions

The field of health protection encompasses the disciplines and services which respond to threats to human health. The profile of health protection has significantly increased in recent years due to emerging infections such as Ebola, Zika virus, COVID-19, Monkeypox and most recently Langya virus. In the UK, health protection is seen as one of three public health pillars alongside health improvement and health-care quality, but in reality the three domains are inseparable and always overlapping. The tools covered in other chapters in this section must be applied to the domain of health protection and the skills specific to health protection are applicable in other domains of public health.

REFERENCES

1. Global Burden of Disease Collaborative Network, Global Burden of Disease Study 2019 (GBD 2019) Demographics 1950–2019, Seattle, WA, Institute for Health Metrics and Evaluation (IHME), 2020.
2. D. S. Shepard., J. A. Walsh, E. Kleinau *et al.*, Setting priorities for the Children's Vaccine Initiative: A cost-effectiveness approach, *Vaccine* **13**(8), 1995, 707–14.
3. L. Schnitzler, L. Janssen, S. Evers *et al.*, The broader societal impacts of COVID-19 and the growing importance of capturing these in health economic analyses, *International Journal of Technology Assessment in Health Care* **37**(1), 2021, e43.
4. J. G. Bartlett, N. Moon, T. W. Chang *et al.*, Role of *Clostridium difficile* in antibiotic-associated pseudomembranous colitis, *Gastroenterology* **75**(5), 1978, 778–82.
5. Antimicrobial Resistance Collaborators, Global burden of bacterial antimicrobial resistance in 2019: A systematic analysis, *The Lancet* **399**(10325), 2022, 629–55.
6. World Health Organization, Food and Agriculture Organization of the United Nations and World Organisation for Animal Health, Taking a multisectoral, one health approach: A tripartite guide to addressing zoonotic diseases in countries, 2019.
7. European Centre for Disease Control, Chlamydia infection: Annual Epidemiological Report for 2019, Surveillance Report, 2020. Available at: www.ecdc.europa.eu/sites/default/files/documents/chlamydia-annual-epidemiological-report-2019.pdf
8. REG 174 Information for UK healthcare professionals. Available at: https://assets.publishing.service.gov.uk/government/uploads/system/uploads/attachment_data/file/1098074/Spikevax_bivalent_Original_Omicron_Information_for_Healthcare_Professionals__Regulation_174_.pdf

9. D. T. Karzon, Smallpox vaccination: The end of an era, *Acta Medica Scandinavica* **197** (S576), 1975, 29–38.

10. UN General Assembly, Transforming our world: The 2030 Agenda for Sustainable Development, 21 October 2015, A/RES/70/1. Available at: https://sustainabledevelopment .un.org/post2015/transformingourworld/publication

11. World Health Organization, Risk reduction and emergency preparedness: WHO six year strategy for the health-sector and community capacity development, Geneva, WHO, 2007, p. 8. Available at: https://apps.who.int/iris/handle/10665/43736

12. Joint Emergency Service Interoperability Programme. Available at: www.jesip.org.uk

13. UN Office for Disaster Risk Reduction, Disaster. Available at: www.undrr.org/terminology/ disaster

Contexts for Public Health Practice

Introduction to Part 2: What Do We Mean by Contexts in Public Health?

Jan Yates, Kirsteen Watson and Stephen Gillam

As we discussed with regard to leadership (see Chapter 7), the context in which public health tools are used has a bearing on the choice of tool and how it is implemented. In the second part of *Essential Public Health: Theory and Practice*, we will consider a range of contemporary contexts in which public health is practised and illustrate how the tools we have described are applied.

Firstly, the individual context. Throughout Part 1 of this book, we have provided examples of where the public health tools we describe have been used. However, you the reader may be left wondering, 'How would I use that skill?' and 'How is that relevant to my job?'

All the editors have had long careers as Consultants in Public Health within the NHS. Our jobs have required us to use all the public health tools at our disposal in the fulfilment of our duties. We use epidemiological tools and demographic information to understand and describe the populations for which we are responsible. We lead teams and multi-agency networks to prioritise and drive changes in health and health improvement policy and practice. We develop strategies to encourage behaviour change in patients, the public and professionals. We focus on and evaluate the quality of screening programmes, their evidence base, equity of provision and safety. We have been part of health protection on-call systems, which respond to incidents and emergencies out of hours that have a potential population health impact. All the tools in Part 1 are part of our daily routines and essential to the outcomes we must achieve.

Many of those who practise public health and need to access these tools are not so explicitly aware of their own public health role, or of the tools they are using. We hope you will be, and the following boxes demonstrate how the public health tools could be applied, by a medical student and a health visitor as examples.

 Can you think of examples of how another professional could apply some of the public health tools? For example, a vascular surgeon, a general practitioner, a hospital manager, an environmental health officer?

As well as there being variety in the professions and roles of those who practise public health, the population for which public health tools are employed varies

Box 1 Examples of the application of public health tools as a medical student

Health needs and information

- You are involved in the completion of death certificates as part of your training and recognise that the correct coding for an individual who died from breast cancer will be obtained by the cancer registration service and used to determine whether the cancer should have been identified earlier through breast screening.
- You use your knowledge of the population demographics in your locality to anticipate a high proportion of Urdu speakers in a clinic and find out in advance how to access translation services.

Evidence-based practice

- You have seen a case of heart failure in a 65-year-old man and you want to find out how to manage the patient based on the current best available evidence for this condition.
- You help the vascular surgeon you are working with prepare a business case for a new lung cancer surveillance service within your hospital and write a section on the evidence of the effectiveness of this in reducing mortality.

Communicable disease control

- You have seen a case of meningococcal meningitis in a 6-year-old school boy and appreciate the need to notify the local public health team to enable contact tracing and appropriate prophylaxis.
- You wash your hands or use alcohol gel between every patient contact and on entry and exit to every ward to reduce the risk of infection – and encourage others to do so.

Leadership and change management

- You are working as a part of team to complete a project as part of your work in paediatrics. There is disagreement on the content of the work and the way it is progressing. You take the lead, put forward a reasonable argument and help your team to complete the assignment on time, which secures good grades.
- You take a special interest in the impact that medical students can have on climate change and convene a student group to consider how you could support one another and encourage others to effect changes in their behaviour.

Health improvement

- During your community placement, you come across a young smoker. You recall evidence on how to best support individuals to stop smoking and take the time to talk to him about the hazards of smoking and signpost him to the local stop-smoking services.
- An obese patient you see in a pre-operative assessment clinic is deemed unsuitable for anaesthesia until they have lost weight. You take the time to question the presiding nurse on the access to weight management services locally for this patient.

Decision-making

- You notice that one of the ward rounds you participate in could be organised more effectively to improve quality of care and discuss with colleagues how you might try a different approach.
- The hospital you are working in sets up a new service to provide a general physician in the emergency department to manage patients who are not severe enough to need hospital emergency care. You recognise that one of the drivers for this new service is the need to reduce the costs of health-care overall in a resource-limited system and a decision has been taken that the benefits of this model are likely to outweigh the costs of employing additional staff.

Box 2 Examples of the application of public health tools as a health visitor working in the community with children or with the elderly

Health needs and information

- You understand that accurate completion of the patient electronic record is required to ensure your service is accurately funded and has sufficient resource to meet all your patients' needs.
- You look at the local health profile for your area and notice there is a relatively low uptake of the MMR vaccine. You take vaccination information with you to your clinics at the local children's centre to ensure you are equipped to answer relevant questions.

Evidence-based practice

- You talk to the mother of a young child who has had repeated ear pain and glue ear about why her child has not been prescribed antibiotics.
- You use an evidence-based stages of change model to support a pregnant mother who wants to stop smoking.

Communicable disease control

- You are contacted by a head teacher who wants to offer some advice to parents about Strep A infection and liaise with the local health protection team to develop some information resources.
- You wash your hands or use alcohol gel between every patient contact and on entry and exit to every home you visit.

Leadership and change management

- You recognise that the way your team schedule their diaries is inefficient and there is a risk that aspects of care for your elderly caseload may be missing. You start discussions about this and form a small group, leading the discussions to redesign the process and mitigate the clinical risks.
- You act as the representative for your union in staff-side discussions about an organisational change process taking place which may affect your employment.

Health improvement

- During your daily work, you come across a young mother who wants to stop smoking but is finding it difficult. You take the time to talk to her about support mechanisms to stop smoking and signpost her to the local stop-smoking services.
- A parent in one of your community clinics seeks advice about how to ensure they can offer healthy foods for weaning to their 1-year-old who only seems to enjoy sweet-tasting foods.

Decision-making

- You are constantly presented with various choices and you develop the ability to analyse the costs and consequences of your actions and arrive at an appropriate decision.
- You are consulted about the closure of a local children's centre site and recognise there is a balance between the need to provide access for as many families as possible and the long-term running costs of multiple service sites. You are able to respond to the consultation with a list of pros and cons to the proposals based on how it will affect your service users.

considerably. There are nuances of implementation when public health is used to describe, improve and protect health and well-being across the life course and we consider these in the first three chapters of Part 2 – with a specific focus on children, adults and older people.

It is also imperative to remember that public health is not practised in a vacuum. It is inseparable from the political, economic, social and environmental factors which influence it, and which it seeks to influence. The last four chapters in Part 2 describe these factors in more detail. We consider the impact and social injustice of inequalities in health in Chapter 14, and linked inextricably to this, the policy (and political) context in which public health must exist in Chapter 15. Chapter 16 highlights the particular role of public health in international development, and in Chapter 17, in tackling significant and substantial challenges to planetary health.

The tools which we have described in Part 1 are all applied in the contexts we describe in Part 2, but the practitioner must be flexible, tenacious and innovative to achieve the optimal public health outcomes in such a complex environment – as you will see.

The Health of Children and Young People
Rebecca Roberts and Rajalakshmi Lakshman

Key points

- A focus on children's public health is important because children represent our future and childhood sets the tone for future health and happiness. What happens in childhood has long-lasting effects on health, making childhood a crucial period for prevention.
- Although child health has improved greatly over time, great disparities still exist between the health of children in different social groups and relative poverty remains a key determinant of child health both in the UK and worldwide. The COVID-19 pandemic has worsened these inequalities.
- Family relationships are an important determinant of many risk factors and play a key role in the transmission of social inequalities.
- Educational settings are important for children's health and well-being and schools should be considered as key partners for the promotion of health and well-being in children.
- Significant challenges facing child public health in the twenty-first century include the rise in emotional and behavioural disorders, childhood obesity, conflict and associated displacement, chronic disease and disability, and climate change.
- The complexity of the underlying determinants of children's health requires a collaborative, cross-disciplinary, integrated approach to prevention and intervention.

11.1 Introduction

Science tells us that a child's experiences from conception through their first five years will go on to shape their next 50. It tells us that the kind of children we raise today, will reflect the kind of world we will live in tomorrow. It tells us that investing in the start of life is not an indulgence, but economically, socially and psychologically vital to a prosperous society.

Jason Knauf, CEO of the Royal Foundation [1]

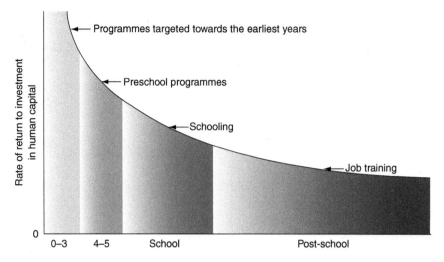

To improve the health of the whole population, it makes sense to focus on children, from a moral, practical and economic perspective. All children have the right to grow up with the best health possible, to be protected from harm and to have access to an education that enables them to fulfil their potential, as enshrined in the UN Convention on the Rights of the Child [2]. Childhood presents an opportunity to promote lifelong health through positive influences and environments, habit formation, biological programming (through epigenetic changes) [3] and education. From an economic perspective, disease prevention is also most effective early in life, as illustrated in Figure 11.1 [4].

The aims of children's public health practice are therefore effectively summarised by the English Department of Health:

> Every child and young person can maximise their potential and future life chances through a collective response that prevents ill health and injury, protects against disease and risks and promotes healthy behaviours and environments. The action must be informed by the voice of children, young people, their parents and caregivers and underpinned by collective system responsibility. [5]

This chapter starts by considering the key differences that make public health practice focused on children unique to that focused on adults and older people, and emphasises the importance of early intervention as part of a life-course approach. The demography of the health of children is described, followed by a description of the major causes of ill health in children and young people, key public health challenges for this age group and their families, and a summary of effective public health interventions to improve health and well-being and reduce inequalities. Three case studies are offered: the impact of the COVID-19 pandemic; childhood obesity; and children and adolescent mental health. These highlight the complexity of these major public health challenges, how the tools described in Part 1 can be used to understand them and the importance of strategic and system-wide approaches.

11.2 What Are the Differences between Children's and Adults' Public Health?

The needs of children and young people should be integral to all public health practice: 'We need everyone in the public services to think family and children and young people at every interaction' [6]. However, there are some areas where there is a distinct difference between adults and children, requiring some specialist understanding (see Box 11.1).

There are opportunities for interventions to improve health and well-being through supporting parenting skills and ensuring home environments are safe and healthy. An entire community shapes a child's experience and thus contributes to their health and well-being, as encapsulated in the idea that 'it takes a village to raise a child' (African proverb). The 'place-based' approach to improving health outcomes consists of interventions at neighbourhood and community level involving the NHS, local government, education and the voluntary and community sectors. Children's public health is therefore child-centred and includes consideration of a wide range of external influences and partnerships.

Some children, such as those with special educational needs and disabilities (SEND), may require additional support. It is important to recognise and have provision to enable these children to reach their potential, particularly in the context

Box 11.1 Important features of child health

- **Context**. The child's world is in large part influenced by their family, parents (including corporate parenting for children in care), friends and education settings where they spend a large part of their day. Hence, most of the interventions to improve child health are delivered through families and communities.
- **Dependence**. The potential vulnerability of children involves consideration of safeguarding and harm prevention. Although some adults also require protection, the universal dependence of children arguably makes it more marked in child public health.
- **Development**. A detailed understanding is required of stages of development, consequent changing needs as children grow, and critical periods for establishing healthy-protective behaviours and preventing exposure to risk factors for ill health.

of on-going growth and development. Some children may be vulnerable to negative adult influences and require support or protection from these adults. Hence, children's public health practice incorporates child safeguarding.

11.3 Importance of the First 1,001 Days

From conception to age 2 years, the human brain and body develops more rapidly than at any other time in life. Although we inherit our genes at conception, what happens during this critical period programmes our physical and mental development through epigenetic changes [7]. Figure 11.2 summarises the key determinants of maternal and child outcomes. There is a compelling body of evidence that physical and emotional development during this period influences health later in life. Table 11.1 presents examples of possible problems during the critical 1,001-day period, interventions to prevent them and health or economic consequences of a lack of support.

Figure 11.2 Key determinants of maternal and child outcomes [6].

'The Healthy Child Programme (0–19)' [8] is a major component of children's public health armoury in England. It aims to improve the health and well-being of children and reduce inequalities through evidence-based interventions [9, 10], including health and development reviews, health promotion, parenting support, screening and immunisation programmes [11].

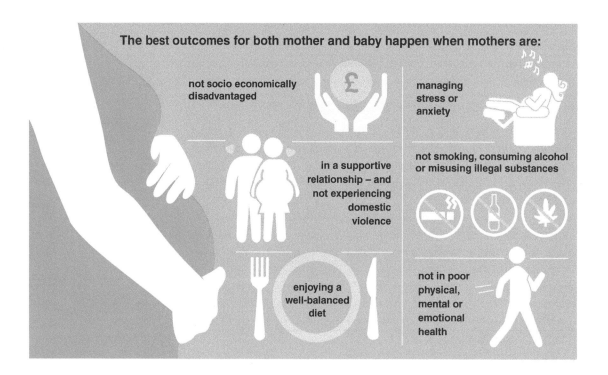

The best outcomes for both mother and baby happen when mothers are:

not socio economically disadvantaged

managing stress or anxiety

in a supportive relationship – and not experiencing domestic violence

not smoking, consuming alcohol or misusing illegal substances

enjoying a well-balanced diet

not in poor physical, mental or emotional health

Table 11.1 Problems, interventions and consequences of inaction in the first 1,001 days

	Problem	Example of policies or interventions	Example of health or economic consequences from lack of support
Maternal	Poor nutrition	Healthy Start Scheme: support for buying fruit, vegetables, milk and vitamins for low-income families	Babies born small or large for gestational age and showing rapid weight gain (crossing weight centile charts) are more likely to develop obesity and cardiovascular disease in later life [12]
	Stress and anxiety in pregnancy	Perinatal mental health support	Poor perinatal mental health
	Smoking	Smoking cessation programmes	Higher risk of miscarriage, still birth and low-birth-weight babies
Child	Adverse childhood experiences (ACEs)*	Early identification and interventions to minimise impact; trauma-informed practice	High numbers of ACEs are associated with greater risk of substance misuse, being a victim of or a perpetrator of crimes or going to prison later in life [13]
	Poor attachment	Promote positive parent–child interaction (e.g. respond, cuddle, relax, play, talk)	Increased risk of behavioural problems Intergenerational parenting difficulties
	Growing up in poverty	Social security system, including child support Debt advice Employment and housing support Taking a holistic whole-family approach	Risks multiple poor outcomes, including poor physical and mental health, reduced educational attainment, increased risk of going into care
	Exposure to environmental smoke or pollution	Legislation to prevent passive smoking or reduce levels of air pollution Fines for leaving car engines on when stationary	Increased rates and poor control of asthma in children
	Poor social-communication skills	Working to improve language acquisition and reading skills in the early years, including by supporting parents to help their children's language development at home	Poor educational attainment and employment prospects
	Lack of physical activity	Local communities providing green spaces, leisure facilities and play areas	Increased rates of childhood obesity

213

Table 11.1 (*cont.*)

	Problem	Example of policies or interventions	Example of health or economic consequences from lack of support
	Poor nutrition	Breastfeeding and introduction of solid foods support for parents National resources such as the UK Start4Life and Change4Life programmes	Increased rates of childhood obesity
Parents	Poor parenting skills	Parenting programmes High-quality education on health, sex and relationships in school curriculum	Higher rates of teenage pregnancy Intergenerational parenting difficulties
	Poor parental mental health	Early identification and enhanced support for vulnerable parents/children	Poor physical and mental health

* ACEs: traumatic events such as exposure to physical, sexual or emotional childhood abuse, family breakdown, exposure to domestic violence or living in a household affected by substance abuse, mental illness or where someone is incarcerated.

11.4 Inequalities Start Early and Are Sustained

Recognising and addressing inequalities is integral to children's public health practice. The influences that lead to health inequalities take their effect throughout life and start early, as discussed in Chapter 14. For example, some areas of the UK have significantly higher proportions of low-birth-weight term babies and higher rates of cardiovascular disease and premature mortality.

Inequalities are sustained throughout the education system, as shown by geographical variation in rates of school readiness, attainment at GCSEs and the proportion of children overweight/obese in primary school. These outcomes are all linked to markers of deprivation in the UK. Figure 11.3 illustrates the advantage of children who grow up in families with a high socioeconomic position; low IQ scores at 22 months of age are improved by age 10. However, children who grow up in families of a low socioeconomic position have worsening IQ by age 10, even overtaken by the children in high socioeconomic position of initial low IQ [14].

Socioeconomic determinants of health and vulnerabilities in children are linked. While it is important to identify and address children's individual risk factors that may make them vulnerable (see Box 11.2), targeting underlying causes of risk factors within families and communities is vital.

There is evidence that those in more deprived sections of the population are more likely to experience clusters of adverse childhood experiences. Furthermore, early adversity can have an intergenerational effect that, if left unchecked, can lead to the perpetuation of disadvantage for subsequent generations [15].

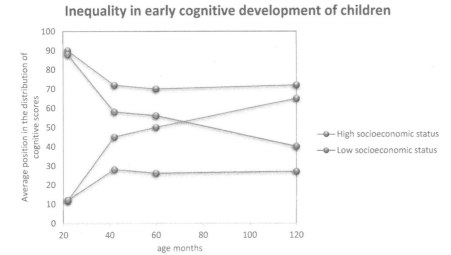

Figure 11.3 Inequality in early cognitive development of children in the 1970 British Cohort Study, at ages 22 months to 10 years. Children of high socioeconomic status maintain or improve their cognitive score compared to children of lower socioeconomic status [14].

Box 11.2

Vulnerable children are defined as children at greater risk of experiencing physical or emotional harm and experiencing poor outcomes.

Groups of vulnerable children include those:

- in care;
- in the criminal justice system;
- with exposure to violence (such as physical, sexual or emotional abuse);
- living with parents with drug or alcohol problems;
- living in unhealthy housing;
- without access to green space;
- living in poverty;
- in workless families;
- who are young carers;
- those with special educational needs, chronic physical or mental illness.

11.5 Demography

Tools and sources such as those outlined in Chapters 1 and 2 can be used to assess the demography and health status of the child population in the UK. According to the 2021 census, there were approximately 10.1 million children aged under 15 years in England and Wales (compared to 9.9 million in 2011), around 17% of the total population. As a proportion, the under-16 population fell from 25% in 1971 to 20% in 2001 and 17% in the most recent 2021 census. This decline, influenced by assumed low fertility rates in the 2020s and 2030s, is projected to continue, while

Figure 11.4 UK population by life stage, mid-2020, mid-2030 and mid-2045 [16].

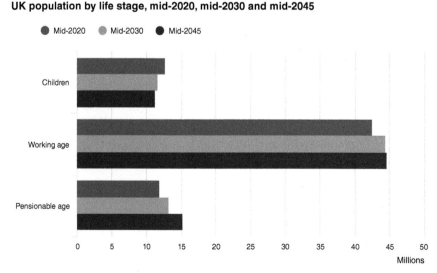

UK population by life stage, mid-2020, mid-2030 and mid-2045

older age groups expand [16] (see Figure 11.4). However, as shown by recent displacement of children and their families due to war, rates of migration may also prove important. There are also regional differences in age distribution.

According to ONS estimates for 2021 [18], there are around 8 million families with dependent children in the UK (around 40% of families). Almost one-quarter of families with dependent children are lone parent families.

11.6 Identifying Causes of Ill Health, Making a Population Diagnosis and Effective Interventions

11.6.1 Mortality and Morbidity in Children

In 2020, it was estimated that globally 5 million children under 5 years died, mostly from preventable and treatable causes, such as pre-term birth complications, birth asphyxia/trauma, pneumonia, congenital anomalies, diarrhoea and malaria. Almost half of those deaths were neonates, aged under 28 days [17]. The difference in mortality rates of children globally vary markedly and are linked to poverty; sub-Saharan Africa and South Asia accounted for more than 80% of the deaths of under-5s in 2020.

There is a difference in causes of death in lower- and higher-income countries (see Chapter 16). For children under 5 years, birth trauma/asphyxia and infectious disease predominate in lower-income countries, whereas perinatal conditions, congenital anomalies and birth asphyxia are the leading causes of death in higher-income countries such as the UK, as illustrated in Table 11.2.

Table 11.2 Main causes of death of children under 5 years in the UK compared to worldwide [18, 19]

UK	Worldwide
Population (2020): 14.2 million children under 18 years (21% total population) 3.9 million children under 5 years (6% total population)	Population (2020): 2.4 billion children under 18 years (30% total population) 678 million children under 5 years (9% total population)
Deaths (2019): Under-5 mortality rate 4/1,000 live births	Deaths (2019): Under-5 mortality rate 38/1,000 live births
Causes of death Most occur in newborns: • prematurity, low birth weight, etc. (perinatal conditions) • congenital anomalies • birth asphyxia Other main causes include: • injury • lower respiratory tract disease	Causes of death Infectious diseases dominate: • pneumonia • diarrhoea • malaria • neonatal infection Other main causes include: • complications of pre-term delivery • birth asphyxia

Injury and violence account for a significant portion of deaths in children aged over 5 years both in the UK and internationally. This includes road traffic accidents, drowning, interpersonal violence and self-harm. There are sex differences, more marked in older children. Injury and poisoning is the leading cause of death in older children (aged 5–19 years) in the UK, with over twice as many deaths in male children compared to female children [20].

Recent global improvements in child mortality have been significant; child mortality halved between 1990 and 2015. Better sanitation, living conditions, nutrition, access to clean water, immunisation, advancement in scientific understanding and health-care, among other factors, have resulted in reduced mortality and morbidity in children throughout the last century (see also Chapter 16).

Significant progress has been made, but ambitions go beyond preventing deaths, to allowing children to thrive and reach their potential and tackling inequities in health within and between countries. There are significant challenges to tackle, as summarised in Table 11.3.

Hence, the focus of children's public health practice varies with location. Routine and bespoke data can provide a helpful insight into some of the current public health challenges and priorities at a national or local level (see also Chapter 2). For example, in England, nationally collated 'Child Health Profiles' identify that the numbers of children living in absolute or relative poverty, children going into care, obesity in Reception and Year 6 children, number of low-birth-weight babies and admissions for emergencies and mental health problems are all increasing [21].

11.6.2 Child Health Promotion, Policy and Collaborative Working

According to the World Health Organization (WHO), the two public health interventions that have had the greatest impact on the world's health are clean water and vaccines. Immunisation and screening programmes are important public health interventions to protect the health of children and identify problems early (see also Chapter 9). Up-to-date UK immunisation schedules and screening programmes for pregnant mothers and newborns can be found on the NHS website, along with helpful information for parents and families and useful tools to aid discussion and encourage uptake and participation.

As with health promotion for adults, child health promotion involves action at national (policy development, legislation) and local level (parenting support, community development, realignment of services). Childhood examples from each of the five pillars of the 1986 Ottawa Charter for Health Promotion [26] include:

- **Building healthy public policy**. For example, health impact assessments for proposed new roads, which consider cycle lanes, pedestrianised areas and child health concerns such as air pollution, asthma and risk of road traffic accidents.

Table 11.3 Key child public health challenges in the UK for the twenty-first century

Social and health inequalities	Child poverty is increasing. The areas with the highest child poverty prevalence have over a third of children living in poverty [22]. Instabilities in the global economies and increasing cost of food and fuel make the situation worse.
Emotional and behavioural/mental health problems	Prevalence is rising in children and young people [23]. Suicide rates are higher for older teenagers (15–19-year-olds) than younger children (10–14-year-olds) and higher in boys than girls.
Childhood obesity and poor nutrition	Prevalence has increased in recent years and this trend may lead to a significant burden of disease and associated financial burden to health services and society (see case study 2 later in this chapter).
Poor vaccination uptake	Childhood vaccination uptake in the UK has been falling in recent years and is below the 95% coverage recommended by the WHO for herd immunity. For example, poor uptake of MMR, due to media scares about links to autism and mistrust of government advice, has resulted in significant risk of outbreaks of measles and greater exposure of pregnant women to rubella.
Chronic disease and disabilities	Disabilities are increasing in prevalence, partly due to improved care and survival of premature and small-for-date babies, and children with complex conditions such as cystic fibrosis and other inherited disorders.
Substance misuse	This includes alcohol, tobacco and recreational drugs. Although smoking rates in England have fallen steadily since 2011, there is a marked socioeconomic disparity with teenagers from the most deprived areas more than twice as likely to smoke regularly than those in the least deprived [24].
Teenage pregnancy	Public health and education policy has been successful in helping to halve the teenage conception rates between 2008 and 2017. However, the UK still has one of the highest rates in Europe, and the impact on health and well-being is substantial, both for teenage mothers and their children [25].
Sexually transmitted infections	Health protection efforts focus mainly on reducing the risk of transmission through safe-sex practices, contraception and encouraging early testing. Health promotion activities in schools are delivered through the relationships and sex education curriculum.
Accidents and injuries	Children living in deprived areas have a higher risk of road traffic injuries. Non-intentional injuries in children, such as falls, poisoning, drowning and burns, are a leading cause of death and disability. Importantly, children have to be protected from intentional harm perpetrated within and outside their families – neglect, abuse, sexual and criminal exploitation.
Conflict and associated displacement	Worldwide there has been a dramatic increase in child refugees, displaced as a consequence of conflict and violence, over the last decade. This has implications for UK universally available public services like education and health (see Chapter 16).
Climate change	Displacement and severe weather events are having a major influence on the physical and mental health of children (see Chapter 17).
Poor air quality	Air pollution is one of the UK's most significant environmental challenges contributing to poor asthma control in children and cardio-respiratory outcomes in adults (see Chapter 17).

- **Creating supportive environments**. For example, promoting active travel to school, planning restrictions on fast food retailers near to schools.
- **Strengthening communities**. For example, enabling parents and children to contribute to decision-making about their health, such as community leisure provision or enabling people to set up a community fridge to cater for local people in food poverty.
- **Re-orienting health services**. For example, ensuring services are child-centred and meet local needs, and access to mental health support via text messaging/ digital solutions.
- **Developing personal knowledge and skills**. For example, programmes to support development of resilience and mindfulness in schools, and relationship, health and sex education in the curriculum.

Chapter 15 describes the ambition in England to see delivery of coordinated, joined-up health and social care services through Integrated Care System (ICS) partnerships. The shift towards collaboration at system level chimes with the approaches to improving children's health described in this chapter: recognising the role of families (providing strong and sustained attachment and a solid foundation in the early years); the value of places (creating environments where conditions allow children to thrive); and the importance of collaboration across systems and working in partnership (such as health and education partnerships). It is envisaged that this approach will significantly benefit families providing more joined-up and synergistic care and support, to prevent children falling between the gaps in services and having to repeat their story multiple times.

11.7 Case Studies of Current Public Health Challenges in the UK

The following three case studies discuss three contemporary examples to illustrate the broad scope of children's public health, associated inequalities and how these relate to the concepts described in the first part of the book.

11.7.1 Case study 1 The COVID-19 pandemic: Indirect impacts on children

It was clear from an early stage in the COVID-19 pandemic that infection caused only very mild illness for the majority of children, so the direct health impacts were minimal. In fact, all-cause child mortality declined in the first year of the pandemic in England, predominantly as a result of reduction in other infectious diseases due to the measures in place to prevent the spread of COVID-19 [27]. However, the health protection measures implemented to control the spread of infection impacted children hugely and arguably disproportionately. Reflections on the full impact of the pandemic on children are on-going and likely to be studied and debated for a long time to come. However, with evidence of widening inequalities in health and other negative impacts, it has certainly created greater and more complex public health challenges. Some of these negative consequences for children and young people in the UK are summarised in Table 11.4.

Table 11.4 Potential negative impact of the COVID-19 pandemic on children and young people in the UK

Disruption to education	The extent of children's contribution to transmission of COVID-19 was initially unknown and educational environments represented opportunities for significant mixing of different households contrary to physical distancing protective measures. Hence, there were several periods of school (and childcare settings) closures during the pandemic. Even when schools were open, they had to operate with strict controls which led to changes in educational experience. Periods of home schooling were enforced when children were recently infected with the virus (or at some stages when children had been in contact with infected individuals). All this led to significant educational disruption and reduced learning.
Social isolation	Many other impacts may have been associated with the closure of schools, including negative impacts on children's access to play/socialising, levels of physical activity, mental health [28] and wider impacts on children's families relating to supporting children at home [29].
Access to health services	Coverage of routine childhood immunisations, such as MMR (measles, mumps and rubella), diphtheria, pertussis and polio, reduced during the pandemic, attributed to a combination of factors, including health protection messaging to 'stay at home' and disruption to health-care services [30]. There was a reduction in access to health-care settings across every age group, but access to emergency care dropped more for children than adults [31].
Exacerbating health inequalities	Even before the pandemic, disadvantaged children were 18 months behind their wealthier peers in learning by the time they finished their GCSEs [32]. When schools closed and learning switched to being predominantly remote, with consequent reliance on access to digital technology, the poorest students' learning time reduced to a greater extent. Even when schools re-opened, disparities remained as attendance of pupils varied with socioeconomic deprivation [33].
Risks to vulnerable children	School closures also left some children more vulnerable and at risk of harm. For instance, children living in households with 'the trio of vulnerabilities' of family issues (parental domestic abuse, parental drug and/or alcohol dependency, and parental mental health issues) were particularly disadvantaged [32]. Disruption of normal protective services and strain on families probably contributed to adverse outcomes, such as a rise in cases of domestic abuse [34].

However, there were also some positive results for public health practice, including the successful collaborative relationships that were enhanced between educational settings and public health specialists. The pandemic has emphasised how important educational settings are for the health of children: not only through learning opportunities, but also the physical activity children participate in during the day or in travelling to and from school, the food they eat, the friends they make, the time it allows their parents to work and the teaching staff who take care of them. School staff should be recognised for their important role in promoting healthy behaviours and well-being of children, integral to the children's public health workforce.

11.7.2 Case study 2 Childhood obesity in England

Obesity is linked to poor physical and mental health outcomes, including reduced life expectancy and risk of chronic disease, and represents a significant economic burden on the NHS (further described in Chapter 12). The threat of the childhood obesity 'epidemic' to public health has been widely recognised and was famously dubbed by former Chief Medical Officer Sir Liam Donaldson as a 'ticking time bomb', referencing the later repercussions for children and society [35]. Excess weight in childhood 'tracks' to adulthood, meaning that overweight children are more likely to become overweight adults. Obesity prevalence is highest in certain groups, also contributing to health inequalities by gender, ethnicity, socioeconomic status, geography and disability.

In England, the National Child Measurement Programme (NCMP) is a nationally mandated public health programme in which the height and weight of children at age 5 years and 11 years are measured and recorded in school. Individual results are shared with parents/carers and the data provide public health surveillance information on children's weight, including trends at local and national level. It is an example of the type of data used by public health professionals to make a 'population diagnosis', or understand the health problems in a region (see Chapters 1 and 2). As described further in Chapter 12, the UK has one of the highest rates of overweight or obese adults in Europe [36] and, despite attempts to tackle it for many years, rates of overweight or obese children continue to increase. In 2022, approximately one in ten children aged 5 years and one in four aged 11 years were obese in England [37].

Obesity is a complex problem. It would be an over-simplification to consider it as just an individual's imbalance between nutritional inputs and energy outputs. The term 'obesogenic environment' [38] refers to the complicated societal and environmental influences on lifestyle which contribute to people gaining excess body weight (see also Chapter 8). Hence, solutions must lie in collaborative, multi-sectoral action and a whole-system approach, rather than simply relying on individual determination to eat more healthily, do more exercise or attend weight management programmes. Obesity prevention strategies must also include measures to reduce weight-based stigma and discrimination, which can threaten the physical and mental health of overweight children and worsen inequalities. Table 11.5 illustrates how action might be planned at different levels and by different agencies to tackle childhood obesity.

Table 11.5 Multi-sectoral response to tackle childhood obesity

Agency/Setting	Example of existing or proposed interventions
National government	Soft drinks levy [39]
	Mandatory sugar reduction in products [39]
	Food labelling/traffic light scheme [40]
	Mandatory calorie labelling on menus [40]
	Healthy Start scheme (vouchers for fresh fruit and vegetables for low-income families) [41]
	Advertising restrictions – TV or online of HFSS* products before 9pm [40]
	Funding national campaigns to encourage healthy weight, e.g. Better Health, Healthier Families [42], Start4Life, Change4Life
	Free school meals for families on low incomes and free fruit/vegetables for all children aged 4–7

Table 11.5 *(cont.)*

Agency/Setting	Example of existing or proposed interventions
Local authorities	Government Food Strategy [43]
	Cooking, nutrition and physical activity in school curriculum
	Healthy schools rating scheme [44]
	Holiday activities and food clubs for children on free school meals
	Childhood obesity strategy [40]
	Advertising ban for HFSS* products (e.g. in bus shelters)
	Planning restrictions on fast food outlets near schools
	Open spaces and green infrastructure embedded into new housing developments
	Improving street safety
	Leisure facilities
	Catering procurement standards
	Services to support breastfeeding and weaning
	Food strategies
	Physical activity strategies
Schools and early years settings	Nutrition and physical activity education
	Physical activity embedded in school day
	Promotion of active travel to school/EYS
	Healthy meals and snacks
	Promoting a 'whole-school' environment to support healthy weight
Media and commercial world	Voluntary reductions in salt, sugar and fat content of food
	Food pricing to promote healthy products
	Social marketing campaigns for healthy eating such as healthier families [42]
	Interactive apps to promote healthier choices, e.g. NHS food scanner app [42]
Communities, neighbourhoods, voluntary organisations	Breastfeeding support
	Healthy weaning [45]
	Community kitchens and fridges (redistribution of food)
	Food banks
	Food poverty alliances
	Community gardens and allotments
	Lunch clubs
	Local sports clubs

* HFSS: high in saturated fat, salt and sugar.

11.7.3 Case study 3 Mental health and emotional well-being in children

Most mental health illnesses start in childhood; over half start before the age of 14 years, and 75% have developed by the age of 18 [46]. They are the leading cause of health-related disabilities in children and young people (CYP) and can have long-lasting adverse impacts, reducing the life chances of those individuals in terms of their physical health, their educational and work prospects, their chances of committing a crime [46] and even the length of their life [47].

Not only is there significant personal cost to individuals affected, but there is also a wider impact on their families, carers and society that results in a very high cost to our economy. Despite this burden of distress, most children and adolescents who experience clinically significant difficulties have not had help sufficiently early in their childhood.

Data used to understand the extent of children's mental health problems in England are captured in various ways. Rates of hospital admissions or referrals for alcohol- or substance-misuse-related conditions, self-harm in CYP and mental health conditions are monitored and available at local, regional and national levels for comparison (see also Chapter 2). However, these represent a small proportion and the more extreme 'tip of the iceberg' of the overall cases.

Large, detailed surveys of children's mental health allow more granular understanding of CYP mental health, including trends over time. The 'Mental Health of Children and Young People in England' survey in 2017 [48] found that around one in nine children of 6–16 years of age had mental health problems. Emotional disorders, such as depression, were the most common. The 2020/21 survey, timed to assess the impact of the COVID-19 pandemic, showed that rates of mental health problems have increased since 2017, with one in six children of 6–16 years of age experiencing problems [23]. Another key finding was an increase in eating disorders in both 11- to 16-year-olds (up from 6.7% in 2017 to 13% in 2021) and 17- to 19-year-olds (up from 44.6% in 2017 to 58.2% in 2021).

A range of other government, academic, voluntary and private sector organisations publish data on children's mental health and well-being. Asking children directly how they feel about issues is important; for example, the 'Big Ask/Big Answer' of 2021 [49] did this, capturing children's views, in their own words, on the impact of the COVID-19 pandemic on their lives. These sources of public health intelligence support understanding of mental health problems facing children and inform strategies to tackle them. Children's voices must be involved in defining the problems and – through co-production – finding solutions.

11.7.3.1 Understanding the Causes of Mental Health Problems and Health Inequalities

The presence of mental health problems in children is associated with a range of factors, including [50]:
- demographics (e.g. age, gender, ethnic group, sexuality);
- family life (e.g. family functioning, parental mental health, qualification status of parent, marital status of parent, family type); and
- socioeconomic circumstances. (e.g. *income-related*: parents' occupations, receipt of welfare benefits, household income; and *location-related*: region, neighbourhood, household tenure, accommodation type).

The balance of risk factors and protective factors in different settings may influence CYP mental health, as illustrated in Figure 11.5.

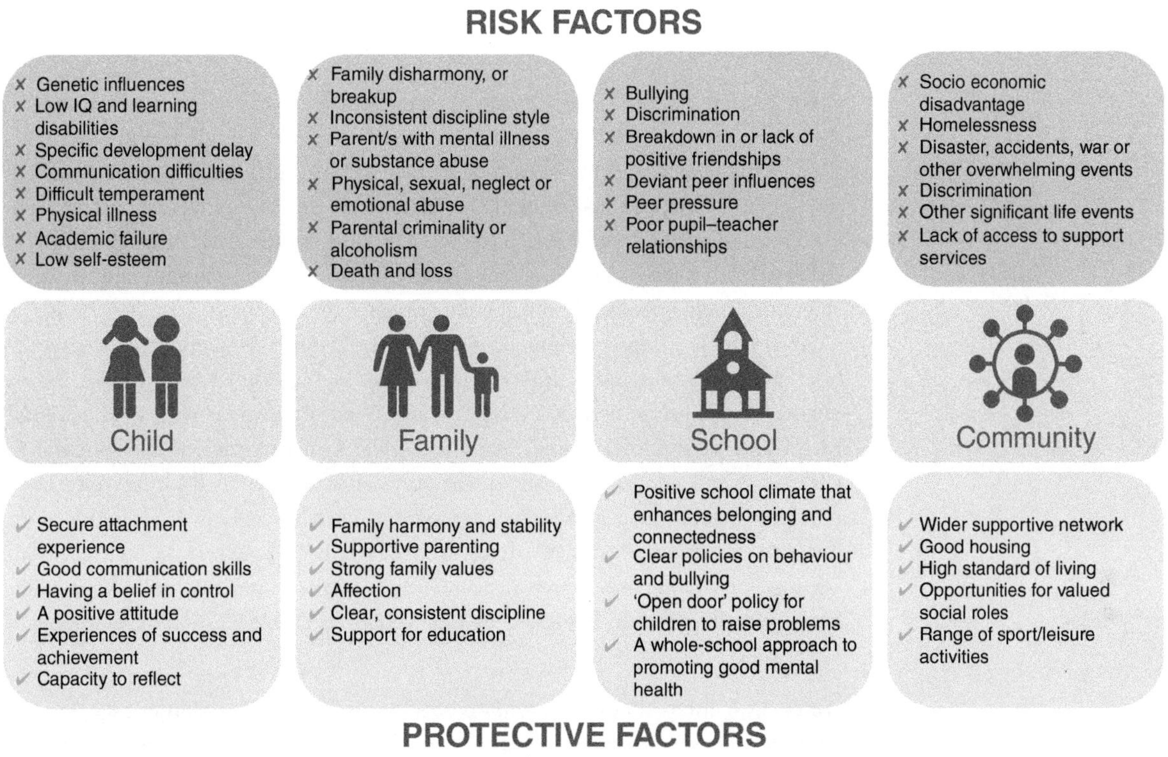

RISK FACTORS

- ✗ Genetic influences
- ✗ Low IQ and learning disabilities
- ✗ Specific development delay
- ✗ Communication difficulties
- ✗ Difficult temperament
- ✗ Physical illness
- ✗ Academic failure
- ✗ Low self-esteem

- ✗ Family disharmony, or breakup
- ✗ Inconsistent discipline style
- ✗ Parent/s with mental illness or substance abuse
- ✗ Physical, sexual, neglect or emotional abuse
- ✗ Parental criminality or alcoholism
- ✗ Death and loss

- ✗ Bullying
- ✗ Discrimination
- ✗ Breakdown in or lack of positive friendships
- ✗ Deviant peer influences
- ✗ Peer pressure
- ✗ Poor pupil–teacher relationships

- ✗ Socio economic disadvantage
- ✗ Homelessness
- ✗ Disaster, accidents, war or other overwhelming events
- ✗ Discrimination
- ✗ Other significant life events
- ✗ Lack of access to support services

Child **Family** **School** **Community**

- ✓ Secure attachment experience
- ✓ Good communication skills
- ✓ Having a belief in control
- ✓ A positive attitude
- ✓ Experiences of success and achievement
- ✓ Capacity to reflect

- ✓ Family harmony and stability
- ✓ Supportive parenting
- ✓ Strong family values
- ✓ Affection
- ✓ Clear, consistent discipline
- ✓ Support for education

- ✓ Positive school climate that enhances belonging and connectedness
- ✓ Clear policies on behaviour and bullying
- ✓ 'Open door' policy for children to raise problems
- ✓ A whole-school approach to promoting good mental health

- ✓ Wider supportive network
- ✓ Good housing
- ✓ High standard of living
- ✓ Opportunities for valued social roles
- ✓ Range of sport/leisure activities

PROTECTIVE FACTORS

Given the demographic, family and socioeconomic factors associated with mental health problems and the risk and protective factors shown in Figure 11.5, it is not surprising that mental health problems are linked to health inequalities. Some groups of children are exposed to clusters of risk factors or adverse child experiences (ACEs), making them more vulnerable. The following list gives examples of groups of children shown to be at greater risk [50]:

Figure 11.5 Risk and protective factors influencing the mental health of children [51].

- looked-after children (children in care);
- LGBTQ+ young people;
- children with special educational needs;
- children with a physical illness;
- homeless children;
- children with parents in prison;
- children with parents who have a mental disorder;
- young people not in education, employment or training;
- young offenders;
- children seeking asylum;
- children with autistic spectrum disorder; and
- young carers.

11.7.3.2 What Works? Preventive Approaches to Tackling CYP Mental Health Problems across the Life Course

Children's mental health prevention strategies must combine prevention of mental disorders (primary prevention, access to early treatment and prevention of secondary complications) and promotion of mental well-being (fostering development of protective factors and resilience) [50]. There must be both universal components, accessible to all children, as well as targeted to those more at risk. Strategies must be delivered in a timely manner across children's lives, recognising the importance of stages of development and critical risk periods.

For mental illness prevention, the first 1,001 days are critical for psycho-neurological development. Interventions need to forge good foundations for all children, with promotion of strong and sustained attachment with their parents/carers and by supporting good parenting skills. At later stages of development in childhood and adolescence, when the prevalence of mental disorders increases, different interventions involving wider settings such as schools are required – for instance, to promote skills in coping with adversity [50]. Access to mental health services for children who develop mental disorders is important throughout childhood, but the demand is higher for older children. Table 11.6 offers examples of

Table 11.6 Interventions to promote good mental health in children [50]

Starting well
Parenting programmes
Promotion of infant attachment
Addressing parental smoking, alcohol and substance misuse
Developing well
Preschool interventions, including social and emotional learning interventions
School-based interventions, including social and emotional learning programmes, self-regulation, play therapy, academic interventions, physical activity promotion, mindfulness, mentoring and family-linked programmes
Promotion of interpersonal skills, emotional regulation, alcohol and drug education
Living well
Social interaction promotion, e.g. volunteering, community engagement, leisure, sport, kindness, gratitude, peer support for parents
Physical activity promotion
Diet
Financial capability
Neighbourhood interventions, including design, functionality, walkability, safety and facilities
Housing interventions
Access to green space
Arts, creativity and music
Positive psychology interventions
Mindfulness, meditation, spiritual interventions

mental well-being promotion interventions from conception to adolescence, demonstrating the different focus as children grow and develop.

A major component of recent government policy in England to tackle poor mental health in children is the promotion of a 'whole-school approach' [52]. This means that schools should adopt a positive and universal focus on well-being, involving the entire school community in the improvement of mental health and well-being outcomes. This approach has many components, such as staff well-being and development, pupil skills training and the mandatory health education curriculum. An additional workforce, Mental Health Support Teams, will bridge the gap between education and health by providing interventions for mild to moderate mental health issues, supporting the development of whole-school approaches, offering consultations to school staff and linking with other agencies to help children get the right support and stay in education [52].

11.8 Conclusions

These examples help to demonstrate the importance of interventions to promote strong foundations for health in infants and young children and for the focus and approach of interventions to change as children grow and their world expands beyond their immediate family. They also highlight the need to have universal promotion of well-being and more targeted approaches for vulnerable children with clusters of risk factors. Work to improve children's health and happiness must be accomplished in a holistic, collaborative manner, aiming to provide a network of support that can be accessed according to need.

REFERENCES

1. Ipsos MORI and Royal Foundation, State of the nation: Understanding public attitudes to the early years, executive summary, November 2020. Available at: https://royalfoundation.com/wp-content/uploads/2020/11/Ipsos-MORI-SON_report_FINAL_V2.4.pdf
2. K. Bäckström, Convention on the Rights of the Child, *International Journal of Early Childhood* **21**, 1989, 35–44.
3. Y. Arima and H. Fukuoka, Developmental origins of health and disease theory in cardiology, *Journal of Cardiology* **76**(1), 2020, 14–17.
4. J. J. Heckman, Schools, skills, and synapses, *Economic Inquiry* **46**(3), 2008, 289–324.
5. V. Pearson, E. De Sousa and A. Furber, What good children and young people's public health looks like, Public Health England, 2019, pp. 1–9. Available at: www.adph.org.uk/wp-content/uploads/2019/06/What-Good-Children-and-Young-Peoples-Public-Health-Looks-Like.pdf
6. Public Health England, Health matters: Giving every child the best start in life, 2016. Available at: www.gov.uk/government/publications/health-matters-giving-every-child-the-best-start-in-life
7. R. L. Boon, Developmental origins of health and disease, *Archives of Disease in Childhood* **91**(12), 2006, 1046.

8. Public Health England. Healthy Child Programme 0 to 19: Health visitor and school nurse commissioning, January 2016. Available at: www.gov.uk/government/publications/healthy-child-programme-0-to-19-health-visitor-and-school-nurse-commissioning

9. House of Commons Health and Social Care Committee, First 1000 days of life, Thirteenth Report of Session 2017–19, 2019. Available at: https://publications.parliament.uk/pa/cm201719/cmselect/cmhealth/1496/1496.pdf

10. Department of Health and Social Care, The best start for life. A vision for the 1,001 critical days, The Early Years Healthy Development Review Report, 2021. Available at: www.gov.uk/government/publications/the-best-start-for-life-a-vision-for-the-1001-critical-days

11. Public Health England, Healthy child programme: Rapid review to update evidence, 2015. Available at: www.gov.uk/government/publications/healthy-child-programme-rapid-review-to-update-evidence

12. World Health Oganization, Report of the commission on ending childhood obesity, 2016. Available at: www.who.int/publications/i/item/9789241510066

13. K. Ford, N. Butler, K. Hughes *et al.*, Adverse childhood experiences (ACEs) in Hertfordshire, Luton and Northamptonshire, 2016. Available at: www.ljmu.ac.uk/~/media/phi-reports/pdf/2016-05-adverse-childhood-experiences-in-hertfordshire-luton-and-northamptonshire.pdf

14. L. Feinstein, Inequality in the early cognitive development of British children in the 1970 cohort, *Economica* **70**(277), 2003, 73–97.

15. Public Health England, No child left behind: Understanding and quantifying vulnerability, 2020, pp. 1–23. Available at: https://assets.publishing.service.gov.uk/government/uploads/system/uploads/attachment_data/file/913974/Understanding_and_quantifying_vulnerability_in_childhood.pdf

16. Office for National Statistics, National population projections: 2020-based interim, 2022. Available at: www.ons.gov.uk/peoplepopulationandcommunity/populationandmigration/populationprojections/bulletins/nationalpopulationprojections/2020basedinterim#changing-age-structure

17. World Health Organization, SDG target 3.2: End preventable deaths of newborns and children under 5 years of age, n.d. Available at: www.who.int/data/gho/data/themes/topics/sdg-target-3_2-newborn-and-child-mortality

18. UNICEF, The state of the world's children 2021: Statistical tables, 2021. Available at: https://data.unicef.org/resources/dataset/the-state-of-the-worlds-children-2021-statistical-tables

19. World Health Organization, The Global Health Observatory, Distribution of causes of death among children aged <5 years (%), 2017. Available at: www.who.int/data/gho/indicator-metadata-registry/imr-details/89

20. Office for National Statistics, Dataset: Leading causes of death, UK. Available at: www.ons.gov.uk/peoplepopulationandcommunity/healthandsocialcare/causesofdeath/datasets/leadingcausesofdeathuk

21. Office for Health Improvement and Disparities, 2023 Child Health Profiles, 2023. Available at: www.gov.uk/government/statistics/2023-child-health-profiles

22. Health Foundation, Map of child poverty, 2023. Available at: www.health.org.uk/evidence-hub/money-and-resources/poverty/map-of-child-poverty

23. NHS Digital, Mental health of children and young people in England 2021 – wave 2 follow up to the 2017 survey, 2021. Available at: https://digital.nhs.uk/data-and-information/publi

cations/statistical/mental-health-of-children-and-young-people-in-england/2021-follow-up-to-the-2017-survey

24. Royal College of Paediatrics and Child Health, State of child health: Smoking in young people, 2021. Available at: https://stateofchildhealth.rcpch.ac.uk/evidence/health-behaviours/smoking-young-people/.

25. Royal College of Paediatrics and Child Health, State of child health: Conceptions in young people, 2021. Available at: https://stateofchildhealth.rcpch.ac.uk/evidence/health-behaviours/conceptions-in-young-people/.

26. World Health Organization, Ottawa Charter for Health Promotion, 1986. Available at: https://apps.who.int/iris/handle/10665/349652.

27. D. Odd, S. Stoianova, T. Williams *et al.*, Child mortality in England during the first year of the COVID-19 pandemic, *Archives of Disease in Childhood* **107**(3), 2022, e22.

28. R. Viner, S. Russell, R. Saulle and E. Al, UCL: Impacts of school closures on physical and mental health of children and young people – a systematic review, 11 February 2021.

29. Office for National Statistics, Parenting in lockdown: Coronavirus and the effects on work-life balance, 2020. Available at: www.ons.gov.uk/peoplepopulationandcommunity/healthandsocialcare/conditionsanddiseases/articles/parentinginlockdowncoronavirusandtheeffectsonworklifebalance/2020-07-22.

30. UK Health Security Agency, COVID-19: Impact on childhood vaccinations: Data to August 2021. Available at: www.gov.uk/government/publications/covid-19-impact-on-childhood-vaccinations-data-to-august-2021.

31. Department of Health and Social Care and Office for National Statistics, Direct and indirect health impacts of COVID-19 in England, 2021, pp. 1–117. Available at: https://assets.publishing.service.gov.uk/government/uploads/system/uploads/attachment_data/file/1018698/S1373_Direct_and_Indirect_Health_Impacts_of_C19_Detailed_Paper_.pdf.

32. Children's Commissioner, Childhood in the time of Covid, 2020, pp. 1–35. Available at: www.childrenscommissioner.gov.uk/report/childhood-in-the-time-of-covid/.

33. Ofqual, Learning during the pandemic: Quantifying lost time, 2021. Available at: www.gov.uk/government/publications/learning-during-the-pandemic/learning-during-the-pandemic-quantifying-lost-time.

34. T. Havard, Domestic abuse and Covid-19: A year into the pandemic, n.d. Available at: https://commonslibrary.parliament.uk/domestic-abuse-and-covid-19-a-year-into-the-pandemic/.

35. L. Donaldson, *Chief Medical Officer Annual Report*, London, Department of Health, 2002.

36. Organisation for Economic Co-operation and Development, OECD statistics: Overweight and obesity among adults, 2021. Available at: www.oecd-ilibrary.org/sites/ae3016b9-en/1/3/4/6/index.html?itemId=/content/publication/ae3016b9-en&_csp_=ca413da5d44587bc564463 41952c275e&itemIGO=oecd&itemContentType=book.

37. NHS Digital, National Child Measurement Programme, England, provisional 2021/22 school year outputs, 2022. Available at: https://digital.nhs.uk/data-and-information/publications/statistical/national-child-measurement-programme/england-provisional-2021-22-school-year-outputs.

38. Government Office for Science, Foresight: Tackling obesities: Future choices – summary of key messages, 2007. Available at: https://assets.publishing.service.gov.uk/government/uploads/system/uploads/attachment_data/file/287943/07-1469x-tackling-obesities-future-choices-summary.pdf.

39. Prime Minister's Office, Childhood obesity: A plan for action, 2017. Available at: www.gov .uk/government/publications/childhood-obesity-a-plan-for-action/childhood-obesity-a-plan-for-action.

40. Department of Health and Social Care, Tackling obesity: Empowering adults and children to live healthier lives, 2020, pp. 1–15. Available at: www.gov.uk/government/publications/ tackling-obesity-government-strategy/tackling-obesity-empowering-adults-and-children-to-live-healthier-lives.

41. National Health Service, Get help to buy food and milk (the Healthy Start scheme), 2022. Available at: www.healthystart.nhs.uk/.

42. National Health Service, Better health, healthier families, 2022. Available at: www.nhs.uk/ healthier-families/.

43. Department for Environment Food & Rural Affairs, Government food strategy, 2022. Available at: www.gov.uk/government/publications/government-food-strategy/govern ment-food-strategy.

44. Department for Education, Healthy schools rating scheme – guidance, 2019. Available at: www.gov.uk/government/publications/healthy-schools-rating-scheme.

45. L. A. Daniels, Feeding practices and parenting: A pathway to child health and family happiness, *Annals of Nutrition & Metabolism* **74**(Suppl. 2), 2019, 29–42.

46. M. Murphy and P. Fogarty, Chapter 10: Mental health problems in children and young people, 2012. Available at: https://assets.publishing.service.gov.uk/government/uploads/ system/uploads/attachment_data/file/252660/33571_2901304_CMO_Chapter_10.pdf.

47. Office for Health Improvement and Disparities, Wellbeing and mental health: Applying all our health, 2022. Available at: www.gov.uk/government/publications/wellbeing-in-mental-health-applying-all-our-health/wellbeing-in-mental-health-applying-all-our-health.

48. NHS Digital, Mental health of children and young people in England, 2017 [PAS], 2018. Available at: https://digital.nhs.uk/data-and-information/publications/statistical/mental-health-of-children-and-young-people-in-england/2017/2017.

49. Children's Commissioner, The Big Answer, 2021. Available at: www.childrenscommissioner .gov.uk/the-big-answer.

50. J. Campion, Public mental health: Evidence, practice and commissioning, Royal Society for Public Health, 2019. Available at: www.rsph.org.uk/our-work/policy/wellbeing/public-mental-health-evidence-practice-and-commissioning.html.

51. Public Health England, The mental health of children and young people in England, 2016. Available at: chrome-extension://efaidnbmnnnibpcajpcglclefindmkaj/https://assets .publishing.service.gov.uk/government/uploads/system/uploads/attachment_data/file/575632/ Mental_health_of_children_in_England.pdf.

52. Department for Education, Guidance: Promoting and supporting mental health and well-being in schools and colleges, 2021. Available at: www.gov.uk/guidance/mental-health-and-wellbeing-support-in-schools-and-colleges.

12

Adult Public Health and Non-Communicable Diseases

Sara Godward

Key points

- Adults aged 15 to 64 years account for a sizeable proportion of the population (over 60%) worldwide and within the UK.
- Non-communicable diseases such as cardiovascular disease and cancer are the leading causes of death in high-income countries. In low-income countries, communicable (infectious) diseases, maternal, perinatal and nutritional conditions and injuries are the leading causes of death, but the prevalence of non-communicable diseases is fast increasing.
- Among adults of working age, in the UK, cancers, cardiovascular diseases, Type 2 diabetes, mental health conditions (predominantly anxiety and depression), overweight and obesity are the significant public health problems.
- Health policies are in place to tackle these conditions, but making a significant impact on the burden of ill health requires effective prevention through the joined-up efforts of local and national government, with the engagement of local communities.

12.1 Introduction

In 2020, approximately 65% of the world's population was estimated to be aged between 15 and 64 years, with a male: female ratio of 1.02. In low-income countries, this age group represents only 55% of the total population [1].

In 2020, 64% of the UK population were aged between 15 and 64 years (see Figure 11.4). Although the total UK population has continued to grow, in 2020 the number of deaths exceeded the number of live births for the first time since 1976. The old-age dependency ratio (number of people of state pensionable age (SPA) and over for every 1,000 people aged 16 to SPA) in the UK was 280 in 2020; and is projected to rise to 352 by 2041 as the population ages [2]. This has led to calls for the

SPA to be raised, with measures to keep people in work at older ages (e.g. investment in health at work, flexible working arrangements, tailored re-training opportunities, etc.) [3].

This chapter considers the major causes of mortality and morbidity for adults and describes the significant burden of these non-communicable diseases, their risk factors and potential public health action. While the conditions discussed are relevant to other age groups, those included – cancers, cardiovascular disease, diabetes, obesity, mental health problems and long COVID – have particular relevance for the large proportion of the population of working age. Public health action for communicable disease is covered in Chapter 10. Box 12.2 also considers the specific opportunities within the workplace to improve health and well-being.

Chapter 8 describes wider opportunities for tackling the underlying structural factors contributing to the development and progression of these diseases, and Chapter 15 describes in further detail the broad-based policy decisions needed to impact on population health. This chapter therefore focuses on specific actions or policies which can be employed to address each of these non-communicable diseases.

12.2 Causes of Mortality and Morbidity

As described in Chapter 1, the average life expectancy at birth has increased globally over the past five decades to 72.8 years in 2019, and healthy life expectancy has increased to 63.7 years [4]. This is largely due to gains in maternal and child health, and major investments and improvements in communicable disease programmes such as for HIV, tuberculosis and malaria: these are discussed further in Chapter 10. The rate of improvement was already slowing before the COVID-19 pandemic led to a fall in life expectancy in 2020. The fall coinciding with COVID-19 was largely seen in the high-income countries and most notably in North America (1.4 years). Although there has been a greater than 10-year improvement in life expectancy in low-income countries recently (compared to a 3-year improvement in high-income countries), there remains a large gap in life expectancy between high- and low-income countries (80.2 and 64. 1 years respectively) [1].

Adult mortality rates have been largely declining over the last 50 years. This is largely attributable to reductions in non-communicable diseases, but the relative importance of a range of causes differs between high- and low-income countries, with non-communicable diseases predominating in high-income countries and communicable diseases, maternal, perinatal and nutritional conditions, and injuries being leading causes of mortality in low-income countries (as described further in Chapter 16) [5]. Population ageing and changes in risk factor distributions in many low-income countries, however, are fuelling an epidemic of non-communicable diseases.

Table 12.1 Mortality among 15–64-year-olds, 2021, England and Wales [6]

Underlying cause of death	Number of deaths (%)
Cancers	13,850 (39)
Diseases of the circulatory system	5,266 (15)
External causes of morbidity and mortality	3,198 (9)
Diseases of the digestive system	3,277 (9)
Diseases of the respiratory system	1,992 (6)
Other causes	7,824 (22)
Total deaths	**35,407 (100.0)**

In the UK, life expectancy at birth was 79.0 years for males and 82.9 years for females in 2018–20, having increased steadily over the previous 20 years, with a slightly higher increase in males than females. The median age at death was 82.3 years for males and 85.8 years for females [1].

The leading causes of mortality among adults aged 15 to 64 years in the UK are shown in Table 12.1. Cancers account for 39% of the deaths, followed by diseases of the circulatory system, which constitute 15% of all deaths [6]. In terms of the burden of ill health in this age group, in addition to living with cancers and cardiovascular diseases, conditions such as obesity, diabetes and mental illness are significant public health challenges. More recently, long COVID, or post COVID syndrome, has also become an important public health issue, affecting 2 million people in the UK in mid-2022 [7].

12.3 Cancer

12.3.1 Burden of Disease

Globally, there are around 17 million cases of cancer each year and 9.6 million deaths. Worldwide, 40% of cancers are of the lung, female breast, bowel and prostate [8].

Although trends vary for individual cancer sites, mortality rates are decreasing for most cancers and are set to fall further, although notably, in the UK, mortality from cancers of the thyroid, liver and anus is set to increase.

12.3.2 Risk Factors

Decreases in many cancers, in particular lung cancer, are largely due to historic reductions in the prevalence of tobacco exposure. Around a third of cancer deaths are attributed to tobacco use. Earlier diagnosis through screening and the availability of more effective treatment also contributes to the fall in, for example, breast cancer. Many of the known risk factors for cancers are avoidable and cancer risk could be decreased further by making changes to individual lifestyles (see Table 12.2).

Table 12.2 Risk factors for cancers [9]

Risk factor	Is a risk factor for
Smoking	Many cancers, particularly lung cancer
Ultraviolet radiation	Malignant melanoma and non-melanoma skin cancer
Physical inactivity	Colon cancer
Obesity	Breast cancer in post-menopausal women, endometrial cancer and colon cancer
Diet	Cancers of the colon, rectum, stomach and prostate
Alcohol	Cancers of the mouth, pharynx, larynx, oesophagus and liver
Infections	Human papillomaviruses linked to cervical cancer, and hepatitis viruses to liver cancer

12.3.3 Prevention

Lifetime risk of a cancer diagnosis is around 50% and around 40% of cancers are considered preventable [9]. Using the terminology of the medical model described in Chapter 10, 'primary' prevention strategies aim to prevent the development of disease, particularly through avoidance or reduction of the risk factors set out in Table 12.2. For example, with the introduction of vaccination for human papillomavirus in 2008 (in girls) and 2019 (boys), a greater than 70% reduction in cervical cancer incidence is anticipated.

'Secondary' prevention refers to interventions to reduce the progression of the disease, and includes raising awareness of signs and symptoms, effective treatment and, importantly, screening (see Chapter 9). Breast cancer screening has been estimated to save around 1,300 [10] lives per year in England due to earlier detection of breast cancer. Mortality rates from cervical cancer have fallen by 75% since the early 1970s when screening was introduced [11]. Studies have shown that screening can reduce bowel cancer mortality by 15% in those screened [12] and a national screening programme for bowel cancer was established in 2010. Introduction of population screening for prostate screening is at present not supported by evidence of effectiveness.

At the 'tertiary' prevention level, the aim is to lessen the impact of an on-going illness or injury. Rehabilitation and palliative care remain important aspects of cancer health-care.

12.3.4 Implications for Policy

In the UK, the Long Term Plan [13] sets out a comprehensive strategy for the British National Health Service (NHS) over the next 10 years. This plans to tackle cancer through prevention, earlier diagnosis and improvements in access to high-quality treatment and care. Core20PLUS5 [14], the NHS approach to reducing inequalities (see Chapter 14 for further details), includes early diagnosis of cancer as one of its five clinical areas. Its stated aim is diagnosis of 75% of cases at stage 1 or 2 by 2028.

12.4 Cardiovascular Diseases

12.4.1 Burden of Disease

Circulatory and heart diseases, often collectively known as cardiovascular diseases (CVD), are one of the leading causes of death in adults of working age in the UK, responsible for more than 19% of deaths in people of working age [6]. Mortality from CVD is falling in the UK, but death rates are still higher than those in some Western European countries. Despite the falling death rates, the burden of mortality and morbidity from CVD is still high, with approximately 7.6 million people in the UK living with heart or circulatory disease [15].

There are socioeconomic and genetic inequalities in cardiovascular mortality rates. The highest mortality rates are concentrated primarily within urban areas with higher historical levels of deprivation, tobacco use and poor diets. A South Asian ethnicity is associated with a higher rate of cardiovascular disease, and a higher prevalence of cardiovascular disease including hypertension contributed to higher death rates from COVID-19 (see Chapter 14).

Overall, CVD is estimated to cost the UK economy £9 billion a year in direct health-care costs and an additional £19 billion due to productivity losses and the informal care of people with CVD [16]. As mortality decreases and morbidity increases, a shift in care from acute medicine to chronic disease management is required and new models of health-care delivery are needed to cope with this.

12.4.2 Risk Factors

Although treatments for these diseases continue to be developed and improved, the proportion of people dying from heart attacks remains high. Since most heart disease is potentially preventable, the focus should be on prevention. Epidemiological studies have identified a number of risk factors for cardiovascular diseases (see Table 12.3).

12.4.3 Prevention

The main intervention to reduce the impact of CVD is the primary prevention of smoking and support to stopping smoking. Ways to achieve this include education programmes, smoking cessation interventions which support smokers to quit, tobacco taxation and legislation to ban smoking in public places. Obesity is also a major risk factor, and interventions should focus on healthier diets (reduced salt, saturated fat, total fat and harmful levels of alcohol consumption, and increased fruit and vegetable consumption) and increased physical activity (see Chapter 8).

Table 12.3 Risk factors for CVD [16]

Non-modifiable risk factors for CVD	Modifiable risk factors for CVD
Older age	High serum cholesterol
Male gender	Hypertension
Ethnicity	Smoking
Family history	Second-hand smoke
Genetic predisposition	Diet high in fat and salt, and low in fruit and vegetables
	Obesity (particularly central obesity)
	Diabetes
	Physical inactivity
	High blood-cholesterol levels

Health policies that create conducive environments for making healthy choices affordable and available are essential for motivating people to adopt and sustain healthy behaviours.

The effects of behavioural risk factors may result in raised blood pressure, and high blood sugar and cholesterol levels. These can be measured in primary care facilities and indicate an increased risk of heart attack, stroke, heart failure and other complications. Early detection and treatment of these risk factors is a form of secondary prevention.

Identifying those at highest risk of CVDs and ensuring they receive appropriate treatment can prevent premature deaths. Access to non-communicable disease medicines and basic health technologies in all primary health-care facilities is essential to ensure that those in need receive treatment and counselling.

While smoking prevalence is largely falling, levels of heavy drinking have not and obesity levels are rising [16]. Around two-thirds of adults are physically active, but activity levels are lower in more deprived areas and in older people. Diabetes (see later) substantially increases the risk of heart disease in both sexes. It also magnifies the effect of other risk factors such as cholesterol levels, hypertension, smoking and obesity. The focus of tertiary prevention is high-quality care and rehabilitation.

12.4.4 Implications for Policy

In 2016, the WHO and the US Centers for Disease Control and Prevention established the 'Global Hearts Initiative' [17]. The initiative is made up of five technical packages, including the MPOWER package for tobacco control, the ACTIVE package for increasing physical activity, the SHAKE package for salt reduction, the REPLACE package to eliminate industrially produced trans-fat from the global food supply and the HEARTS technical package to strengthen the detection and management of CVD in primary health-care.

Since CVD is both one of the largest contributors to inequalities in life expectancy and largely preventable, it follows that significant efforts on targeted prevention will tackle inequalities. Many high-income countries already have a national programme of CVD health checks and Core20PLUS5 [15], the NHS approach to reducing inequalities, includes hypertension case finding and optimal management and cholesterol management as one of its five clinical areas (see Chapter 16).

12.5 Type 2 Diabetes

12.5.1 Burden of Disease

The rising number of people diagnosed with diabetes is due to the ageing population and the increasing prevalence of obesity. Type 1 diabetes is a disease of insulin deficiency, usually caused by destruction of the pancreas. Type 2 diabetes involves insulin resistance, whereby the body can no longer respond to insulin efficiently. Most (90%) is Type 2 diabetes, which is both preventable and can be brought into remission [18].

Diabetes is a significant cause of morbidity and mortality. People with diabetes have a lower life expectancy and they are more likely to develop coronary heart disease and stroke. Diabetes is the leading cause of blindness among those of a working age in the UK and the NHS spends at least 10% of its budget each year on diabetes care [19]. If undiagnosed, untreated or not managed effectively, diabetes has a high risk of complications. Often, complications begin before diagnosis (50% of individuals have evidence of complications on diagnosis of Type 2 diabetes). However, if managed effectively, complications of diabetes can be reduced considerably and life expectancy can be increased.

12.5.2 Risk Factors

Due to its aetiology, Type 1 diabetes almost always occurs in individuals under the age of 40 years, whereas Type 2 diabetes generally tends to occur in those over the age of 40. Changing lifestyle factors are resulting in Type 2 diabetes being detected in younger individuals. In the UK, the prevalence of diabetes is at least six times higher among individuals from Asian communities and about three times higher in individuals from African and African-Caribbean communities (see Table 12.4). Diabetes often appears before the age of 40 among these individuals. A genetic predisposition is known to exist in both types of diabetes, although the disease is determined by complex gene–environment interactions. Around 80-90% of individuals with Type 2 diabetes are overweight [19].

Table 12.4 Risk factors for diabetes [19]

Ethnicity (African-Caribbean or South Asian)
Genetic predisposition
Overweight and obesity
Physical inactivity

12.5.3 Prevention

The pattern of risk factors means that effective primary prevention should focus on increasing physical activity levels, improving diet and nutrition, and reducing overweight and obesity. Secondary prevention includes increased awareness of symptoms, follow-up and regular testing of individuals known to be at increased risk of developing diabetes, the opportunistic testing of people with multiple risk factors for diabetes, and screening for retinopathy.

The risk of complications due to diabetes is high, which makes tertiary prevention important. Early detection and treatment of microvascular complications (retinopathy, nephropathy, neuropathy) can prevent impairment. Control of hypertension, reduction of cholesterol levels and smoking cessation in people with diabetes reduces their risk of developing both microvascular complications and cardiovascular disease, and regular recall and review of people with diabetes improves the subsequent outcomes.

12.5.4 Implications for Policy

In 2021, the WHO, together with the Canadian government, launched the Global Diabetes Compact [20] to galvanise efforts to both reduce the risk of diabetes and ensure that all people diagnosed with diabetes have access to equitable, comprehensive, affordable and quality treatment and care, including during humanitarian emergencies. The highest increases in diabetes globally are expected in Africa. The number of people suffering from the disease is predicted to rise to 55 million by 2045 – a 134% spike compared with 2021. At 70%, the continent also has the world's highest number of people who do not know they have diabetes. COVID-19 increased the risk of death in people with diabetes (an estimated 25% of COVID-19 deaths were linked), which has led to calls for earlier treatment and better care. In low-income countries, the lower costs of primary prevention over management mean that investment in knowledge and skills among professionals, raising awareness of the causes and symptoms in the wider population and lobbying for better labelling by the food and beverage industries is of particular benefit [21].

Initiatives like the NHS Diabetes Programme [19] focus on secondary prevention (i.e. treatment and care):

1. ensuring patients have access to specialist multidisciplinary foot-care teams with an aim of reducing amputations;
2. ensuring patients have access to diabetes inpatient specialist nursing teams in hospitals to improve the quality of their care;

3. reducing variation in the achievement of the three NICE recommended treatment targets (HbA1c (blood sugar), cholesterol and blood pressure) for adults and one treatment target (HbA1c) for children; and
4. expanding provision of structured education (including digital options) to better support patient self-management.

12.6 Obesity

12.6.1 Burden of Disease

Obesity is caused by a sustained imbalance between the energy intake (higher) and energy expenditure (lower). The main measures for assessment of obesity are described in Box 12.1.

Box 12.1 Assessment of body weight and obesity

1. **Body mass index (BMI).** This is measured as weight (kg) divided by height squared (m), and classified into four categories, as shown in Table 12.5.

Table 12.5 Body mass index

Classification	BMI (kg/m^2)
Underweight	<18.5
Healthy weight	18.5–24.9
Overweight	25.0–29.9
Obese	30.0 or more

The risk of morbidity and mortality rises with increases in BMI over 25, the risk of co-morbidities being very severe in individuals with morbid obesity (i.e. BMI of 40 or more), particularly among individuals with central obesity (see below).

2. **Waist circumference.** 'Central obesity' refers to the excess accumulation of fat in the abdominal area, which increases fat around organs such as the liver and pancreas. Higher central obesity is correlated with higher diabetes risk, with cut-off points indicating risk of co-morbidities as follows:

    80 cm (31.5 inches) for all women;

    94 cm (37 inches) for most men;

    90 m (35 inches) for South Asian men.

3. **Waist–hip ratio.** This is calculated as the waist circumference (m) divided by the hip circumference (m).

Values of 0.95 or more among men and 0.85 or more among women are correlated with a higher risk of diabetes.

Obesity is a significant public health problem globally [22], where around 13% of adults are obese, at least 40% are overweight or obese, and there is an increasing trend of rising obesity in both adults and children (see also Chapter 11). The prevalence of obesity in the UK has risen year on year from 15% in 1993 to nearly 30% in 2018 [16]. The relative increase is much higher among women than men. Obesity contributed to higher death rates in the COVID-19 pandemic [23].

Obesity is associated with increased mortality and morbidity and a decreased quality of life. Health problems associated with obesity are shown in Table 12.6.

Metabolic syndrome is the medical term for a combination of diabetes, high blood pressure (hypertension) and obesity.

Table 12.6 Effect of obesity on health

Greatly increased risk of:	Moderately increased risk of:	Slightly increased risk of:
Type 2 diabetes	Coronary heart disease	Breast cancer in post-menopausal women, colon cancer
Insulin resistance	Hypertension	Polycystic ovaries
Gall bladder diseases	Stroke	Risk of anaesthetic complications
Dyslipidaemia	Osteoarthritis (knees and hips)	Impaired fertility
Breathlessness	Hyperuricaemia and gout	Low back pain
Sleep apnoea	Psychological factors	Reproductive hormone abnormalities

12.6.2 Risk Factors

Table 12.7 lists risk factors associated with a higher risk of obesity. Although at the metabolic level, obesity usually derives from an individual's imbalance between nutritional inputs and energy outputs, as described in Chapter 11, this is an over-simplification that hides a complex problem with significant structural and multidimensional contributory factors. The rise in global obesity has been linked to environmental and behavioural changes (e.g. sedentary lifestyles, easy access to high-calorie, low-cost foods) brought about by economic development, modernisation and urbanisation.

Table 12.7 Risk factors for obesity [22]

Older age
Female sex
Lower socioeconomic status
Black Caribbean and Black African ethnicity (obesity is low in Chinese populations)
Physical inactivity

12.6.3 Prevention

The *population* approach to primary prevention for obesity seeks to lower the risk of becoming overweight or obese in the whole community. It consists largely of two elements: promoting a balanced diet and increasing physical activity levels in the community.

The *high-risk* approach to primary prevention concentrates on individuals who have an increased chance of becoming overweight or obese, such as individuals from lower socioeconomic classes, individuals from South Asian communities (increased risk of diseases caused by obesity), Black Caribbean and Black African individuals (higher prevalence of obesity), people with physical disabilities affecting mobility and people with learning difficulties.

For secondary prevention in those already overweight or obese, for weight management to be effective and sustainable, a combination of advice on diet and physical activity, and motivation and support to make and maintain these changes, are essential. This underpins the design of public sector-commissioned local weight management programmes. For some individuals, drug treatment and surgery may be additional options to consider.

12.6.4 Implications for Policy

Policy to tackle obesity is multifactorial [24]. It includes efforts in primary prevention (e.g. legislation on food content, advertising and labelling, infrastructure projects promoting active travel, and universal but tailored educational programmes) and nutrition training for health professionals. Chapter 11 presents a useful case study on strategies for tackling childhood obesity. Investment in secondary prevention includes emphasis on brief interventions and expanded provision of weight management programmes. Tertiary prevention may include surgery.

In an attempt to curb the increased prevalence of obesity, from October 2022 the UK government aims to restrict the promotion of food and drinks high in fat, salt or sugar (HFSS) in large and medium retailers [25].

12.7 Mental Health

12.7.1 Burden of Disease

Definitions of mental health include concepts such as psychological well-being, autonomy, competence, intergenerational dependence, and actualisation of one's intellectual and emotional potential. Although it is difficult to define mental health comprehensively, it is generally agreed that mental health is broader than a lack of mental illness.

The WHO defines 'mental health' as 'a state of well-being in which the individual realises his or her own abilities, can cope with the normal stresses of life, can work productively and fruitfully, and is able to make a contribution to his or her community' [26]. The term 'mental illness' refers to health conditions characterised by alterations in thinking, mood or behaviour associated with distress and/or impaired functioning.

Mental health conditions are common and increasing worldwide. The WHO estimates that mental health conditions now constitute 1 in 5 years lived with disability and that a quarter of all people suffer from mental health and behavioural conditions at some time during their lives, with a prevalence of about one in eight among the adult population at any given time [26]. Even higher prevalence is expected in more recent years as a consequence of events including the COVID-19 pandemic, political and economic pressures and continuing humanitarian crises. While effective prevention and treatment options exist, most people with mental health conditions do not have access to effective care. Many people also experience stigma, discrimination and violations of human rights.

Common mental health conditions in people of working age include anxiety disorders, social depression, bipolar disorder, post-traumatic stress disorder, schizophrenia and neurodevelopmental disorders.

At any one time, individual, family, community and structural factors may combine to either protect or undermine mental health. Although most people are resilient, people who are exposed to adverse circumstances – including poverty, violence, disability and inequality – are at higher risk. Protective risk factors include individual psychological and biological factors, such as emotional skills, as well as genetics.

Mental health conditions are often co-morbid with other mental or physical health conditions. For example, up to two-thirds of people with a physical long-term condition also have anxiety and/or depression.

Globally, among people aged 15–49, self-harm accounted for 6% of deaths and years of life lost in 2019 [5]. The rates are higher in high-income countries. The trend is falling in both, but in Australia, for example, suicide is the leading cause of death in people between the ages of 15 and 44 [27]. The rate among Aboriginal and Torres Strait Islander peoples is twice that of their non-Indigenous counterparts, the rate is twice as high in people living rurally and 75% are male. It is estimated that the impact of suicide deaths is felt by up to 135 people, including family members, work colleagues, friends and first responders at the time of death [28].

12.7.2 Risk Factors

Table 12.8 describes key risk factors for poor mental health. Age is an important determinant of mental illness and the prevalence of some mental health conditions (e.g. depression) rises with age. There is little difference in the overall prevalence of mild to moderate mental health conditions by sex [27]. This is also true for severe mental health conditions, except depression, which has a higher prevalence among females, and substance misuse, which has a higher prevalence among males. The sex

Table 12.8 Risk factors for mental health problems
Age
Female sex (for depression)
Exposure to violence, conflict and disasters
Stressful life events
Ethnic minority status
Low socioeconomic status
Genetic predisposition

difference in some mental health conditions could be due to a higher exposure to domestic and sexual violence among women. In 2021, nearly 1.5 million (5.5%) adults aged 16 to 74 in England and Wales reported a domestic-abuse-related crime, continuing the trend of a year-on-year increase of around 6%. In 96% of sexual assaults, the victim was female [29].

Research suggests the existence of a genetic predisposition to mental health conditions such as schizophrenia, depression and dementia. However, common mental health conditions are twice as high among the lowest socioeconomic categories as compared to the highest category in both high- and low-income countries. Conditions such as schizophrenia are reported to be higher among British-born ethnic-minority populations. Explanatory factors suggested include increased vulnerability due to social isolation and fewer social networks [30]. Mental health and behavioural conditions such as schizophrenia, depression and suicide show an association with life events (job insecurity, bereavement, relationship breakdown, change of residence, business failure, etc.), particularly if they occur in quick succession. War, civil strife and natural disasters affect several million people worldwide and have a huge effect on the mental health of the people affected. Common mental health conditions reported include mental distress, post-traumatic stress disorder, depression and anxiety.

12.7.3 Prevention

The importance of good mental health and well-being for the individual and society is increasingly recognised and our understanding has been strengthened by our experiences with the COVID-19 pandemic. As described earlier, good mental health is more than the absence of mental illness. Promotion of good mental health is multifactorial.

There is a need to increase prevention activities universally and to offer targeted and more support to particular groups (i.e. an approach of proportionate universalism).

Primary prevention could include community development projects to improve green and blue spaces, promote social networks and social capital, create opportunities for high-quality employment, and education programmes to raise awareness of mental health issues and build skills in resilience. Secondary and tertiary prevention might include improved access to talking therapies, debt reduction advice, support by telephone or online, medication and back-to-work programmes.

At national level, legislation can be enacted to reduce discrimination and to set aside funding for mental health promotion, support and services.

A significant shift will require multi-agency working (health and social care; the voluntary and private sectors; housing, employment and training; and the community), with the same objective in mind across all sectors and levels, maintained for a sufficient period to embed change.

Chapter 11 presents a case study outlining potential risks for adverse mental health in children and interventions which aim to improve mental health in children and offer support and care where required.

12.7.4 Implications for Policy

In many parts of the world, mental health and mental health conditions receive a low priority in terms of funding for health-care, and a low relative priority compared to physical health, with only a minority of people receiving any treatment. According to the WHO, although mental health and behavioural conditions constitute 12% of the global burden of disease, the mental health budgets of many countries are less than 1% of their total expenditures [26].

The WHO's Comprehensive Mental Health Action Plan 2013–2030 [31] recognises the essential role of mental health in achieving health for all people. The plan includes four major objectives:

- to strengthen effective leadership and governance for mental health;
- to provide comprehensive, integrated and responsive mental health and social care services in community-based settings;
- to implement strategies for promotion and prevention in mental health; and
- to strengthen information systems, evidence and research for mental health.

New South Wales in Australia offers an example of a targeted and holistic approach to improving Aboriginal mental health and well-being in recognition of the higher and specific cultural needs of this group [32].

12.8 Other Approaches

Examples of approaches to tackling individual lifestyle factors or the wider determinants of health are described elsewhere (see Chapters 8 and 14). Another approach for adults of working age can be to focus on the workplace. There is clear evidence [33] that good work improves health and well-being across people's lives and protects

Box 12.2 Examples of health and well-being interventions in the workplace

- A workplace may be able to improve workers' access to health checks or vaccinations (e.g. through hosting clinics or allowing time off during the working day to attend appointments).
- A workplace could allow employees to train as workplace health champions, raising awareness of the impact of common conditions such as the menopause, offering brief interventions and raising awareness among co-workers of signs and symptoms of disease or signposting for support.
- Some employers may offer initiatives to encourage healthy behaviours through incentives (e.g. including fruit in vending machines, support to active travel, etc.).

against social exclusion, but in addition the workplace in which working-age adults spend most of their waking hours is an opportunity for health improvement. Productivity is influenced by the health of individuals, which is in turn affected by conditions in the workplace.

Most employers recognise the symbiotic relationship between health and work, although smaller businesses tend to focus more exclusively on their legal responsibilities and be less proactive in promoting their employees' health [34]. Employers have legal obligations to provide a safe workplace that prevents work-related illness and accidents [35], but also provide a setting with existing communication mechanisms that can be used to promote and endorse health messages in addition to training about the specific safety messages for the role (see Box 12.2).

In adults of working age, poor health that leads to loss of employment is likely to worsen health and that of their families and efforts should be directed at all levels of prevention for the benefit of the individuals and their families and the cost to society.

12.9 Conclusions

This chapter has described the epidemiology and prevention of some common diseases and conditions which present public health challenges among adults aged 15 to 64 years. We have noted the risk factors in common that contribute to multiple causes of ill health (e.g. smoking and obesity), that some diseases are often co-morbid (e.g. long-term mental and physical health conditions) and that occurrence of one can increase the risk of another (e.g. diabetes and stroke).

It is recognised that prevention is a key component of any strategy to tackle these issues, and that in tackling prevention, inequalities can also be addressed. This chapter has considered approaches which focus on addressing a specific disease or group of similar diseases (e.g. cardiovascular health checks and cancer screening). This chapter also identifies the significant merits of concerted and integrated efforts across organisations and sectors to tackle complex health conditions simultaneously at different levels (e.g. mental health and well-being).

REFERENCES

1. The World Bank Databank, Health nutrition and population statistics. Available at: https://databank.worldbank.org/home.aspx
2. Office for National Statistics, National life tables – life expectancy in the UK: 2018 to 2020, released 25 September 2021. Available at: www.ons.gov.uk/peoplepopulationandcommunity/birthsdeathsandmarriages/lifeexpectancies/bulletins/nationallifetablesunitedkingdom/2018to2020
3. The Centre for Social Justice, Ageing confidently: Supporting an ageing workforce, 2019. Available at: www.centreforsocialjustice.org.uk/wp-content/uploads/2020/01/CSJJ7421-Ageing-Report-190815-WEB.pdf
4. The Global Health Observatory, Healthy life expectancy (HALE) at birth (years), World Health Organization. Available at: www.who.int/data/gho/data/indicators/indicator-details/GHO/gho-ghe-hale-healthy-life-expectancy-at-birth
5. The Institute for Health Metrics and Evaluation, Global burden of disease. Available at: www.healthdata.org/gbd/2019
6. Office for National Statistics, Deaths registered in England and Wales, 2021. Available at: www.ons.gov.uk/peoplepopulationandcommunity/birthsdeathsandmarriages/deaths/datasets/deathsregisteredinenglandandwalesseriesdrreferencetables
7. Office for National Statistics, Census 2021 – Prevalence of ongoing symptoms following coronavirus (COVID-19) infection in the UK: 1 December 2022. Available at: www.ons.gov.uk/peoplepopulationandcommunity/healthandsocialcare/conditionsanddiseases/bulletins/prevalenceofongoingsymptomsfollowingcoronaviruscovid19infectionintheuk/1december2022
8. Cancer Research UK, Worldwide cancer statistics. Available at: www.cancerresearchuk.org/health-professional/cancer-statistics/worldwide-cancer
9. World Health Organization, Preventing cancer. Available at: www.who.int/activities/preventing-cancer
10. National Health Service, How to decide if you want breast screening, September 2021. Available at: www.nhs.uk/conditions/breast-screening-mammogram/how-to-decide-if-you-want-breast-screening/
11. Cancer Research UK, Cervical cancer statistics. Available at: www.cancerresearchuk.org/health-professional/cancer-statistics/statistics-by-cancer-type/cervical-cancer
12. Bowel Cancer UK, The screening gap. Available at: www.bowelcanceruk.org.uk/news-and-blogs/research-blog/the-screening-gap/
13. National Health Service, NHS long term plan. Available at: www.longtermplan.nhs.uk/
14. NHS England, Core20PLUS5 (adults) – an approach to reducing healthcare inequalities. Available at: www.england.nhs.uk/about/equality/equality-hub/national-healthcare-inequalities-improvement-programme/core20plus5/

15. British Heart Foundation, Heart statistics, August 2022. Available at: www.bhf.org.uk/what-we-do/our-research/heart-statistics

16. Chief Medical Officer, Health trends and variation in England, London, Department of Health, 2020. Available at: www.gov.uk/government/publications/chief-medical-officers-annual-report-2020-health-trends-and-variation-in-england

17. World Health Organization, Global Hearts Initiative: Working together to promote cardiovascular health, September 2016. Available at: www.who.int/news/item/15-09-2016-global-hearts-initiative

18. Diabetes UK. Available at: www.diabetes.org.uk

19. NHS England, NHS Diabetes Prevention Programme (NHS DPP). Available at: www.england.nhs.uk/diabetes/diabetes-prevention/

20. World Health Organization, The WHO Global Diabetes Compact. Available at: www.who.int/initiatives/the-who-global-diabetes-compact

21. Diabetes Africa. Available at: https://diabetesafrica.org/

22. World Health Organization, Obesity. Available at: www.who.int/health-topics/obesity

23. Office for National Statistics, Census 2021 – Obesity and mortality during the coronavirus (COVID-19) pandemic, England: 24 January 2020 to 30 August 2022, October 2022. Available at: www.ons.gov.uk/peoplepopulationandcommunity/birthsdeathsandmarriages/deaths/articles/obesityandmortalityduringthecoronaviruscovid19pandemicengland24january2020to30august2022/24january2020to30august2022

24. Centers for Disease Control and Prevention, Nutrition, physical activity, and obesity prevention strategies. Available at: www.cdc.gov/obesity/resources/strategies-guidelines.html

25. UK Department of Health and Social Care, Restricting promotions of products high in fat, sugar and salt by location and by price: government response to public consultation, 19 July 2021. Available at: www.gov.uk/government/consultations/restricting-promotions-of-food-and-drink-that-is-high-in-fat-sugar-and-salt/outcome/restricting-promotions-of-products-high-in-fat-sugar-and-salt-by-location-and-by-price-government-response-to-public-consultation

26. World Health Organization, Mental health. Available at: www.who.int/health-topics/mental-health

27. Lifeline, Australia: Data and statistics. Available at: www.lifeline.org.au/resources/data-and-statistics/

28. J. Cerel, M. M. Brown, M. Maple *et al.*, How many people are exposed to suicide? Not six, *Suicide & Life-Threatening Behavior* **49**(2), 2019, 529–34.

29. Office for National Statistics, Census 2021 – Domestic abuse prevalence and trends, England and Wales: Year ending March 2021, 24 November 2021. Available at: www.ons.gov.uk/peoplepopulationandcommunity/crimeandjustice/articles/domesticabuseprevalenceandtrendsenglandandwales/yearendingmarch2021

30. Mental health Foundation, Black, Asian and minority ethnic (BAME) communities, 30 September 2021. Available at: www.mentalhealth.org.uk/explore-mental-health/a-z-topics/black-asian-and-minority-ethnic-bame-communities

31. World Health Organization, Comprehensive Mental Health Action Plan 2013–2030. Available at: www.who.int/publications/i/item/9789240031029

32. NSW Government, Australia, NSW Aboriginal mental health and Wellbeing Strategy 2020–2025. Available at: www.health.nsw.gov.au/mentalhealth/resources/Pages/aborig-mh-wellbeing-2020-2025.aspx

33. World Health Organization and J. Burton, WHO healthy workplace framework and model: Background and supporting literature and practices, 2010. Available at: https://apps.who .int/iris/handle/10665/113144

34. Department for Work & Pensions, Research and analysis – Summary: Sickness absence and health in the workplace: Understanding employer behaviour and practice, 20 July 2021. Available at: www.gov.uk/government/publications/sickness-absence-and-health-in-the-workplace-understanding-employer-behaviour-and-practice/sickness-absence-and-health-in-the-workplace-understanding-employer-behaviour-and-practice-summary

35. Health and Safety Executive, Health and safety guidance. Available at: www.hse.gov.uk/

13

Public Health and Ageing
Lincoln Sargeant and Louise Lafortune

Key points

- The population of older people has been increasing in number and as a proportion of populations worldwide.
- The prevalence of physical and cognitive frailty increases with age and, as a result, older people lose the intrinsic capacity and functional ability that enable them to live full and independent lives as they age.
- Prevention strategies need to focus on maintaining independence rather than avoidance of specific conditions.
- While primary, secondary and tertiary prevention play a role in avoiding, delaying and mitigating the impact of physical and cognitive decline, many older people will need support through health and social care.
- Informal carers, who are often relatives, provide the majority of social care for older people, with more formal arrangements possibly becoming necessary as functional ability or health status deteriorate.
- Policy responses to ageing populations need to promote independent living and financial and physical security, as well as health and social care provision, in order to encourage older people to be active participants in society.

13.1 Introduction

The proportion of the population living into old age has been increasing worldwide. For the first time in history, there are more older people than children under 5 years of age. The task for public health is to understand the relationships between ageing, health and the environment (physical, social and economic) in which people live, to promote healthy ageing and prevent the disability and subsequent dependency that is often associated with growing old.

This chapter examines the factors that lead to ageing populations and explores the health, social and economic consequences of the change in the population structure. It then goes on to outline strategies that can lead to healthy ageing and other public health actions that could help to manage the challenges posed – and the opportunities afforded – by the relative and absolute increase in the number of older people.

13.2 The Demography of Old Age

Falling fertility rates and increased infant survival since the late nineteenth and early twentieth centuries have contributed to a larger proportion of the population surviving to middle age. The population structure resembles a pyramid in a young population, but becomes more cylindrical as the population ages (see Chapter 2).

Adult survival has also increased since the mid-twentieth century following improvements in the prevention and treatment of major premature causes of death such as heart disease. More people survive to age 65. Improved life expectancy has also occurred in the older age groups, although there is great inequity in longevity according to economic and social groups. For example, it is estimated that more than 70% of the rise in the maximum age at death in Sweden, which rose from about 101 years during the 1860s to about 108 years during the 1990s, was attributable to reductions in death rates above age 70 [1]. Together, these trends have led to relative and absolute increases in the population at older ages, most marked in the oldest old.

Another phenomenon occurring in the mid-twentieth century indicates that further marked increases in the older population can be expected in developed countries in the next few decades. A rapid increase in fertility rates beginning with the end of the Second World War lasting into the 1960s gave rise to the 'baby boom' generation. This generation has now reached the 'young old' age category and will further exaggerate the ageing population profile in those developed countries, bringing with it changing expectations of health and social care provision.

'Old age' is often defined as beginning at age 65 years, but there is no biological rationale for this cut-off. It may be possible to define old age in terms of economic activity. In the UK, 65 years has been the age of retirement for men since 1908, but before then it was 70 years. Between 1970 and 2020, the average age of retirement has decreased slightly in men and women across European and many low-income countries. There is pressure, however, to increase, if not abolish, retirement ages and to increase the age at which state pensions are awarded. For instance, the pension age in the UK is now expected to reach 67 by 2028. In many emerging economies, populations carry on working into old age as state provision for older people is minimal or non-existent. Nevertheless, old age is often categorised as shown in Box 13.1.

Box 13.1 Old-age categories

Young old – 65 to 74 years
Middle old – 75 to 84 years
Oldest old – 85 years and over
Supercentenarians – 110 years and over

The economic activity of the working population supports children and economically inactive adults such as retired older people. Dependency ratios are used to summarise the balance of economically active to inactive members of a society. The total dependency ratio is the ratio of the number of persons aged 65 and over (age when they are generally economically inactive) and the number of persons aged between 15 and 64. The value is expressed per 100 persons of working age (15–64). One constituent of this, the old-age dependency ratio, averaged 30.4% for OECD countries in 2020 and is projected to be over 52% in 2050. A high dependency ratio has the potential to limit the available funds for pensions and health-care of older people, and can have a profound impact on societies, especially those in lower-income countries, where the rate of ageing has been faster than in the West.

However, experience of old age varies greatly. People over 65 years can, and do, continue to contribute economically and are not necessarily dependent on the 'working-age population'. Pension and retirement ages are changing in many societies (where they exist). Many older individuals support economically active younger family members through childcare, provide social care as unpaid carers for frail or disabled family members, and contribute to their community in a myriad of ways. Furthermore, the on-going COVID-19 pandemic has meant that in some cases older people have been supporting adult children through the economic downturn.

13.3 Ageing and Health

Ageing is related to ill health in one of three main ways:

- Some conditions are associated with ageing in that they can be expected to occur with all individuals as they age. High-frequency hearing, for example, declines predictably with age.
- Ill health can occur in older people because resilience decreases with age. For example, a fall in an older person is more likely to lead to fractures because of bone loss than in a young person.
- Some diseases are very closely associated with ageing, such as Alzheimer's disease. Influences over the life course determine health in old age.

As described in Chapters 10 and 11, events during foetal life affect the risk of conditions such as diabetes and heart disease later in life, but there is evidence that these influences can be modified or interrupted by adopting healthy lifestyle choices at any stage [2].

Cognitive and physical frailty increase with age and have adverse consequences in terms of morbidity and mortality, and also disability and possible need for help with daily activities (see Box 13.2). This means that increasing proportions of people, as they age, need more support to perform activities of daily living, such as bathing and dressing (Box 13.3).

Box 13.2 Healthy ageing

Functional ability comprises the health-related attributes that enable people to be and to do what they have reason to value. It is made up of the intrinsic capacity of the individual, relevant environmental characteristics and the interactions between the individual and these characteristics.

Intrinsic capacity is the composite of all the physical and mental capacities of an individual.

Environments comprise all the factors in the extrinsic world that form the context of an individual's life. These include – from the micro-level to the macro-level – home, communities and the broader society.

Disability data identify problems towards the severe end of the spectrum and later on in life. In contrast, distinguishing between environment changes and decline in intrinsic capacity, which generally starts small and much earlier in life, allows for earlier interventions to foster healthy ageing [3].

Box 13.3 Activities and instrumental activities of daily living

Activities of daily living
- Dressing, including putting on shoes and socks
- Walking across a room
- Bathing or showering
- Eating, such as cutting up food
- Getting in or out of bed
- Using the toilet, including getting up or down

Instrumental activities of daily living
- Using a map to figure out how to get around in a strange place
- Preparing a hot meal
- Shopping for groceries
- Making telephone calls
- Taking medications
- Doing work around the house or garden
- Managing money, such as paying bills and keeping track of expenses

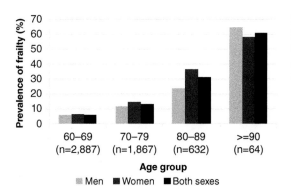

Figure 13.1 Weighted
prevalence of frailty in the
English Longitudinal Study of
Ageing, by age and sex
(2008–09) [4].

Figure 13.1 shows the weighted prevalence of frailty by age and sex from the English Longitudinal Study of Ageing [4]. Among frail individuals, difficulties in performing activities or instrumental activities of daily living were reported by 57% or 64%, respectively, versus 13% or 15%, respectively, among the non-frail individuals. Data from a study published in 2022 suggest that the prevalence of frailty in adults aged 50+ in England was estimated to be 8.1% (95% CI 7.3–8.8%), with substantial geographic variation and higher prevalence of frailty in urban than rural areas, and coastal compared with inland areas [5].

The strong association of ill health and disability with age has led to concerns that as the population ages, so will the burden of ill health. It should be noted that whereas the health-care costs of ill health are concentrated at the end of life, irrespective of the age of death, the support and social care burden arises when disability sets in.

There is limited data on the overall effect of a longer life span on time spent in ill health. The worst-case scenario (see Figure 13.2) is that with increased life expectancy a greater proportion of time is spent in ill health. The Office for National Statistics estimates that, for the period 2017–19, healthy life expectancy at age 65 for UK men was 72% of overall life expectancy at that age. For women, the proportion was 58.5% [6].

Strategies for healthy ageing have aimed at keeping people in good health as long as possible. In 2015, the World Health Organization adopted the term 'healthy ageing' to signal that the ageing process can be so [3]. Healthy ageing is not merely a disease-free state that distinguishes between healthy and unhealthy individuals. It is based on life-course and functional perspectives, and defined as 'the process of developing and maintaining the functional ability that enables well-being in older age'. This clearly includes broader themes than just health.

Key factors for promoting healthy ageing relate to the role of the social and neighbourhood environment. Both individual and neighbourhood deprivation are associated with poor health, but the associations are not straightforward and specific mechanisms are not understood. A systematic review found that neighbourhood

Figure 13.2 Scenarios for
healthy life expectancy.

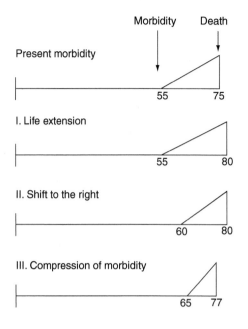

socioeconomic composition was the strongest and most consistent predictor of a variety of health outcomes, in particular the positive association between the physical environment, perceived or objective, and physical activity [7].

13.4 Prevention

Promoting healthy ageing has many facets, but any public health approach to healthy ageing needs to consider the major preventable health threats in old age. The major chronic conditions are listed in Box 13.4 [8], most of which are described in more detail in Chapter 12. Multi-morbidity is a common feature in old age and frailty rather than age predicts risk of hospitalisation, care home admission and death. The focus of prevention therefore needs to be on promoting independence rather than avoiding, delaying or ameliorating the impact of specific disease conditions.

13.4.1 Primary Prevention

Prevention of chronic disease starts with promotion of healthy lifestyles in earlier life, but is also beneficial in old age. Studies have identified modifiable predictors for 5-year mortality risk in older people living in the community [9, 10]. Physical inactivity, a history of smoking, low body mass index and high blood pressure were among the modifiable factors identified to increased risk of death. Promoting physical activity in older people is an effective primary prevention strategy for conditions such as heart

> **Box 13.4 Health conditions affecting older people [8]**
>
> - Cardiovascular disease (such as coronary heart disease)
> - Hypertension
> - Stroke
> - Diabetes
> - Cancer
> - Chronic obstructive pulmonary disease (COPD)
> - Musculo-skeletal conditions (such as arthritis and osteoporosis)
> - Mental health conditions (mostly dementia and depression)
> - Blindness and visual impairment
>
> Note: The causes of disability in older age are similar for men and women, although women are more likely to report musculo-skeletal problems.

disease, diabetes and dementia. Other primary prevention strategies such as blood pressure control are also highly effective in older people in preventing heart disease, stroke and dementia.

Malnutrition in older people is also a concern. The causes in this age group are complex, but poor nutrition may be a symptom of social isolation, functional disability and poverty [11]. Vitamin D is important for bone health, but may have other beneficial effects. Ensuring adequate nutrition, social engagement and intellectual stimulation are important primary prevention measures in older people.

Primary prevention is also relevant for acute illnesses in older people. During the winter months, the number of deaths among older people reaches higher levels than observed in the summer months. This 'excess winter mortality' is mainly due to acute respiratory illnesses, of which influenza is the most important. Primary prevention of excess winter mortality among older people can be achieved through vaccination against influenza.

13.4.2 Secondary Prevention

For other conditions, the opportunity for primary prevention in old age may be limited. In this context, secondary prevention may be appropriate where the condition can be detected and treated at an early stage, such as screening. For example, colorectal cancers develop slowly and prevention in older people often depends on early diagnosis through screening. Not all attempts at early diagnosis meet the criteria for screening (see Chapter 9), but may be valuable in helping older people and their carers to manage their independence and quality of life. For, example, early identification of frailty can be helpful in planning for future health and care needs.

13.4.3 Tertiary Prevention

Where primary or secondary prevention are not possible, the aim is to reduce the complications of disease. Many chronic illnesses have their onset in middle age, but have their greatest impact in old age. Ameliorating or preventing complications of these illnesses as well as rehabilitation are the mainstay of prevention for many older people. Appropriate management of diabetes, for example, aims to reduce disability that can result from lower-limb amputations and blindness.

As mentioned above, disability from physical and cognitive impairment limit the potential of older people to enjoy optimal health. The older population is susceptible to injury from falls and this is a major cause of disability and mortality in those aged over 75 years. Falls-prevention strategies make use of rehabilitation to reduce the disability that can occur with fractures that result from falls in this age group [12]. Dementia, the leading cause of cognitive impairment in the older population, is also a key threat to healthy ageing. The Lancet Commission on dementia prevention, intervention and care in its 2020 report identified 12 modifiable risk factors that could prevent or delay up to 40% of dementias [13].

13.5 Case Studies of Public Health and Ageing

These case studies explore two contemporary examples to illustrate the specific complexities and challenges of improving health and well-being in older people and reducing inequalities, and how these relate to the concepts described in the first part of the book.

13.5.1 Case study 1 Frailty

The challenges of prevention in the elderly can be illustrated by frailty prevention. Frailty is not an illness, but a syndrome that combines the effects of natural ageing with the outcomes of multiple long-term conditions, a loss of fitness and reserves. It describes the composite deficits that make someone less able to cope with physical and cognitive impairments, resulting in greater need for support to live independently. It is characterised by low physiological reserves, vulnerability to illness and high risk of disability, institutionalisation and death. About 13% of older people living in the community are thought to be frail [14].

Frailty prevention may focus on individual components or conditions that contribute to it, such as falls and dementia. Falls are estimated to occur in about 30% of the over-65 population. Although less than one fall in ten results in a fracture, a fifth of fall incidents require medical attention [15].

A Cochrane review [16] reported that exercise interventions reduced both the rate of falls and the risk of falling. Increasing physical activity and addressing other cardiovascular risk factors such as treating high blood pressure can prevent

Alzheimer's disease, as well as vascular dementia [13]. Primary prevention of frailty will therefore encompass several domains, including multicomponent exercise, nutrition, cognitive training and management of long-term conditions. There is some evidence that falls-prevention strategies can be cost saving [17].

Frailty indices have been developed that allow the identification of pre-frailty stages and detection of people at the early stages of frailty. These are based on the number of deficits a person has or on the number of frailty features exhibited [18]. There are also randomised controlled studies in which interventions that included physical activity components improved physical outcomes in pre-frail and frail older people [19]. Although there is no single agreed screening tool for frailty, research indicates that there is a pre-clinical state that can be identified and that effective interventions exist than can change the trajectory of frailty development, offering opportunities for secondary prevention.

Tertiary prevention seeks to reduce the risk of disability, hospitalisation, loss of independence and death that result from frailty. A holistic approach that incorporates physical activity, nutrition, cognitive and psychological rehabilitation, and social interventions is needed to prevent adverse outcomes from frailty. It also involves ameliorating the impact of issues such as falls that can accelerate the progress of frailty. For example, after a hip fracture, many older people are not able to return to independent living, with about 20% requiring nursing-home care. Mortality is high, with estimates of up to 40% within the first year after the fracture [20]. A Cochrane review found that rehabilitation after surgery by a multidisciplinary team and supervised by an appropriate medical specialist results in fewer cases of 'poor outcome' (death or deterioration in residential status) [17].

13.5.2 Case study 2 Loneliness and isolation

The effect of social isolation on health and well-being of older people has been increasingly recognised as an important modifiable factor [21]. Loneliness and social isolation are related but distinct concepts. Social isolation is concerned with social connections that can be objectively assessed, while loneliness is a subjective feeling. Both objective and subjective measures of social isolation are associated with increased risk of mortality [22]. The interaction between objective measures of social isolation and all-cause and cardiovascular disease mortality may be mediated in part through feelings of loneliness and depression. Loneliness in turn can influence behaviours such as physical activity and smoking and is associated with an increased risk of depression. These contribute to the adverse health outcomes experienced by people who report feeling lonely.

Although social isolation can predispose to loneliness, the quality of social contacts is more important than quantity in determining whether someone feels lonely. However, having a wide range of opportunities to build and maintain social networks increases the chances of having emotionally satisfying relationships that reduce our risk of loneliness. Primary prevention depends on having social environments that promote participation. This includes physical spaces where people can come together around shared interests and the ability to move easily between the social amenities in the community. For older people with mobility issues, removing barriers so they can access opportunities for social interaction would be an important primary prevention measure. Other barriers to social participation are more challenging than improving physical access and transport links. For example, perceptions of community safety and belonging will influence whether people feel they can form connections with others in their neighbourhood.

Identifying people at risk for social isolation and loneliness is possible, but there are no accepted tools that would be suitable for population screening. Since the response to social isolation is individual and it is not understood what may trigger feelings of loneliness in one person compared to another, there is no agreed 'treatment' that can be offered to a screen-detected person. A formal screening programme is unlikely, but awareness of social isolation, loneliness and the risk they pose to physical and mental health is important for older people and those who provide services and support for them. Older people at risk or experiencing social isolation and loneliness can be supported to engage in interventions to reverse or reduce the risk.

The evidence suggests that group-based interventions are more effective than one-to-one activities and digital technologies have the potential to help older people form virtual communities and to connect or reconnect with others of shared interest over large distances [23]. These measures may be especially useful for those with established feelings of loneliness and can help prevent sequelae such as depression. Tertiary prevention can also involve addressing the physical risks of social isolation, such as ensuring that older people have contacts to ensure they are safe and attending to their physical needs. Domiciliary care can address these risks, as well as providing emotional support for older people living on their own.

13.6 Health and Social Care

The increasing prevalence of cognitive and physical frailty with age means that older people are more likely than younger age groups to use health and social care services. According to the English Longitudinal Study of Ageing (ELSA), the need for help because of limitations in activities of daily living or mobility increases with age, with 71% of frail individuals receiving help, in contrast to only 31% in non-frail individuals [4]. Assistance with activities of daily living (see Box 13.3) included help with shopping or doing work around the house or garden in 98% of frail people, and help with intimate activities such as dressing and bathing in 67%. The support needed can be provided formally by health and social services, voluntary organisations and community projects, or informally by spouses, extended family, neighbours and friends. For those aged 75 and over, caring was mostly provided by the younger generations, such as children, children-in-law or grandchildren. In addition to family, privately paid employees, social- or health-service workers and friends or neighbours provided some help [4].

In the Medical Research Council Cognitive Function and Ageing Study (CFAS) [24], the prevalence of severe cognitive impairment rose from 1.2% in men and 1.8% in women aged 65–69 years, to 17.1% and 35.0%, respectively, in those aged over 90 years. Among those with dementia and another health condition, there was an overall increase in the use of services, particularly for day-to-day care workers, home helps and day centres. This was associated in the newer cohort with an increased use of unpaid carers [25].

The burden of providing care for older people is considerable. The 2011 census in the UK reported an estimated 5.8 million unpaid carers, half of whom were caring for someone over 75 years old and 22.1% of whom were over 65 [26]. Close to 40% of carers were caring 20 or more hours per week. Of these carers, 5.6% were older adults providing more than 50 hours a week. In addition to the time required to care for an older relative, there are health consequences for the carer. Carers were two-and-a-half times more likely than the general population to report being in bad health [27].

The rate of institutionalisation increases from 20% in the first year after diagnosis of dementia to 50% after 5 years [28]. A systematic review of predictors of institutionalisation in people aged 65 years and over found that, among community dwellers, the highest rate of institutionalisation was 17% over 6 years. Predictors of institutionalisation were increased age, low self-rated health status, functional and cognitive impairment, dementia, prior nursing-home placement and a high number of prescribed medications [29].

A major concern for older people, their families and for governments is the cost of funding care and support in old age. Older people risk spending the majority of their income and assets, including their homes, to pay for social support and residential care. In several countries, there is active debate about the most sustainable models for funding long-term social care. Funding for social care through taxation or social insurance schemes is established in some European countries, while in others individuals and their families are expected to bear the brunt of the cost for social support and care.

This picture should be balanced with the on-going economic and social contribution that older people make. Many continue in paid employment past retirement age. Many volunteers are themselves formal and informal carers for children and other older people. The presence of disabilities or frailty does not mean that older people do not still contribute to their families and communities. They simply adapt to allow for changes in their circumstances as they age.

13.7 End-of-Life Care

The majority of deaths in most developed countries occur in old age. It is important to recognise and deliver high-quality care to older people with terminal conditions in a way that relieves suffering and maintains the autonomy and dignity of the individual and their families. Cancer, heart failure and dementia are among the most common conditions requiring palliative care among older people.

Most people in the European region die in hospital rather than at home. However, there are variations with age and postcode. In the UK, the hospital as place of death is highest among the middle old, while among the oldest old it is the care home [30]. There is evidence that those who live in deprived neighbourhoods are less likely to die in a hospice or receive hospice-at-home care [30]. Older people lack access to specialist palliative care in many countries. In the UK, the majority of specialist palliative services beds are provided by voluntary agencies. The location of such services is often determined by historical factors rather than by needs assessment. Studies from Australia, the USA and the UK suggest that people with terminal conditions other than cancer are less likely to be admitted to hospices where specialist palliative services are offered [31, 32]. This diverts the provision of specialist care towards younger cancer patients. Heart failure, despite having a 5-year prognosis that is comparable to or worse than several cancers, is more likely to be overlooked as a reason for specialist palliative care.

13.8 Policy Responses

The increasing prevalence of disability associated with old age puts significant pressure on health systems to provide adequate care and support. Women typically outlive their spouses and this places them at great risk, especially where social-support systems are not well developed. In lower-income countries, there is a double burden of disease, where diseases associated with old age are emerging alongside traditional health problems of infectious diseases and malnutrition.

The recent UN Decade of Ageing builds on and responds to global commitments and calls for action in its global multi-sectoral strategy to change the view of population ageing from a challenge to an opportunity [33] (see Box 13.5). To foster

> ### Box 13.5 UN Decade of Ageing [33] advocates four areas for action
> - change how we think, feel and act towards age and ageing;
> - ensure that communities foster the abilities of older people;
> - deliver person-centred integrated care and primary health services responsive to older people; and
> - provide access to long-term care for older people who need it.

healthy ageing and improve the lives of older people and their families and communities, fundamental shifts will be required not only in the actions we take, but also in how we think about age and ageing.

In addition to prevention and provision of adequate health and social care support, including the needs and training of carers, the WHO advocates steps to increase participation of older people in the wider society. This can be achieved through an emphasis on lifelong learning and on opportunities for economic and social participation through formal or informal work and voluntary activities. In order for older people to age actively, broader issues of housing, transport and income support must also be considered. Security issues are also highlighted to defend the rights of older people and to protect against elder abuse. These concerns may become particularly pressing at the end of life if the older person's autonomy is not respected in decisions about their health and financial affairs.

Social expectations and attitudes are changing with respect to old age, particularly as the 'baby boom' generation ages. Some of the key challenges for policy-makers are: intergenerational attitudes; financial concerns; the ability and willingness of future societies to provide care and support for its frail, older populations; and attention to challenging debates, such as assisted death and euthanasia. In addition to quality of care, considerations of quality of life have also been prominent. Technologies such as the Internet have increased access to health information and enabled the older population to make more informed choices about their health. An important choice in this population concerns the timing and circumstances of their death.

There is a constant need to provide appropriate evidence to underpin policy. This is particularly challenging in the case of older people. The presence of co-morbidity often means that older people are excluded from clinical trials of interventions that could prevent ill health in this population. The Medical Research Council Cognitive Function and Ageing Study (MRC CFAS) found that individuals who refused participation in the follow-up phase were more likely to have poor cognitive ability and had fewer years of full-time education compared with those followed up [34]. This suggests that long-term studies of ageing and health may under-represent disadvantaged and disabled people.

13.9 Conclusions

Longevity is an important goal for public health, but it brings about a new set of challenges. Health in old age, as at any age, is not 'merely the absence of disease'. However, age is strongly associated with disease and disability. The role of prevention may be progressively limited at increasing ages and this means that public health must seek to support, care and enable where prevention is not possible. However, policies need to balance investment in immediate care and support against investment in developing and implementing strategies for primary, secondary and tertiary prevention.

The phenomenon of ageing also illustrates the wider determinants of health that must be addressed if older people are to remain active and independent participants in their communities. This demands flexibility in approaching the definition and expectations of 'old age'.

REFERENCES

1. J. R. Wilmoth, L. J. Deegan, H. Lundstrom and S. Horiuchi, Increase of maximum lifespan in Sweden, 1861–1999, *Science* **289**(5488), 2000, 2366–8.
2. F. Mzayek, J. K. Cruickshank, D. Amoah *et al.*, Birth weight was longitudinally associated with cardiometabolic risk markers in mid-adulthood, *Annals of Epidemiology* **26**(9), 2016, 643–7.
3. World Health Organization, World report on ageing and health, 2015. Available at: www .who.int/publications/i/item/9789241565042
4. C. Gale, C. Cooper and A. Sayer, Prevalence of frailty and disability: Findings from the English Longitudinal Study of Ageing, *Age and Ageing* **44**(1), 2015, 162–5.
5. D. R. Sinclair, A. Maharani, T. Chandola *et al.*, Frailty among older adults and its distribution in England, *Journal of Frailty & Aging* **11**(2), 2022, 163–8.
6. Office of National Statistics, Health state life expectancies at age 65 years in the UK, 2022. Available at: www.ons.gov.uk/peoplepopulationandcommunity/healthandsocialcare/ healthandlifeexpectancies/bulletins/healthstatelifeexpectanciesuk/2017to2019#health-state-life-expectancies-at-age-65-years-in-the-uk
7. I. H. Yen, Y. L. Michael and L. Perdue, Neighborhood environment in studies of health of older adults: A systematic review, *American Journal of Preventive Medicine* **37**(5), 2009, 455–63.
8. World Health Organization, Fact sheets: Ageing and health, October 2022. Available at: www.who.int/news-room/fact-sheets/detail/ageing-and-health
9. M. D. L. O'Connell, M. M. Marron, R. M. Boudreau *et al.*, Mortality in relation to changes in a healthy aging index: The health, aging, and body composition study, *Journals of Gerontology – Series A Biological Sciences and Medical Sciences* **74**(5), 2019, 726–32.
10. E. Puterman, J. Weiss, B. A. Hives *et al.*, Predicting mortality from 57 economic, behavioral, social, and psychological factors, *Proceedings of the National Academy of Sciences USA* **117** (28), 2020, 16273–82.
11. K. Norman, U. Haß and M. Pirlich, Malnutrition in older adults: Recent advances and remaining challenges, *Nutrients* **13**(8), 2021, 2764.
12. National Institute for Health and Care Excellence (NICE), Assessment and prevention of falls in older people, June 2013. Available at: www.nice.org.uk/guidance/cg161/evidence/ falls-full-guidance-190033741
13. G. Livingston, J. Huntley, A. Sommerlad *et al.*, Dementia prevention, intervention, and care: 2020 report of the Lancet Commission, *The Lancet* **396**(10248), 2020, 413–46.
14. N. Veronese, C. Custodero, A. Cella *et al.*, Prevalence of multidimensional frailty and pre-frailty in older people in different settings: A systematic review and meta-analysis, *Ageing Research Reviews* **72**, 2021, 101498.

15. N. Salari, N. Darvishi, M. Ahmadipanah *et al.*, Global prevalence of falls in the older adults: A comprehensive systematic review and meta-analysis, *Journal of Orthopaedic Surgery & Research* **17**(1), 2022, 334.

16. L D. Gillespie, M. C. Robertson, W. J. Gillespie *et al.*, Interventions for preventing falls in older people living in the community, *Cochrane Database of Systematic Reviews* **9**, 2012, CD007146.

17. H. H. Handoll, I. D. Cameron, J. C. Mak *et al.*, Multidisciplinary rehabilitation for older people with hip fractures, *Cochrane Database of Systematic Reviews* **11**(11), 2021, CD007125.

18. A. Clegg, J. Young, S. Iliffe *et al.*, Frailty in elderly people, *The Lancet* **381**(9868), 2013, 752–62.

19. T. Kidd, F. Mold, C. Jones *et al.*, What are the most effective interventions to improve physical performance in pre-frail and frail adults? A systematic review of randomised control trials, *BMC Geriatrics* **19**(1), 2019, 184.

20. S. M. Dyer, M. Crotty, N. Fairhall *et al.*, Fragility Fracture Network (FFN) Rehabilitation Research Special Interest Group: A critical review of the long-term disability outcomes following hip fracture, *BMC Geriatrics* **16**(1), 2016, 158.

21. Public Health England and UCL Institute of Health Equity, Reducing social isolation across the lifecourse, 2015. Available at: https://assets.publishing.service.gov.uk/government/uploads/system/uploads/attachment_data/file/461120/3a_Social_isolation-Full-revised.pdf

22. R. Naito, D. P. Leong, S. I. Bangdiwala *et al.*, Impact of social isolation on mortality and morbidity in 20 high-income, middle-income and low-income countries in five continents, *BMJ Global Health* **6**(3), 2021, e004124.

23. European Observatory on Health Systems and Policies, J. Marczak, R. Wittenberg *et al.*, Preventing social isolation and loneliness among older people, *Eurohealth* **25**(4), 2019, 3–5.

24. C. Brayne, F. E. Matthews, M. A. McGee and C. Jagger, Health and ill-health in the older population in England and Wales: The Medical Research Council Cognitive Function and Ageing Study (MRC CFAS), *Age and Ageing* **30**(1), 2001, 53–62.

25. H. Bennett, S. Norton, F. Bunn *et al.*, The impact of dementia on service use by individuals with a comorbid health condition: A comparison of two cross-sectional analyses conducted approximately 10 years apart, *BMC Medicine* **16**, 2018, 114.

26. Office for National Statistics, Census analysis: Unpaid care in England and Wales, 2011 and comparison with 2001, 2011. Available at: www.ons.gov.uk/peoplepopulationandcommunity/healthandsocialcare/healthcaresystem/articles/2011censusanalysisunpaidcareinenglandandwales2011andcomparisonwith2001/2013-02-15

27. R. Del-Pino-Casado, E. Priego-Cubero, C. López-Martínez and V. Orgeta, Subjective caregiver burden and anxiety in informal caregivers: A systematic review and meta-analysis, *PLoS One* **16**(3), 2021, e0247143.

28. M. Luppa, T. Luck, E. Brähler *et al.*, Prediction of institutionalisation in dementia. A systematic review, *Dementia and Geriatric Cognitive Disorders* **26**(1), 2008, 65–78.

29. M. Luppa, T. Luck, S. Weyerer *et al.*, Prediction of institutionalisation in the elderly: A systematic review, *Age and Ageing* **39**(1), 2010, 31–8.

30. E. Chukwusa, P. Yu, J. Verne *et al.*, Regional variations in geographic access to inpatient hospices and place of death: A population-based study in England, UK, *PLoS One* **15**(4), 2020, e0231666.

31. K. L. Quinn, P. Wegier, T. A. Stukel *et al.*, Comparison of palliative care delivery in the last year of life between adults with terminal noncancer illness or cancer, *JAMA Network Open* **4** (3), 2021, e210677. Erratum in: *JAMA Network Open* **4**(4), 2021, e218238.

32. M. Romanò, Barriers to early utilization of palliative care in heart failure: A narrative review, *Healthcare (Basel)* **8**(1), 2020, 36.

33. United Nations, EHO's work on the UN Decade of Healthy Ageing (2021–2030). Available at: www.who.int/initiatives/decade-of-healthy-ageing

34. F. E. Matthews, M. Chatfield, C. Freeman *et al.*, Attrition and bias in the MRC Cognitive Function and Ageing Study: An epidemiological investigation, *BMC Public Health* **4**, 2004, 12.

Health Inequalities and Public Health Practice

Anne Swift

Key points

- The health status of different groups (as with individuals) demonstrates variation; some of this variation is to be expected because of chance and differential exposures to disease risk factors.
- When these differences are systematic (not caused by random chance), they are described as health disparities. These may be attributable to the distribution of the wider determinants of health. If so, these differences are usually then referred to as 'health inequalities' or 'health inequities', seen as unfair and become a matter of social justice and political action.
- For meaningful change, health, well-being and reducing inequalities must be explicit, long-term priorities on the political agenda.
- Action can be taken at every level, from individuals through to whole systems.

14.1 Introduction

> Health inequalities are the systematic, avoidable and unfair differences in health outcomes that can be observed between populations, between social groups within the same population or as a gradient across a population ranked by social position. [1]

The above definition was the result of a literature review on the nature of health inequalities – its main finding was that the only element on which all authors could agree was that health was the outcome of interest! The wording given here, however, incorporates important elements of health inequalities from a public health perspective:

- **systematic differences** – not random chance;
- **avoidable** – these are not inevitable differences in health outcomes;

- **unfair** – generally this means that the differences in health outcomes are related to characteristics that should have no association with that health outcome and that these poorer outcomes are therefore unjustly, disproportionately affecting particular groups.

There is a range of characteristics of populations within which significant health inequalities can be demonstrated. Often, socioeconomic status (SES; also expressed as relative deprivation by geography, typically using the Indices of Multiple Deprivation; see Box 14.1 and Chapter 2) is the major factor differentiating groups experiencing different outcomes. However, other factors can also be implicated, such as those characteristics protected under UK equality legislation, social exclusion – populations often termed 'inclusion health groups' – and geographical differences (further described in Box 14.4).

Box 14.1 The English Indices of Multiple Deprivation (IMD) (2019)

- ranks small areas in England (average population 1,500) from 1 (most deprived) to 32,844 (least deprived);
- is a composite measure including income, employment, education, crime, housing and the environment; and
- is widely used in health inequalities research and service delivery.

That differences in health outcomes exist between groups is unsurprising and, in some cases, seems subject to 'natural law' – for example, the increased risk of mortality from cardiovascular disease in those aged over 80 years compared to under 20, or higher rates of lung cancer in smokers compared to those who have never smoked. Such 'common sense', arguably unavoidable differences are termed **'health disparities'** – a term usually understood to be value-neutral. By contrast, more complex differences in health outcomes which seem to derive from differences in opportunities or systemic bias are deemed 'unfair' and are referred to as **'health inequalities'** or **'health inequities'**. Both equality and equity relate to fairness, but have subtly different meanings:

- **Equality** refers to the distribution of resources, goods and/or services equally between everyone; treating everybody the same regardless of need.
- **Equity** refers to resource distribution on the basis of need; those who have higher levels of need receive greater resources.

There are general patterns of usage of these terms: geographically, the term health inequality tends to be favoured in Europe, while health inequity is used (more correctly) in the Americas to describe differences that are unjust and unfair (in which case health **inequality** may be used to describe simple differences in outcomes without implying an element of injustice).

This chapter delves further into how we describe health inequalities and different measures and data that illustrate these differences. Causes and mechanisms of inequality are explored, followed by examples of inequality across groups with certain population characteristics, including: ethnicity; gender, sexual orientation and gender identity; disability; and socially excluded groups. Finally, approaches and strategies for reducing health inequalities are presented, with potential actions described at the micro-, meso- and macro-levels.

14.1.1 Describing Health Inequalities

Inequality can be framed as inequality of *opportunity* **or** of *outcomes*. However, equality of opportunity is difficult to measure, provide or ensure, as it is shaped by hidden privileges and disadvantages, themselves affected by underlying structural societal factors. Outcomes are therefore more likely to be genuine metrics of equality, with the added benefit of measuring what we are ultimately interested in.

Measuring differences in health outcomes across different populations can be challenging. Some of the most robust and stark metrics are also those that capture the most extreme outcomes (such as mortality statistics) and therefore risk understating health and well-being and the burden of illness on the population. Life expectancy (LE) is frequently used to describe differences between populations, since this is a clear and well-established metric that provides meaningful comparators across time, place and person (see Figure 14.1).

Disability Free Life Expectancy (DFLE) is also a useful measure which incorporates morbidity from disease later in life.

In Figure 14.2, DFLE is plotted against relative deprivation. There is a clear relationship between deprivation percentile and length of healthy life; those who are in the most deprived groups are less likely to survive much beyond retirement age, while only those in the most affluent areas are likely to be able to not only live to see retirement, but be healthy enough to fully enjoy it.

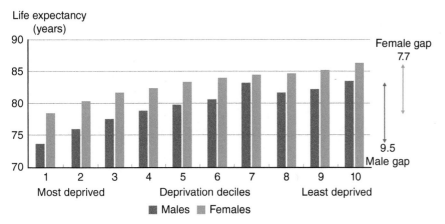

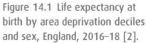

Figure 14.1 Life expectancy at birth by area deprivation deciles and sex, England, 2016–18 [2].

Figure 14.2 Life expectancy and Disability Free Life Expectancy at birth by area deprivation deciles, 2009–13, England [2].

(a) Males

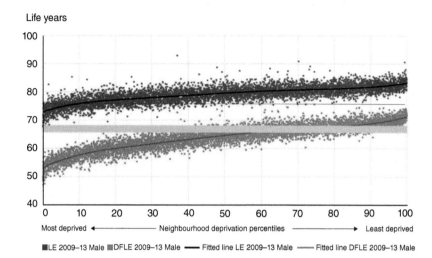

(b) Females

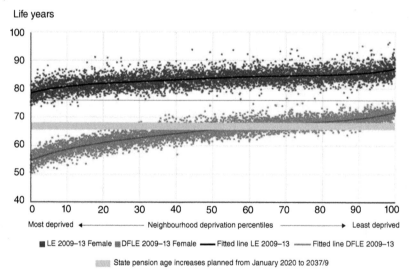

Variation in UK life expectancy is also seen by gender – women tend to live longer than men, although this gap is closing (mainly due to cohort effects of smoking, since women in general took up smoking later than men and are therefore experiencing health impacts later). Geographical variations in life expectancy are some of the most well-known health inequalities, with stark differences described across single cities such as London and Glasgow (Figure 14.3).

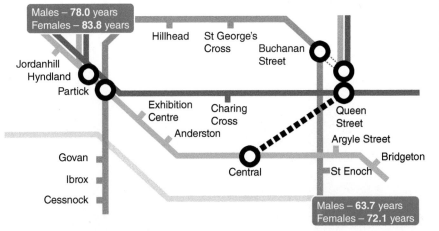

Figure 14.3 Life expectancy differences between areas six railway stations apart in Glasgow, Scotland [3].

As described in Chapters 2 and 11, the infant mortality rate (IMR) is a sensitive indicator of the well-being of a society and reflects both environmental influences (such as infectious diseases) and maternal health and well-being. Factors such as lack of antenatal care, unhealthy maternal weight, smoking or alcohol use in pregnancy, and maternal stress are key in determining perinatal outcomes.

Analysis of IMR by deprivation, social class and income all demonstrate the same patterns: the more affluent the group, the lower the risk of infant deaths. As the majority of the UK population has become less well-off in comparison to those at the very top, we see gains in LE and IMR stalling or even reversing.

Maternity-related deaths demonstrate stark inequalities in health between groups defined in other ways, too. Pregnancy outcomes for women in minority ethnic groups in the UK are generally poorer than for White women. In the case of Black women, this translates to more than four times as many women dying in pregnancy, while neonatal deaths vary significantly by ethnic group [4] (see Figure 14.4). Neonatal death rates increase with deprivation across all ethnic groups; some ethnic groups are much more affected by the higher rates of neonatal deaths associated with deprivation.

14.1.2 Causes and Mechanisms of Inequalities

What are the mechanisms and pathways that lead from occupying a particular place in society to the inequalities in health outcomes that we see? In 1980, the Black Report offered four potential explanations for health inequalities [5]:

1. **Artefact.** Younger people (with better health) are more likely to enter occupations that are of higher social status as routine and manual work becomes more automated and mechanised – thus the poorer health of those in the lower social classes is a function of a greater average age. However, the age-standardisation of data eliminates age as a potential confounder of this relationship.

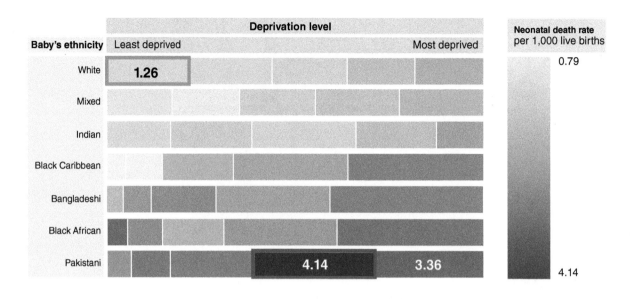

Figure 14.4 Neonatal deaths in the UK, 2016–20 [4].

2. **Selection** (i.e. those with poorer health do less well economically). A causal association between health and social class is accepted, but social class is the dependent variable. While there may be an element of health or disability impacting social mobility, it is unlikely to be a significant enough effect to account for the major health differences seen between social classes.

3. **Cultural/behavioural**. Health impacts are the result of people making entirely free choices about health behaviours. This explanation does not accept that structural factors beyond individuals' control influence health behaviours.

4. **Structural/materialist**. Cultural and behavioural factors are merely intermediates in the chain of causation since these health 'choices' are determined largely by the level of control that individuals and communities have over their lives. It is the larger structural and societal factors that ultimately determine this level of control and therefore ultimately create differences in health outcomes.

It might seem logical to assume that the factors that most influence the health of an individual or a population are those that relate directly to health outcomes, such as genetic risks, access to high-quality health-care and health-related behaviours, such as smoking, diet and physical activity. While these are all relevant to health and ill health, the *causes of variation in these factors* are more influential in determining risks of health and illness and therefore in determining health inequalities. The government-commissioned 'Marmot Review', *Fair Society, Healthy Lives* [6], built on decades of work, including the Whitehall studies [7] and work on the social determinants of health for the World Health Organization [8], to conclude that, above all, health inequality in the UK required action on the social and economic environment and in particular giving children the best start in life. As Michael Marmot puts it, '... people's ability to take personal responsibility is shaped by their circumstances. People cannot take responsibility if they cannot control what happens to them' [9].

These 'causes of the causes [of health and illness]' are termed the social (or wider) determinants of health and are the non-medical factors that influence health outcomes: the social, economic and environmental conditions in which we are born, grow, live, work and age [6]. Moreover, as described in Chapter 11, inequalities and limiting factors tend to accumulate from birth and persist across the life course. These are those structural forces which the Black Report concluded were the key to understanding inequalities. This view, sometimes termed the 'wealth to health' model, is the one most often encountered in public health considerations of health inequalities. Other professional groups such as economists may have different perspectives on the direction of the association between deprivation and health outcomes (Box 14.2).

Box 14.2 The economist's view

Selection or reverse causation argues that the poor health of some groups is caused at least in part by the characteristic defining that group (such as deprivation).

Suggested mechanisms for this include those who are healthier being more able to improve their social status through marrying 'up', the negative impact on education and therefore earning potential of poor health in childhood, and adulthood loss of income and status through ill health and disability.

Broadly, international comparisons show that less equal societies, with greater difference in income, wealth and power across their population, do less well over a range of health and social outcomes. In turn, the distribution of such resources is underpinned by global forces, political priorities and societal values [10]. Thus, the structural forces or barriers that affect an individual's lifestyle, choices and opportunities are largely outside their control.

These are depicted in the well-known 'rainbow' model published by Dahlgren and Whitehead in 1991 (see Chapter 1, Figure 1.3) and the Pencheon and Bradley model of the driving forces affecting health from Chapter 8 which is reproduced again below (Figure 14.5), which demonstrates the interactive and complex nature of these determinants (see also Chapter 8).

At the individual level, the social determinants of health differentially affect our ability to lead a flourishing life. The balance between the accumulation and depletion of these capabilities over the individual's life course depends on the interrelationships between material circumstance, psycho-social conditions and access to essential services.

As the outermost layer of the Dahlgren and Whitehead 'rainbow', socioeconomic conditions (or when translated to the individual, SES) impact directly and indirectly

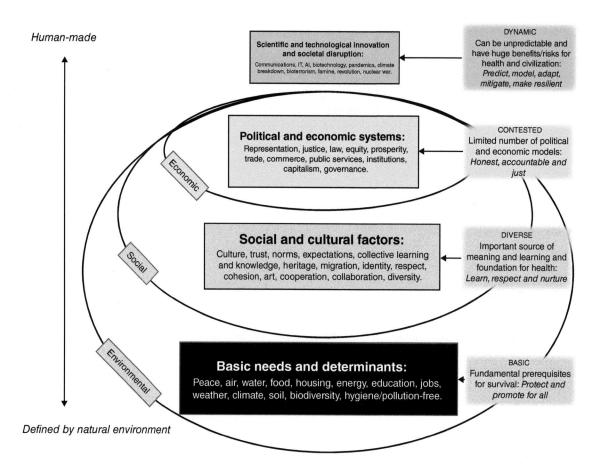

Human-made

Scientific and technological innovation and societal disruption:
Communications, IT, AI, biotechnology, pandemics, climate breakdown, bioterrorism, famine, revolution, nuclear war.

DYNAMIC
Can be unpredictable and have huge benefits/risks for health and civilization: *Predict, model, adapt, mitigate, make resilient*

Political and economic systems:
Representation, justice, law, equity, prosperity, trade, commerce, public services, institutions, capitalism, governance.

CONTESTED
Limited number of political and economic models: *Honest, accountable and just*

Economic

Social and cultural factors:
Culture, trust, norms, expectations, collective learning and knowledge, heritage, migration, identity, respect, cohesion, art, cooperation, collaboration, diversity.

DIVERSE
Important source of meaning and learning and foundation for health: *Learn, respect and nurture*

Social

Basic needs and determinants:
Peace, air, water, food, housing, energy, education, jobs, weather, climate, soil, biodiversity, hygiene/pollution-free.

BASIC
Fundamental prerequisites for survival: *Protect and promote for all*

Environmental

Defined by natural environment

Figure 14.5 The Pencheon and Bradley model of determinants of health.

on all the other mechanisms and causes stemming from them. Even when particular mechanisms and causal pathways are addressed, they tend to be replaced by others that maintain the relationship between SES and health inequalities. This is the basis of Link and colleagues' theory of fundamental causes (Box 14.3) [11], with other authors adopting the concept and arguing that racism in all its forms (structural, institutional and interpersonal) is a fundamental cause of racialised inequalities [12].

McCartney and colleagues [13] propose framing this as a matter of differential power, arguing that this is the common element represented by access to the long list of flexible resources, including available money, social support, knowledge and influence.

Michael Marmot also describes the problem as one of differential power and conceptualises a model of three pertinent types of power [9] (see Figure 14.6).

He also emphasises that thinking of inequalities in terms of a binary – the 'haves' and 'have nots', poverty and affluence – is an oversimplification that both allows inequalities to remain a marginal issue and avoids an uncomfortable truth: that societies with greater wealth inequality do less well however they are measured. It

Box 14.3 Fundamental cause theory [11]

A fundamental cause of health inequalities has four defining features:

1. it is linked to multiple diseases;
2. it affects these disease outcomes through multiple risk factors;
3. it is related to access to resources that can help to prevent disease or minimise sequelae of disease once it occurs; and
4. mechanisms linking the fundamental cause and disease change over time, but the association is maintained.

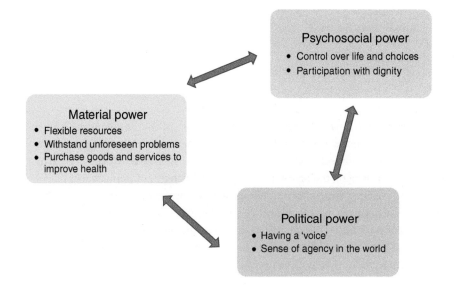

Figure 14.6 Types of power operating to determine individuals' levels of agency in their lives [9].

is not only those at the bottom who suffer: it is the whole population (with the exception of those at the very top – the 1%). The steepness of this social gradient, Marmot and others argue, is the real determinant of well-being of a society [14].

14.2 Dimensions of Inequality – Populations and Groups

Health inequalities are frequently framed as health outcomes varying by SES. While it is a key driver of health inequality, SES is not the only variable associated with differences in health status between groups (see Box 14.4). It is beyond the scope of this chapter to provide an exhaustive list of these observed inequalities, but some key illustrative examples will be given.

Box 14.4 Examples of characteristics known to influence health outcomes in the UK

'Protected characteristics' under UK Equality Act 2010:	Socially excluded groups considered under the heading 'inclusion health':
Sex	People experiencing homelessness
Ethnicity	People in the criminal justice system
Disability	Sex workers
Age	Gypsy, Roma and Traveller communities
Sexual orientation	Migrants and refugees
Gender reassignment	People who use substances
Religion	Victims of modern slavery
Marital status	
Pregnancy and maternity	

Considering groups of people as a whole is problematic as it necessarily requires overlooking individual differences in favour of descriptors that characterise a 'type' of person – someone who identifies as gender different from that assigned at birth, for example, or someone whose skin colour is not perceived by most as 'White'. While acknowledging the problems and potential dangers of stereotyping, there are clear, well-defined and unfair differences between health outcomes of groups in the UK. These must not be ignored while we maintain a thoughtful approach to the dangers of *essentialism* (assuming groups have inherent unchanging common characteristics) and the reification of diverse and varied categories of people and their – possibly minimal – shared characteristics [12].

We also cannot treat these groupings as mutually exclusive. The legal scholar Kimberle Crenshaw first described in 1989 how the experiences of Black women are marginalised in the context of anti-discrimination law [15]. Crenshaw argues that within minoritised groups, those who lack other privileges (e.g. on the basis of sex or class) are further marginalised and experience multiple burdens of discrimination and inequality. This *intersectionality* is an important phenomenon to bear in mind when looking at examples of unequal health outcomes.

14.2.1 Ethnicity

The 2021 UK census demonstrated an increase in all 'high-level' ethnic population groups other than 'White' (Figure 14.7), although more than 81% of the population of England and Wales identify in this latter category [16].

Ethnic identity has an increasingly recognised association with health outcomes both in the UK and internationally, although the data are not always easy to interpret.

Inequalities in pregnancy outcomes by ethnicity are stark. Between 2016 and 2020, Black African mothers in the most income-deprived 20% of the UK population experienced a stillbirth rate of 8.1 per 1,000 live births compared to the least deprived White mothers, in whom the rate was 2.78 per 1,000 live births. Stillbirth rates increased with deprivation across all ethnic groups, but the rate in the least deprived 20% of Black African mothers was still higher than that of the most deprived White mothers [4]. There is also a more than four-fold difference in maternal mortality rates among women from Black ethnic backgrounds and an almost two-fold difference among women from Asian ethnic backgrounds compared to White women [17] (see Figure 14.8).

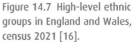

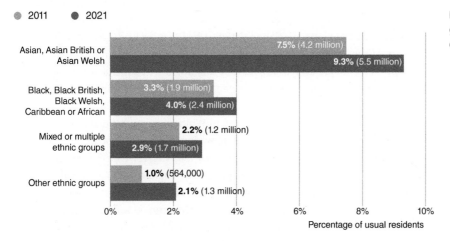

Figure 14.7 High-level ethnic groups in England and Wales, census 2021 [16].

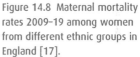

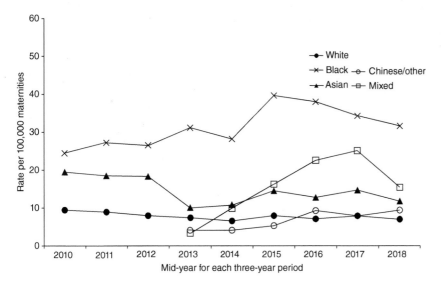

Figure 14.8 Maternal mortality rates 2009–19 among women from different ethnic groups in England [17].

Significant inequalities also exist by ethnicity in accessing mental health services, experience of care and mental health outcomes. Adults of Caribbean and/or African heritage are more likely than any other ethnic group to be detained under the Mental Health Act, while minority ethnic groups (in White majority countries) are over-represented in all crisis and secure services. Despite evidence from the UK Adult Psychiatric Morbidity Survey 2014 that Black populations report higher prevalence of all mental illnesses (including common mental health conditions such as depression and anxiety) compared to the whole population, they are under-represented in treatment services overall and in particular low-intensity community-based services such as Improving Access to Psychological Therapies (IAPT) in the NHS. Black people are more likely to be diagnosed with psychosis (in particular schizophrenia) in majority White population countries (the UK, the USA, the Netherlands), but not in countries with a majority Black population [18]. As far back as the early 1980s, this was potentially attributed to misdiagnosis of psychosis in Black people experiencing acute distress due to life events [19], thereby inflating the true incidence of psychosis in these populations. It has been suggested that once adjusted for social factors – such as those linked to overt racism – the rates of psychosis seen in minority ethnic groups are almost equivalent to those seen in White majority populations.

Echoing discussions of power and autonomy in the genesis of health inequalities earlier in this chapter, Jongsma and colleagues [20] suggest that the disparities in psychosis risk seen in ethnic minority populations could arise as a function of multiple social and cultural barriers in achieving autonomy and control over one's environment and life experiences. Williams and Mohammed state a similar conclusion: 'Multiple aspects of racism relate to each other and combine, additively and interactively, with other psycho-social risks and resources to affect health' [21]. The COVID-19 pandemic was another clear demonstration of racialised health inequalities becoming apparent in real time. Higher morbidity and mortality were seen in groups of other than White ethnic identity in the first wave, as is well known, but this continued. In the early 2022 third wave of the pandemic, people of Bangladeshi and Pakistani origin were more likely to die compared to the White British population [22] (Figure 14.9).

Nazroo [12] makes a case for a 'big picture', sociologically informed view of the complexity of these inequalities, suggesting cutting through the suggested mid-level mechanisms and proposed biological differences is racism as a fundamental cause. He considers racism at three interacting levels: the structural (macro), institutional (meso) and interpersonal (micro). He suggests that it is in fact these ingrained hierarchical beliefs that drive not only the inequities themselves, but also the many explanations posited – for example, the focus on attempting to find a genetic cause for the ethnic disparity in COVID morbidity and mortality early in the pandemic.

A further category of internalised racism has been described [23] through which the discriminated-against integrate the racist ideas of being 'less-than' into their

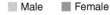

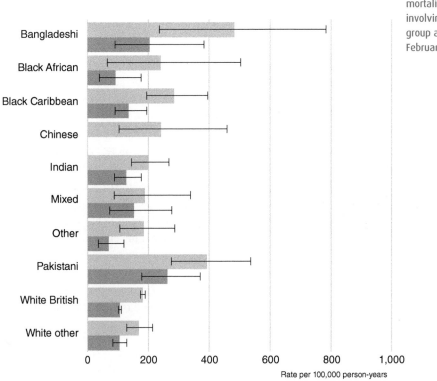

Figure 14.9 Age-standardised mortality rates of deaths involving COVID-19 by ethnic group and sex, England, January–February 2022 [22].

identity, creating self-fulfilling prophesies (e.g. of educational failure, criminality or drug use), increased autonomic stress through negative emotional reactions, racial trauma and a wider 'syndrome' described by Meyer [24] as 'minority stress'. These combine to create a physical, emotional and mental load that has the potential to significantly disrupt mental and physical health.

Many of the concepts and mechanisms producing racialised health inequalities described above also apply to other groups in society.

14.2.2 Gender, Sexual Orientation and Gender Identity

Despite an apparent life expectancy advantage, women experience a significant health disadvantage worldwide. Near-universally enacted inequalities in power, assets and caring responsibilities combined with labour-market inequalities and the burden of unpaid work leave women more likely to have fewer resources [25]. Acknowledgement of the prioritisation of men in health research and health-care provision has allowed discussion of women's health needs as distinct from men's – from the negative health impacts of juggling multiple roles [26], to a lack of consideration of menopause as a topic worthy of scholarship. Only in the 2020s have we seen specific strategies for improving women's health discussed in the UK.

14.2.2.1 Sexual Orientation and Gender Identity

Sexual orientation may refer to multiple elements of an individual's experience, including sexual identity, romantic and/or sexual attraction or behaviours. The 2021 census provided the first comprehensive population-level data on sexual orientation in the UK, achieving a 92.5% response rate of the eligible population aged 16 years or older; 1.5 million people – 3.2% of the population – self-identified as 'Gay or Lesbian, Bisexual, or Other'. In contrast, 89.4% identified as 'straight/ heterosexual'.

Gender identity refers to an individual's sense of their own gender, which may or may not be the same as the sex assigned at birth. 2021 census data (94% question response rate) revealed that 0.5% of the population of England and Wales over the age of 16 (262,000 people) identify as a gender identity different from that assigned at birth, with roughly equal numbers of transmen and transwomen responding.

People who identify as a minority sexual identity experience significant health inequalities compared to the heterosexual population, including higher rates of various long-term conditions (Figure 14.10), multi-morbidity and mental illness

Figure 14.10 Odds ratios for long-term conditions by sexual orientation (sexual minority and heterosexual), adjusted for deprivation, ethnic group, region and age (N = 1,341,339) [27].

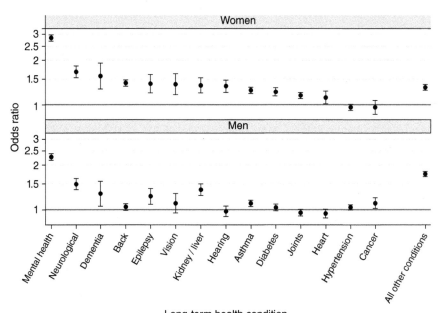

[27, 28]. Trans people have a particularly high risk of mental health difficulties, with 70% of gender-diverse people having experienced depression in the last year (compared to 52% of LGB people and 20% of the general population), and nearly half (46%) of trans people having considered taking their own life in the last year (compared to 31% of non-trans LGB people) [29].

The mechanisms underlying these patterns include higher levels of behaviours that risk health, including smoking, alcohol use and having an unhealthy weight [30, 31], although as discussed in this chapter and Chapter 8, these in turn are influenced by social determinants. Many of these 'causes of the causes' are similar to those described above in relation to ethnicity, such as minority stress, internalised discrimination and reduced access to services, as a result of fear or poor previous experiences of health-care.

In response to growing awareness of these inequalities, the UK government published an 'LGBT Action Plan' in 2018, promising action to better monitor these disparities and work to address the causes. Globally, there remain many countries in which identifying as a minority sexual or gender identity is explicitly unacceptable, including 70 which criminalise adult same-sex relationships [32] and several countries in which the death penalty can be invoked for adults who have participated in consensual same-sex acts.

14.2.3 Disability

Disability, defined by the UK Equalities Act 2010, is any physical or mental impairment that has a 'substantial and long-term negative impact' on a person's ability to undertake normal day-to-day activities. Data from the UK Family Resources Survey 2019–20 indicate that around one in five people in the UK are disabled [33]. These include restrictions on mobility and problems with fatigue and stamina – the two most common types of disability in the UK – but also intellectual disability, long-term medical conditions, and specific learning disabilities such as autism spectrum disorder and Attention Deficit (Hyperactivity) Disorder. Mental health impairment is the single most common disability among working-age adults.

Beyond the significant impacts of the impairment itself, disabled people experience inequalities in quality of life, general health and well-being, and service provision. For example, 15% of disabled people reported feeling 'often or always' lonely in 2021, compared to around 4% of non-disabled people [34] (see Figure 14.11).

Intellectual disability (ID), which may be mild, carries a particularly heavy additional burden since the life expectancy of those with ID is on average around 20 years less than those without ID, after adjustment for causes linked to the intellectual impairment. Much of this avoidable burden of mortality is related to health-care

Figure 14.11 The proportion of disabled people who felt lonely 'often or always' in 2021 has increased compared with 2014 [34].

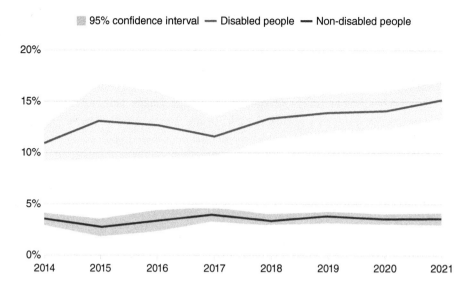

staff's lack of understanding of the needs and normal behaviours of people with ID, together with over-medication and lack of high-quality physical health-care [35]. The life expectancy gap is reducing through efforts to address these issues, but much remains to be done.

14.2.4 Inclusion Health – Socially Excluded Groups

Groups who are not generally included in mainstream society (e.g. those who are homeless, who work in the sex industry or are refugees; see Box 14.4 for more examples) on average experience much worse health than the general population. Brief consideration of the social determinants of health yields clear reasons for poor health outcomes in these groups, yet the impacts are stark: the average age at death for a homeless man in the UK in 2021 was 45.4 years – 34 years of life lost, compared to the average UK male life expectancy of 79.5 years. More than half of these deaths are related to drug poisoning, suicide and alcohol – so-called 'deaths of despair' – but at least a third die from readily treatable conditions, such as infections and long-term conditions [36].

People in contact with the criminal justice system experience very poor health; people in prison are 50% more likely to die than the general population, but this is even higher – more than twice and three times as high, respectively – for ex-prisoners and offenders in the community [37] (see Figure 14.12). Prisoners are four times more likely to be smokers and mental health problems are very common.

There are many other groups which experience significant health inequalities and there is not the scope to consider them all here. In common though are the mechanisms underlying these observations which have been discussed at length both in this chapter and Chapter 8.

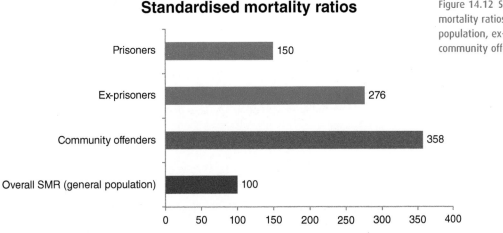

Standardised mortality ratios

Figure 14.12 Standardised mortality ratios for UK prison population, ex-prisoners and community offenders [37].

14.3 Approaches to Reducing Health Inequalities

When considering approaches to improving the situation, we need to consider the bigger picture of the social determinants and driving forces of health and inequalities as a whole. Lynch [38] proposes that in 'medicalising' inequalities – framing the problem as one of just health – we risk making it even more difficult to solve and ignoring the importance of other social factors such as education, employment, housing and wider social policy areas. Some authors posit that UK policy and rhetoric has moved from discussions of the upstream social determinants of health (SDoH) to a behavioural, personal responsibility model – so-called 'lifestyle drift' [39]. Such an approach ignores 50% of the levels of influence on health described in the highly influential Dahlgren and Whitehead 'rainbow' model, first published in 1991 [40].

Actions and approaches aimed at reducing health inequalities can be categorised at the level of the system into micro-level actions (e.g. during a health-care encounter with an individual), meso-level (such as at the local health system or community level) and macro-level (policy-making and political decisions). These are summarised in Box 14.5 and are described further below. The health improvement model described in Chapter 8 also describes levels of action, with further specific examples for public health practitioners.

14.3.1 Micro-Level Interventions: What Can Individual Health-Care Professionals Do?

In the UK, various attempts have been made to generate ideas and resources for individual health-care workers to address inequalities. The areas for potential action tend to cluster under four headings:

Box 14.5 Actions to influence health inequalities

Micro-level – individuals

- education and training of self and others on the SDoH;
- advocacy, support and signposting for individual patients and families;
- influencing and advocacy within the hyperlocal setting;
- working in partnership with other agencies and sectors to coordinate activity on SDoH; and
- active consideration of power dynamics within interactions with patients, communities and agencies.

Meso-level – health systems

- include health inequalities reduction explicitly in organisational aims and contracts;
- ensure systems are developed to collect, analyse and act on pertinent data;
- mindfully allocate resources and workforce – adopt proportionate universal approaches;
- prioritise prevention;
- explore and develop opportunities to act as an anchor institution within the community;
- partner with and support the work of other agencies in acting on SDoH; and
- adopt community-centric, assets-based and whole-systems approaches to development of public health and health services.

Macro-level – policy-makers

- consider the impacts on health and health inequalities in all policy-making;
- develop a national strategy for action on the social determinants of health;
- whole-systems working, policies and accountability;
- develop the social determinants of health workforce;
- nurture disruptive and radical leadership for action; and
- develop public engagement, understanding and empowerment on the social determinants.

14.3.1.1 Education and Training

There is growing enthusiasm for **education** about social determinants of health, social justice and health inequalities in health professional training [41], although there seems to be little in the way of large-scale change, particularly in undergraduate medical curricula [42]. Behind these calls for curriculum change lies a sense that doctors and other health-care professionals have a duty to 'do something' about the upstream causes of poor health (e.g. [43], [44]) although this is not a universally accepted component of the medical role [45]. Greater understanding of the social determinants and the inequalities faced by particular groups may, however, go some way to **improving access to health-care** for minority populations (e.g. LGBTQ, Travellers) and better care by **dispelling persistent myths** (e.g. Black people having higher pain tolerance and (literally) thicker skin).

Workplace-based training in equality and diversity is commonplace; training encouraging greater self-awareness around '**unconscious bias**' may also support individual practitioners in developing their understanding of attitudes and behaviours towards people different from themselves.

14.3.1.2 Actions with Individual Patients

It can be helpful for all health professionals to consider themselves – their time, attention and energy – in terms of scarce resources and consider how these **resources are allocated** (as described further in Chapter 5). People tend to be drawn to those who share similar characteristics, but if this tendency is allowed to affect patient care (e.g. through more time, empathy or attention being given to patients similar in background or status to the professional), this has clear potential to increase inequalities.

Gathering information – including social history and population-level data – can inform thinking around potential support, as well as improve understanding of these issues at population level. Awareness and use of **social prescribing** may also be appropriate ways to support individuals' needs, which may facilitate direct action on the wider determinants of health. Advice on debt management or housing, referral to social activities that reduce isolation or support with finding employment are examples of this type of help. Health professionals may also act as **advocates for individual patients** in situations where the formal support of a professional could influence a decision affecting the wider determinants of health, such as benefits applications or housing appeals. There is a public sector duty to refer if people who are homeless or at risk of homelessness are encountered in practice.

14.3.1.3 Advocacy

Apart from advocating for individuals and families in their care, professionals are in a strong position to **advocate for local and national policies** that support inclusion of diverse groups and recognise the powerful effects of the social determinants of health. Evidence shows us what works to reduce health inequalities: the Acheson Inquiry recommendations delivered in the 1997–2001 Labour government's strategy on health inequalities were comprehensive, across government and the NHS, with clear metrics and an underlying comprehension of the nature of the problem [46] (see Box 14.6). Closer to home, health professionals can **advocate for better training and education** on the social determinants of health, for improved care pathways that are designed to accommodate those who are sometimes excluded (usually

Box 14.6 What works in reducing health inequalities?

The 1998 Acheson Inquiry [46] findings were incorporated into the then Labour government's strategy on health inequalities.

This was a comprehensive, cross-government strategy, with clear metrics (improved life expectancy and a reduction in life expectancy variation) and four overall areas for action:

1. supporting families;
2. engaging the community in tackling deprivation;
3. improving prevention and health-care; and
4. tackling the social determinants of health.

Policies included Sure Start children's centres to support early-years development and parenting, increasing public spending on social programmes and providing additional NHS funding for areas with significant deprivation, the introduction of a national minimum wage, and tax and benefit changes to reduce child poverty.

Although widely declared *not* to have 'worked' by the end of the time the strategy was active (2010), further analysis with longer-term data indicate that inequalities did in fact reduce during the strategy implementation and have started to increase again since the strategy actions have ceased [47]. Buck [48] takes the following lessons: that at population level inequalities are persistent and stubborn to shift; that we need to create sustained focus to make any change; that a coherent and multifactorial approach across government and the NHS is required; and that we must take the long view in establishing whether a programme has been successful or not. We must also make sure that we learn from the efforts of the past before 'inventing the future'.

unintentionally) and for **working conditions** that support health workers' own rights to a standard of living that promotes health. It is also imperative that systems develop **data collection systems** so that population-level health disparities can be measured and tracked, and the impact of actions can be monitored. This is another area in which health professionals can act as powerful advocates within their own organisation.

14.3.1.4 Working in Partnership

By **leading across systems** - not just within single organisations - public health leaders and health professionals can influence the wider determinants and improve the coherence of work in different sectors, including non-health-care.

More locally, clinicians can **work in partnership** with leaders and managers within their own services and organisations to ensure that wider determinants of health are considered in decision-making and that services are designed and commissioned with an understanding of health inequalities in mind.

14.3.2 Meso-Level: What Can Health Systems Do?

Access to high-quality health-care is one force driving inequalities, but it is arguably far from the most important. Health-care systems do, however, bear the impacts of avoidable illness and from an economic as well as an ethical perspective, systems therefore have an interest in reducing the population health-care burden. Many of the individual interventions described above can only be performed in the context of a health-care organisation. At the level of the organisation and the system itself, there are further possibilities.

Systems and organisations set priorities; by including an **explicit intention to reduce health inequalities** and holding people to account, work undertaken across the system is much more likely to include elements that will have an impact. For example, the NHS Core20PLUS5 framework is NHS England's approach to supporting health systems to prioritise areas that will impact on health inequalities. 'Core 20' refers to the one-fifth most deprived of the population as defined by the Indices of Multiple Deprivation (IMD; see Box 14.1); 'Plus' allows local systems to identify local priorities, such as minority ethnic communities or inclusion health groups; and '5' reminds systems of the five clinical areas identified as priorities for reducing inequality: maternity, severe mental illness, respiratory disease, early cancer diagnosis, and hypertension and lipid management [49].

Enabling and encouraging the **collection of relevant data** allows the measuring and monitoring of inequalities. Fundamental data such as ethnicity are starting to be more reliably collected across the NHS, but characteristics such as sexual orientation and gender identity are very poorly recorded, despite there being an NHS information standard in place.

The **allocation of resources and the health-care workforce** by organisations can impact on health inequalities by reversing the tendency for deprived areas (with the most need) to have the lowest concentrations of health-care staff and services, the 'inverse care law' famously first noted by Julian Tudor-Hart in the 1970s (see Chapter 6).

The recognition that large health organisations are major employers, consumers of resources and producers of waste in the places where they are situated offers another avenue for impacting on the social determinants of health, in what are being termed **'anchor' institutions** (because they are large and unlikely to move). As such, hospitals and health systems are beginning to recognise the externalities associated with their health-care activity. Healthy workforce policies and practices, adopting ethical procurement practices that prioritise the local economy where possible and supporting the development of community resources and facilities are examples of opportunities.

Beyond their own direct activities, organisations can also support the work of **other local agencies** to disrupt and act on the social determinants of health, such as supporting local housing and employment initiatives.

14.3.4 Macro-Level: What Can Policy-Making and Politics Do?

Health inequalities are not inevitable. They can, and have, changed over time in response to policy (see Box 14.6) – evidence demonstrates that inequalities can be reduced (and exacerbated) by policy decisions. However, it is neither simple nor quick to achieve measurable change, meaning that there needs to be long-term commitment to tackling health inequalities not only from the government of the moment, but also from society as a whole. The improvements seen in the 2000s were the result of comprehensive, evidence-informed cross-government strategy (including but not focusing solely on health-care) with clear outcome metrics and efforts to maintain focused action over time. This is further discussed in Chapter 15 with respect to policy.

The 2020 update to the Marmot report recommended that the lessons of those years be learned, suggesting the following priorities [2]:

Implementation of action on health inequalities and their social determinants
1. Develop a national strategy for action on the social determinants of health with the aim of reducing inequalities in health.
2. Ensure proportionate universal allocation of resources and implementation of policies.
3. Early intervention to prevent health inequalities.
4. Develop the social determinants of health workforce.
5. Engage the public.
6. Develop whole-systems monitoring and strengthen accountability for health inequalities.

Similarly, the King's Fund describes the 'concerted, systematic and sustained' action needed to impact on outcomes [50]:
(1) An enduring **national mission** to tackle inequality
  (a) Stronger focus on preventive care and risk factor clustering
  (b) Clear national outcomes that can be delivered locally
(2) Local and national partnerships – **systems working**
  (a) Openly available, high-quality data available
  (b) Distilling what works and sharing it
  (c) Tackling health inequalities as central 'business as usual' for the NHS
(3) Local leadership for **disruption**
  (a) Challenging current 'downstream' health-care norms and moving money to reinforce prevention and the importance of the social determinants of health
  (b) Prioritising and empowering communities to mobilise assets

14.4 Conclusions

Unfair differences in health outcomes between groups are neither inevitable nor impervious to action, but a wide-ranging and concerted effort at all levels of public life is required to impact on the social factors that produce these inequalities. We have a good understanding of the determinants and mechanisms that underlie consistent observations of health inequalities – what is needed now is action. There is potential at every level for individuals to act on the social determinants of health and health inequalities; any given action may necessarily only have a tiny impact, but, through coherent and persistent efforts, things can change for the better.

REFERENCES

1. G. McCartney, F. Popham, R. McMaster and A. Cumbers, Defining health and health inequalities, *Public Health* **172**, 2019, 22–30.
2. M. Marmot, J. Allen, T. Boyce *et al.*, *Health Equity in England: The Marmot review 10 years on*, Institute of Health Equity/The Health Foundation, 2020.
3. Public Health Scotland, Measuring health inequalities, 2021. Available at: www .healthscotland.scot/health-inequalities/measuring-health-inequalities
4. E. Draper, I. Gallimore, L. Smith *et al.*, MBRRACE-UK perinatal mortality surveillance report, UK perinatal deaths for births from January to December 2020, Leicester, The Infant Mortality and Morbidity Studies, Department of Health Sciences, University of Leicester, 2022.
5. D. Blane, An assessment of the Black Report's explanations of health inequalities, *Sociology of Health & Illness* **7**(3), 1985, 423–45.
6. M. Marmot, P. Goldblatt, J. Allen *et al.*, *Fair Society, Healthy Lives: The Marmot Review*, London, Institute for Health Equity, 2010.
7. M. G. Marmot, S. Stansfeld, C. Patel *et al.*, Health inequalities among British civil servants: The Whitehall II study, *The Lancet* **337**(8754), 1991, 1387–93.
8. M. Marmot, S. Friel, R. Bell *et al.*, Closing the gap in a generation: Health equity through action on the social determinants of health, *The Lancet* **372**(9650), 2008, 1661–9.
9. M. Marmot, *The Health Gap: The Challenge of an Unequal World*, London, Bloomsbury, 2015.
10. NHS Health Scotland, Health inequalities policy review for the Scottish Ministerial Task Force on Health Inequalities, 2013.
11. J. C. Phelan, B. G. Link and P. Tehranifar, Social conditions as fundamental causes of health inequalities: Theory, evidence, and policy implications, *Journal of Health and Social Behavior* **51**(Suppl. 1), 2010, S28–S40.
12. J. Nazroo, Race/ethnic inequalities in health: Moving beyond confusion to focus on fundamental causes, Institute for Fiscal Studies, 2022.
13. G. Mccartney, E. Dickie, O. Escobar and C. Collins, Health inequalities, fundamental causes and power: Towards the practice of good theory, *Sociology of Health & Illness* **43**(1), 2021, 20–39.
14. R. Wilkinson and K. Pickett, *The Spirit Level: Why More Equal Societies Almost Always Do Better*, London, Penguin, 2009.
15. K. Crenshaw, Demarginalizing the intersection of race and sex: A Black feminist critique of antidiscrimination doctrine, feminist theory and antiracist politics, *University of Chicago Legal Forum* **1989**(1), 1989, article 8.

16. Office for National Statistics, Ethnic group, England and Wales: Census 2021, 2022. Available at: www.ons.gov.uk/peoplepopulationandcommunity/culturalidentity/ethnicity/bulletins/ethnicgroupenglandandwales/census2021

17. M. Knight, K. Bunch, R. Patel *et al.*, *Saving Lives, Improving Mothers' Care: Lessons Learned to Inform Maternity Care from the UK and Ireland Confidential Enquiries into Maternal Deaths and Morbidity 2018–20*, Oxford, National Perinatal Epidemiology Unit, University of Oxford, 2022.

18. C. Morgan, P. Fearon, J. Lappin *et al.*, Ethnicity and long-term course and outcome of psychotic disorders in a UK sample: The ÆSOP-10 study, *British Journal of Psychiatry* **211** (2), 2017, 88–94.

19. M. Lipsedge and R. Littlewood, *Aliens and Alienists: Ethnic Minorities and Psychiatry*, London, Routledge, 1997.

20. H. E. Jongsma, S. Karlsen, J. B. Kirkbride and P. B. Jones, Understanding the excess psychosis risk in ethnic minorities: The impact of structure and identity, *Social Psychiatry and Psychiatric Epidemiology* **56**(11), 2021, 1913–21.

21. D. R. Williams and S. A. Mohammed, Racism and health I, *American Behavioral Scientist* **57** (8), 2013, 1152–73.

22. Office for National Statistics, Updating ethnic contrasts in deaths involving the coronavirus (COVID-19), England: 10 January 2022 to 16 February 2022, 2022. Available at: www.ons.gov.uk/peoplepopulationandcommunity/birthsdeathsandmarriages/deaths/articles/updatingethniccontrastsindeathsinvolvingthecoronaviruscovid19englandandwales/10january2022to16february2022

23. E. J. R. David, T. M. Schroeder and J. Fernandez, Internalized racism: A systematic review of the psychological literature on racism's most insidious consequence, *Journal of Social Issues* **75**(4), 2019, 1057–86.

24. I. H. Meyer, Minority stress and mental health in gay men, *Journal of Health and Social Behavior* **36**(1), 1995, 38–56.

25. L. Platt, *Understanding Inequalities*, 2nd ed., Cambridge, Polity Press, 2019.

26. E. Riska, Women's health: Issues and prospects, *Scandinavian Journal of Public Health* **28** (2), 2000, 84–7.

27. C. L. Saunders, S. Maccarthy, C. Meads *et al.*, Long-term conditions among sexual minority adults in England: Evidence from a cross-sectional analysis of responses to the English GP Patient Survey, *BJGP Open* **5**(5), 2021, BJGPO.2021.0067.

28. J. Semlyen, M. King, J. Varney and G. Hagger-Johnson, Sexual orientation and symptoms of common mental disorder or low wellbeing: Combined meta-analysis of 12 UK population health surveys, *BMC Psychiatry* **16**(1), 2016, 67.

29. Stonewall, LGBT in Britain: Health Report, 2018.

30. L. Shahab, J. Brown, G. Hagger-Johnson *et al.*, Sexual orientation identity and tobacco and hazardous alcohol use: Findings from a cross-sectional English population survey, *BMJ Open* **7**(10), 2017, e015058.

31. J. Semlyen, T. J. Curtis and J. Varney, Sexual orientation identity in relation to unhealthy body mass index: Individual participant data meta-analysis of 93,429 individuals from 12 UK health surveys, *Journal of Public Health (Oxford)* **42**(1), 2020, 98–106.

32. House of Lords Library, Human rights of LGBT people worldwide, n.d. Available at: https://lordslibrary.parliament.uk/human-rights-of-lgbt-people-worldwide/

33. Department for Work and Pensions, Family Resources Survey: Financial year 2019 to 2020, 2021. Available at: www.gov.uk/government/statistics/family-resources-survey-financial-year-2019-to-2020

34. Office for National Statistics, Outcomes for disabled people in the UK: 2021, 2022. Available at: www.ons.gov.uk/peoplepopulationandcommunity/healthandsocialcare/disability/articles/outcomesfordisabledpeopleintheuk/2021

35. P. Heslop, P. S. Blair, P. Fleming *et al.*, The confidential inquiry into premature deaths of people with intellectual disabilities in the UK: A population-based study, *The Lancet* **383** (9920), 2014, 889–95.

36. R. Aldridge, D. Menezes, D. Lewer *et al.*, Causes of death among homeless people: A population-based cross-sectional study of linked hospitalisation and mortality data in England [version 1; peer review: 2 approved], *Wellcome Open Research* **4**(49), 2019.

37. Revolving Doors, Rebalancing Act 2017. Available at: https://revolving-doors.org.uk/publications/rebalancing-act/

38. J. Lynch, Reframing inequality? The health inequalities turn as a dangerous frame shift, *Journal of Public Health* **39**(4), 2017, 653–60.

39. K. Qureshi, It's not just pills and potions? Depoliticising health inequalities policy in England, *Anthropology & Medicine* **20**(1), 2013, 1–12.

40. G. Dahlgren and M. Whitehead, The Dahlgren-Whitehead model of health determinants: 30 years on and still chasing rainbows, *Public Health* **199**, 2021, 20–4.

41. S. Gillam, V. Rodrigues and P. Myles, Public health education in UK medical schools: Towards consensus, *Journal of Public Health (Oxford)* **38**(3), 2016, 522–5.

42. H. Dixon, A. Povall, A. Ledger and G. Ashwell, Medical students' experiences of health inequalities and inclusion health education, *The Clinical Teacher*, 2021.

43. D. Bhugra, All medicine is social, *Journal of the Royal Society of Medicine* **107**(5), 2014, 183–6.

44. T. D. Bhate and L. C. Loh, Building a generation of physician advocates: The case for including mandatory training in advocacy in Canadian medical school curricula, *Academic Medicine* **90**(12), 2015, 1602–6.

45. T. S. Huddle, Political activism is not mandated by medical professionalism, *American Journal of Bioethics* **14**(9), 2014, 51–3.

46. D. Acheson (Chair) *et al.*, Independent inquiry into inequalities in health report, 1998. Available at: www.gov.uk/government/publications/independent-inquiry-into-inequalities-in-health-report

47. B. Barr, J. Higgerson and M. Whitehead, Investigating the impact of the English health inequalities strategy: Time trend analysis, *British Medical Journal* **358**, 2017, j3310.

48. D. Buck, Reducing inequalities in health: Towards a brave old world? The King's Fund, 2017. Available at: www.kingsfund.org.uk/blog/2017/08/reducing-inequalities-health-towards-brave-old-world

49. NHS England, Core20PLUS5 (adults) – an approach to reducing healthcare inequalities. Available at: www.england.nhs.uk/about/equality/equality-hub/national-healthcare-inequalities-improvement-programme/core20plus5/

50. T. Lewis, D. Buck and L. Wenzel, Equity and endurance: How can we tackle health inequalities this time? The King's Fund, 2022. Available at: www.kingsfund.org.uk/publications/how-can-we-tackle-health-inequalities

15

Health Policy

Richard Lewis and Stephen Gillam

Key points

- The development and implementation of health policy is influenced by people or organisations, the wider political context and circumstances, the process by which policy is made and the content of the policy itself (i.e. what it is designed to achieve).
- Rational, bureaucratic models of policy-making exist, but they underplay the contingent, ad hoc nature of these processes in practice.
- Policy-making is a political process and can only ever be partially evidence-based because policy is concerned with what ought to be as well as what is.
- Health policy in high-income countries tends to be dominated by discussions about the provision of health-care rather than wider public health and its determinants.
- Health-care policy has become more focused on management since the late twentieth century and in England has been characterised by constant reform.
- Understanding how policy is created and developed can help those working in public health to influence its development and implementation locally.

15.1 Introduction

The World Health Organization defines health policy as 'the decisions, plans and actions that are undertaken to achieve specific health care goals within a society' [1]. Broadly speaking, this refers to a set of overarching principles, goals, plans, rules or legislation that influence the actions of those involved in health and health-care. This can occur at a national level, or more locally with the development of local health policies – for example, by local commissioners, or those within a clinical environment (e.g. clinical guidance or public health practice such as screening programmes).

Health policy can help to set out agreed priorities, principles and consensus; define agreed plans of action; and identify desired processes or outcomes. For effective practice, it is valuable to have an understanding of the way in which health policy is developed, how it is utilised to effect change and how it can be influenced and shaped by practitioners in public health.

The development of local policies, strategies and actions based on health needs is covered in Part 1 of this book, specifically in Chapters 1, 4, 5, 6 and 8. This chapter focuses on the interplay of health policy and politics at a national level, and:

- explores the process by which health policy is created and the context in which it is developed and influenced;
- considers the interplay between policy and its implementation; and
- offers a narrative of the evolution of national health policy and politics in England over the last 30 years.

15.2 What Do We Mean by Policy and How Is It Made?

A common-sense approach would equate public policy with the formal decisions or explicit proposals of governments or public agencies. In practice, the process of policy-making is subtler and more complex. Policy may emerge from a series of apparently unrelated decisions and governments or public agencies do not control the outcomes of intended policies with any great certainty. In fact, government policy may be as much about what they choose not to do as about what they choose to do [2].

At a national level, the policy process is the means by which particular policies emerge and are pursued by governments and government agencies. There are many competing explanations of how policy is created [3]. However, a simple and useful way of understanding how policy is made is as the consequence of the inter-relation of 'actors' (those people or organisations that populate the process), the wider context, the process by which policy is made and the content of the policy itself (i.e. what it is designed to achieve) [4] (see Figure 15.1).

Early theories of the policy process as a system were dominated by two opposing schools of thought: the 'rationalists' and the 'incrementalists'. 'Rational' models have their roots in the ground-breaking work of Max Weber, for whom bureaucracies were

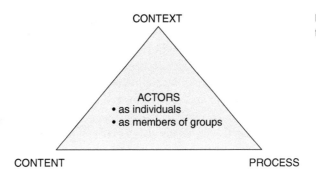

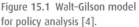

Figure 15.1 Walt–Gilson model for policy analysis [4].

Figure 15.2 Adapted from
Walt's four key stages of
rational policy development [6].

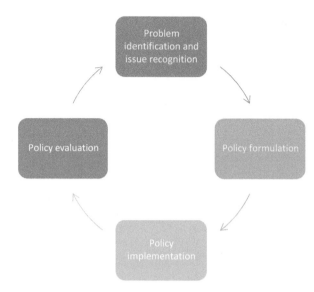

the prime means of organising societal activities [5]. Rationalists describe the policy process in terms of a series of *linked, but distinct phases* and types of activity that together produce a 'policy'. Such an approach is based on the application of a logical and apparently sequential set of functions and technical skills to ensure that an appropriate response is generated to a 'policy problem' [6, 7] (see Figure 15.2).

This 'rational' approach to the policy process is attractive in that it identifies different types of activities that may be involved (and reflects the way in which policy-makers often conceive of the process). However, it has been criticised for implying that the process is a well-ordered translation of objectives into action. Increasingly, this model of comprehensive rationality has been challenged by the notion of 'bounded rationality' – it is simply not reasonable to expect policy-makers to be able to take all information into account in reaching decisions, to make the right choices nor to have sufficient control over the system [8]. More realistically, they look to make decisions that are satisfactory or 'good enough' – or to 'satisfice' (sufficing and satisfying), to use Simon's terminology [9].

Moreover, critics such as Lindblom oppose the very notion that objectives (i.e. the policy 'ends') can be identified separately from any consideration of the policy 'means' [10]. In actual decision-making, he suggests, policy-makers do not, *nor should they*, set prior aims, but instead seek only to move from the status quo in small steps and by reaching agreement among competing interest groups. Human beings, he felt, simply do not possess the ability to process all necessary information to make 'rational' decisions. In this view, 'muddling through' by negotiation between different interest groups is often the most productive approach.

15.3 The Context for Policy-Making

Policies exist in a 'context' – the environment within which any policy is located, which reflects both constraints and opportunities. Leichter identified four distinct sets of contextual factors that impact on national health policy (see Box 15.1) [11].

At a more practical level, context also includes factors such as the formal and informal relationships between health-care organisations and local interest groups, the wider economy and the local population's health status.

One important contextual factor of particular interest to students of health policy is that of 'professionalism'. Professionals wield power by virtue of their specialist knowledge, and their ability to control the supply of their membership and regulate their own affairs. As a result, professionals enjoy high degrees of autonomy and discretion. The medical profession exercises three distinct forms of autonomy:

- 'economic' (determining remuneration);
- 'political' (influencing policy); and
- 'clinical' (controlling clinical performance) [12].

Changes in one area are not necessarily accompanied by declining influence elsewhere.

Alford's classic study of the New York health system published in 1975 identified key interest groups within the policy process [13]. 'Professional monopolisers' (the medical profession) were the dominant power, challenged only by 'corporate rationalisers' (managerial interests) who sought to exert control over the medical professionals. The interests of community groups and patients exercised little power within the health-care system and were described by Alford as 'repressed'. Importantly, Alford suggested that professional power allowed the medical interest group to control the ideological and cultural environment that supported their dominant position.

The position of the medical profession within the British policy process has been described as a 'state-licensed elite' [14]. The predominance of medical interests since the formation of the NHS has been described as a form of 'ideological corporatism',

---

Box 15.1 Contextual factors that impact on national health policy [11]

- **situational** factors – transient conditions, such as war, that allow governments to introduce policies otherwise considered out of bounds;
- **structural** factors – relatively unchanging elements in society, such as the political regime;
- **cultural** factors – reflecting the values within society; and
- **environmental** factors – those that impinge on states from their contact with other countries.

where governments and the profession share a similar world view and organised medical interest groups enjoy significant policy influence and autonomy. However, a number of conflicts have emerged between government and the medical profession. For example, the introduction of market-based reforms to the NHS since the 1980s (part of a trend towards 'new public management' that is discussed further below) has been a source of on-going dispute between the government and the British trade union and professional body for doctors and medical students, the British Medical Association. Successive governments have also changed the contractual terms which bound both independently contracted and employed professionals to the NHS. The fact that many of these reforms were pursued amid significant opposition from professional interests suggests that the prevailing corporatist accommodation between government and professions is weaker now than it once was [15].

15.4 Implementation as Part of the Policy Process

In rational models of the policy process, as illustrated in Figure 15.2, implementation features as a distinct phase that occurs once formal 'policy' has been created. Implementation is seen as simply a 'technical' or 'managerial' process unconnected to the more vital issue of policy content and the initial decision to act (or not to act). This 'top-down' conceptualisation of the policy process (where managers faithfully execute policy coming down from a political policy-making cadre) has been challenged by empirical studies. These studies suggest that policy implementation is fundamentally intertwined with 'policy-making'. In this view, policy also emerges 'bottom up' from the actions (or inaction) of those responsible for implementation. There is also a frequent lack of correspondence between policy objectives and their outcomes – the so-called 'implementation deficit'. Top-down models of policy-making exaggerate the power of politicians and civil servants; bottom-up models highlight spontaneity and adaptation.

Support for the bottom-up approach is based on two propositions:
- the selection of policy solutions may occur during implementation (i.e. policies may not always be clearly defined prior to their operationalisation); and
- the behaviour of implementers may adapt the policy content or its outcome.

For example, a study by Lipsky identified a key role for 'street-level bureaucrats' who were able to alter policy outcomes through the way in which they chose to respond to pressures from above [16]. An examination of Dutch policy on heart transplants, for example, showed that national policy was deliberately subverted by health-service providers who did not agree with the proposed policy [17]. In another example, a national policy in New Zealand in the early 1990s to introduce user charges to hospital outpatient services proved unpopular with the hospital managers and staff who had to collect them, and these were progressively withdrawn and finally abandoned two years after introduction [7].

Health-care organisations may therefore pursue their own strategies and policy agenda and are unlikely to see themselves as passive implementers of government policy. A number of factors may influence the ability of the centre to control the actions of the lower levels of the health system such as the source of funds and who controls them, legislation that sets out where authority lies, and the ability of government to enforce operating rules [7].

In the UK, NHS organisations have their own collective interest groups (such as the NHS Confederation and NHS Providers) that actively promote policy and seek to influence government opinion. This means that ministers' ability to achieve change on the ground is often more constrained than they might wish. Finally, doctors influence policy both collectively – via their trade union, the British Medical Association – and individually. Politicians are all too aware of the power of a profession that makes contact with 6 million people a week.

15.4.1 Recent Health Policy in England

This section considers briefly some of the main features of health policy in England since 1990. The reforms introduced in 1990 by the Conservative government heralded a period of heated policy debate that continues to this day, especially with increasing and unsustainable demands on the NHS, which are becoming ever-more prominent in the media since the COVID-19 pandemic. Note that in the post-devolution era, England, Wales and Scotland have adopted significantly different health policies.

Prior to the reforms of 1990, management of the NHS had been characterised by bureaucratic governance, with administrators working alongside professional clinical leaders in a form of 'consensus management'. The 1990 reforms introduced greater dynamism (and controversy) into the sector, significantly through a division between the 'purchasers' of health-care and increasingly autonomous providers. Purchasers were given the responsibility to meet their populations' needs by securing the right mix of services from the best available providers. This aimed to foster competition among providers, which it was anticipated would lead to increased efficiency and quality. This 'purchaser-provider' split became an enduring feature of English NHS policy, with subsequent NHS reorganisations in England all seeking to find a magic formula to balance market forces with the needs of a (largely) publicly owned bureaucracy much cherished by the population.

These market reforms were consistent with a broader international movement from the 1970s called 'new public management' (NPM). NPM was a governmental response to what was seen (by some at least) as inefficient public provision of services that delivered poor levels of efficiency and a lack of consideration of patients' views. Instead, new policy instruments became popular, such as perform-ance management, competition, greater disaggregation of and freedom to operate for service providers, and an emphasis on private sector management styles, techniques and reward systems [18]. It is notable that the 1990 reforms were presaged by the introduction of 'general management' to the NHS, following a report by a private sector businessman, Sir Roy Griffiths.

While NHS policy remained a key political battlefield in UK party politics, the degree of convergence between Conservative and Labour parties was perhaps surprising. The period between 1990 and 1997 saw reforms that were stronger in rhetoric than in practice (central government found it hard to 'let go' of a policy area so important to voters). The arrival of Tony Blair's Labour government saw not the dismantling of the 'internal market', but its refinement, as a way to improve access and quality of care for patients. The Labour government's reforms of the NHS comprised three overlapping strategies [19]:

- The first dimension of reform was to improve the provision of care through increased investment in service provision (in the shape of more health professionals, equipment and buildings). As a consequence, health spending rose from around 7% of gross domestic product (GDP) in 2000 to reach about 10% by 2010, a proportion approaching that of the European average.
- The second dimension of reform involved setting national standards and targets and creating a regulatory infrastructure to monitor these standards (such as the quality regulator now known as the Care Quality Commission).
- The third dimension of reform involved the further development of market forces, in particular by giving patients the right to choose their provider, creating foundation trusts with greater freedoms from central government control. New payment systems were introduced which rewarded providers according to the volume of services and which supported competition between providers (including an increasing proportion of private sector providers).

Intrinsic to the creation of markets was the notion that the centre-local relationship between government and the NHS should shift, with less hands-on control by Whitehall. In Labour's language, this was part of a wider movement to 'new localism' founded in the belief that concentrating decision-making within central government was not only wrong in principle, but inefficient in an ever-more complex world and prone to policy failure [20].

The trend towards harnessing competition and 'market forces' and the reduction in central government control was continued by the 2010 coalition government and perhaps reached its apotheosis in the 2012 Health and Care Act, which strengthened powers of the independent regulator, Monitor, to prevent anti-competitive behaviour and created new commissioning arrangements and liberalisation of market entry for private providers. The NHS Commissioning Board (later known as NHS England, the NHS headquarters in England) was established as an independent body and the government replaced (in theory at least) top-down direction of the NHS with a 'mandate' that set out the objectives it wished NHS England to achieve.

While the 2012 Health and Social Care Act looked to be a determined continuation on the path to marketisation, in fact it proved a high-water mark for NHS competition among suppliers of care. The furore that resulted from these proposals – from sections of the public, trade unions (including the BMA) and, importantly, Liberal Democrat coalition partners – demonstrated clearly that the introduction of market principles to the NHS remained a deeply controversial issue (and some more radical elements of the initial policy were removed or watered down in Parliament).

However, a significant change in economic circumstances led to a change in policy direction. From 1997, significant improvements in waiting times had been achieved, but these were enabled by large and continuous increases in NHS budgets. Between 1996 and 2010, the NHS received real-terms annual growth in funding of 6.4%. But the economic crash of 2008 brought immense pressure on NHS (and other public sector) funding, resulting in a historically low settlement of only 0.85% per year over the next decade [21]. Consequently, large gaps in funding and services were predicted, driven in particular by the increasing numbers of people with long-term conditions [22].

In this context, policy attention shifted from access and waiting times to trying to proactively manage chronic disease and preventing future hospitalisations. This latter challenge appeared better suited to 'joining up' or integrating services between different health-care organisations, creating a 'pathway' of care for patients with joined-up care between the hospital and community. Thus, austerity brought forward a change in policy [23]. As a result, a greater focus on integrated care emerged, involving collaboration between primary, community, hospital and social care. There was a particular emphasis on avoiding emergency admissions to hospital, although pilots were mostly unsuccessful in this regard [24].

Alongside these experiments with new integrated care models, a return to collaborative strategic planning replaced elements of the NHS market [23]. Sustainability and Transformation Partnerships (STPs) were introduced in 2016 to oversee the development and delivery of health and social care for defined populations. The 2022 Health and Care Act then replaced STPs with 42 Integrated Care Boards and Integrated Care Partnerships. Integrated Care Boards are comprised of local health-care providers with new duties to collaborate and a shared accountability for the collective spend on NHS services. Chapters 1 to 6 in Part 1 outline the theory behind how information, evidence and data is used to inform priorities, decisions and spending by these local integrated partnerships. Competition within NHS markets appears to be, for now at least, no longer the driving force of NHS policy after three decades of experiment.

15.5 Recent Developments in Public Health Policy

The public health system has been through many changes over recent years, but is critical to improving health in communities. Evidence suggests that health services have contributed only a third of recent improvements in life expectancy [25]. Health inequalities are pervasive in many countries, but are particularly stark in the UK (see Chapter 14) and as is described throughout this textbook, the COVID-19 pandemic further aggravated socioeconomic, geographical and ethnic inequalities. Addressing the unequal distribution of wider determinants of health (such as income, education, employment and housing) has the potential to achieve greater improvements (see Chapter 8).

Health policy-makers tend to focus on the levers they can pull – such as preventive health-care, health promotion and pharmaceutical interventions – to limited effect. Yet decades of advocacy, beginning with the Black Report in 1980, have evidenced the bolder policies required [26]. Progress to reduce inequalities and their impact is possible with political will [27]. As described in Chapter 14, substantial investment is required in public services welfare, a fairer system of wages and taxation, better infrastructure (e.g. transport and digital connectivity), stronger labour protection, measures to tackle systemic racism and action to reduce profits from unhealthy commodities (e.g. alcohol, ultra-processed foods, tobacco and gambling). Research suggests the British public support such measures [28].

Broadly speaking, Labour governments committed to Beveridge's model of the welfare state have been readier to support interventions designed to tackle inequalities [29]. By contrast, libertarian Conservative regimes have downplayed their usefulness. In this view, expanding the 'nanny state' may impede the wealth-creating individualism that best alleviates poverty. Recent policy developments are illustrative.

The coalition government under David Cameron stated a commitment to reduce inequalities [30]. Michael Marmot's review, *Fair Society, Healthy Lives*, was to provide the basis of implementation [31]. However, against a background of fiscal austerity, little progress was made on key policy priorities (see Box 15.2). Indeed, in a follow-up report 10 years on, Marmot found regional inequalities in health and wealth had worsened, with stalling life expectancy attributed in part to the impact of cuts to public services in different parts of the country [32].

The government of Boris Johnson pledged to reduce regional inequalities in life expectancy. Yet a medical model of health persisted with an emphasis on access to

Box 15.2 Health Equity in England – priorities [31]

- give every child the best start in life;
- enable all people to maximise their capabilities and have control over their lives;
- create fair employment and good work for all;
- ensure a healthy standard of living for all; and
- create and develop healthy and sustainable places and communities.

screening, diagnostics and lifestyle modification as the principal means to narrow gaps. The 'Levelling Up' White Paper extolled the merits of regional devolution, but without sufficient additional investment for public services [33].

As described specifically in Chapters 8 and 10–14, policies addressing the social determinants of health require working across many sectors (health, education, criminal justice, local government, transport, etc.) and more effective inter-departmental working. This requires what is often referred to as a 'whole-systems approach'. Commonly understood characteristics of whole-systems working include that:
- services are responsive to the needs of whole populations;
- all stakeholders accept their interdependency;
- partnerships are advanced by sharing a vision of the service priorities; and
- users of the system do not experience unnecessary gaps or duplication.

The coalition government moved the local public health function from health authorities into local government with the aim that they would have greater influence over NHS and social care services, children's services, education, leisure, transport and housing policy through new Health and Wellbeing Boards.

Public Health England (PHE) was set up in 2013 as an executive agency of the Department of Health to set public health policy, and strengthen emergency preparedness and health protection. The centralisation of expertise aimed to allow for more coordinated action on national priorities, but proximity to government proved problematic. Ideological opposition has stalled the implementation of minimum unit alcohol pricing and sugar taxes, for example.

In the wake of the immediate phase of the COVID-19 pandemic, PHE was subsequently disbanded in 2021: its health protection functions were formally transferred into the UK Health Security Agency, while its health improvement functions were transferred to the Office for Health Improvement and Disparities (OHID) in the Department of Health and Social Care. At the time of writing, it is too soon to know whether these changes will have their desired effect, but the history of recent reorganisations of the NHS and health policy-making bodies suggest that reorganisations unaccompanied by political will or resources seldom achieve their aims.

Replacement of the term 'heath inequalities' with the more anodyne 'health disparities' is symbolically significant. In the mid-1990s, civil servants were instructed to substitute 'health variations' to dampen persistent public interest in health inequalities. These manipulations have only served to give this politically charged topic greater prominence.

The amount of time people spend in poor health has actually increased as life expectancy has stalled and health inequalities have increased. Successive Conservative administrations have been charged with 'malign neglect' of a public health system that is 'broken'; a royal commission may be required to fix it [34].

15.6 Conclusions

Health policy is primarily concerned with the provision of health-care to those already sick. Public health and preventive policies tend to be marginalised. This reflects the political sensitivity attached to health-care services and the supposed priorities of the electorate.

In England, there has been a significant 'policy churn' since the 1990s, with successive governments pursuing reforms of the organisations that deliver NHS services and the incentives they face. In particular, 'new public management' has been adopted in an attempt to increase efficiency. While there is economic evidence suggesting that greater competition may enhance quality in specific circumstances [35], other commentators believe that competition between providers may impede the delivery of integrated care to patients [36].

At the time of writing, policy-makers are now placing great faith in local partnerships rather than competition for improving health and reducing health inequalities. This policy is also backed by only limited evidence at the present time [37] and generating research and evidence will be an important element of their implementation and evolution, to inform and support efforts towards more effective, cost-effective, efficient, patient-centred and joined-up care.

REFERENCES

1. World Health Organization, Quality of care. Available at: www.who.int/health-topics/quality-of-care#tab=tab_1health-ethics-governance/diseases/covid-19
2. T. Dye, *Top Down Policymaking*, London, Chatham House Publishers, 2001.
3. P. A. Sabatier, *Theories of the Policy Process*, Cambridge, MA, Westview Press, 2007.
4. G. Walt and L. Gilson, Reforming the health sector in developing countries: the central role of policy analysis. *Health Policy and Planning* **9**(4), 1994, 353–370.
5. M. Weber, *The Theory of Social and Economic Organization*, New York, NY, Free Press, 1963.
6. G. Walt, *Health Policy: An Introduction to Process and Power*, London; Zed Books, 1994.
7. K. Buse, N. Mays, and G. Walt, *Making Health Policy*, 2nd ed., Maidenhead, McGraw-Hill Education, 2012.
8. P. Cairney, *Understanding Public Policy: Theories and Issues*, 2nd ed., London, Red Globe Press, 2020.
9. H. Simon, *Administrative Behaviour*, 3rd ed., London, MacMillan, 1976.
10. C. E. Lindblom, The science of muddling through, *Public Administration Review* **19**(2), 1959, 79–88.
11. H. M. Leichter, *A Comparative Approach to Policy Analysis: Health Care Policy in Four Nations*, Cambridge, Cambridge University Press, 1979.

12. M.-A. Elston, The politics of professional power: Medicine in changing health service. In J. Gabe, M. Calnan and M. Bury (eds.), *The Sociology of the Health Service*, London, Routledge, pp. 58–88.

13. R. R. Alford, *Health Care Politics*, Chicago, IL, University of Chicago Press, 1975.

14. S. Harrison, D. J. Hunter and C. Pollitt, *The Dynamics of British Health Policy*, London, Unwin, 1990.

15. E. Ferlie, *Analysing Health Care Organizations: A Personal Anthology*, New York, NY, Routledge, 2016.

16. M. Lipsky, Towards a theory of street-level bureaucracy. In W. D. Hawley, M. Lipsky, S. B. Greenberg *et al.* (eds.), *Theoretical Perspectives on Urban Politics*, Englewood Cliffs, NJ, Prentice-Hall, 1976, pp. 196–213.

17. A. De Roo and H. Maarse, Understanding the central-local relationship in health care: A new approach, *International Journal of Health Planning & Management* 5(1), 1990, 15–25.

18. C. Hood, A public management for all seasons, *Public Administration* 69, 1991, 3–19.

19. S. Stevens, Reform strategies for the English NHS, *Health Affairs* 23(3), 2004, 37–44.

20. G. Stoker, New localism, progressive politics and democracy. In A. Gamble and T. Wright (eds.), *Restating the State*, Oxford, Blackwell, 2004.

21. R. Crawford and C. Emmerson, *NHS and Social Care Funding: The Outlook to 2021/22*, London, Nuffield Trust and Institute for Fiscal Studies, 2012.

22. NHS England, NHS five year forward view, London, 2014. Available at: www.england.nhs.uk/publi cation/nhs-five-year-forward-view/

23. R. Q. Lewis, More reform of the English National Health Service: From competition back to planning? *Journal of Health Service* 49(1), 2019, 5–16.

24. R. Q. Lewis, K. Checkland, M. A. Durand *et al.*, Integrated care in England: What can we learn from a decade of national pilot programmes? *International Journal of Integrated Care* 21(4), 2021, 5.

25. J. Bunker, The role of medical care in contributing to health improvement within society, *International Journal of Epidemiology* 30(6), 2001, 1260–3.

26. D. Black, J. N. Morris, C. Smith *et al.*, Inequalities in health: Report of a research working group, Department of Health and Social Services, 1980.

27. C. Bambra, K. E. Smith and J. Pearce, Scaling up: The politics of health and place, *Social Science & Medicine* 232, 2019, 36–42.

28. K. E. Smith, A. K. Macintyre, S. Weakley et al., Public understandings of potential policy responses to health inequalities: Evidence from a UK national survey and citizens' juries in three UK cities, *Social Science & Medicine* 291, 2021, 114458.

29. R. Klein, *The New Politics of the NHS*, 7th ed., London, Longman, 2013.

30. Department of Health, *Healthy Lives, Healthy People: Our Strategy for Public Health in England*, London, The Stationery Office, 2010.

31. M. Marmot, Strategic review of health inequalities in England post-2010, Marmot review final report, University College London. Available at: www.ucl.ac.uk/gheg/marmotreview/Documents

32. M. Marmot, Health equity in England: The Marmot review 10 years on, Institute of Health Equity/Health Foundation, February 2020.

33. R. Ralston, K. Smith, C. H. O'Connor and A. Brown, Levelling up the UK: Is the government serious about reducing regional health inequalities? *British Medical Journal* **377**, 2022, e070589.

34. G. Scally, The UK's public health system is broken, *British Medical Journal* **378**, 2022, o2210.

35. M. Gaynor, C. Propper and S. Seiler, Free to choose? Reform or choice, and consideration sets in the English National Health Service, *American Journal of Economic Affairs* **106**(11), 2016, 3521-57.

36. N. Mays, Is there evidence that competition in health care is a good thing? No, *British Medical Journal* **343**, 2011, d4337.

37. H. Alderwick, A. Hutchings and N. Mays, A cure for everything and nothing? Local partnerships for improving health, *British Medical Journal* **378**, 2022, e070910.

16

International Development and Public Health

Gillian Turner and Jenny Amery

Key points

- In 2015, world leaders committed to the Sustainable Development Goals (SDGs), including, 'Ensure healthy lives and promote well-being for all at all ages', incorporating the concept of Universal Health Coverage (UHC) – that is, protecting poor people from large out-of-pocket expenditure on health, and improving equity of access to effective health services.
- Almost all preventable child and pregnancy-related deaths occur in low- or low-middle-income countries. Poorer people are most likely to suffer from communicable diseases. Non-communicable diseases are increasing in lower-income countries.
- The majority of people living in extreme poverty live where state institutions are weak or ineffective, including in middle-income countries. International agencies need to assist such countries to progress towards UHC, while focusing efforts on low-income countries or those in humanitarian crisis.
- Different models of financing and organising health services are appropriate for different contexts. There is no one 'right' model.
- Better data systems are needed to monitor the impact of health policies and health spend; to measure health-service quality; to enable early detection of diseases of epidemic potential; and to identify and combat resistance to key antibiotics.
- Greater coordination between the multiplicity of global health agencies is urgently needed to increase their impact.
- More research is needed into the prevention and management of diseases of poverty and ways of reaching the poorest people with proven cost-effective life-saving interventions.

16.1 Introduction

This chapter extends the consideration of the changing global burden of diseases and discusses what is required to mount an effective response to public health challenges, particularly in countries where people are living in extreme poverty (less than $1.90 per day [1]). It considers the role of international development assistance and the responsibilities of the international community in improving the health of poor people.

16.2 The Links between Poverty and Health

Poor health often results from poverty: malnutrition, limited or no access to clean water, sanitation, housing, health and education services; in turn it contributes to poverty and impedes economic growth [2]. A person who is repeatedly ill cannot earn a decent living or contribute to the workforce. Unmet need for modern family-planning methods results in early and repeated pregnancies, closely spaced births, and increased risks of illness and death for the child and mother. Undernourished and frequently sick children do not learn well and often drop out of school early. When a family member falls sick, poor households may have to make huge payments for health-care, sell their livestock, land or other assets, become indebted to money lenders or enter bonded labour agreements, which may keep the family in poverty. Poverty and ill health cause misery and loss of hope. A lack of access to health-care also means opportunities to stop the spread of communicable diseases are missed, resulting in increased illness in the wider community.

There are wide differences between health outcomes for the richest and poorest within countries and while mortality rates have fallen across quintiles, the discrepancy between the richest and poorest has been sustained [3]. Table 16.1 shows inequalities in under-5 mortality rates for low- and middle-income countries combined (excluding China) in 1990, 2000 and 2016. The gap between the lowest and

Table 16.1 Estimates and 90% uncertainty intervals for quintile-specific under-5 mortality rate in 1990, 2000 and 2016, for all low-income and middle-income countries (excluding China) combined [3]

	Under-5 mortality rate (deaths per 1,000 live births)		
	1990	2000	2016
First quintile (poorest)	142·2 (138·6–146·2)	115·3 (112·2–118·5)	64·6 (61·1–70·1)
Second quintile	135·9 (132·6–139·4)	108·9 (106·2–112·0)	58·0 (54·9–63·1)
Third quintile	120·6 (118·0–123·5)	97·3 (95·2–99·6)	51·1 (48·6–55·3)
Fourth quintile	104·1 (101·4–107·0)	83·2 (81·1–85·7)	42·5 (40·2–46·1)
Fifth quintile (richest)	70·2 (68·0–72·5)	57·8 (56·1–59·7)	31·3 (29·5–34·2)
Ratio of first to fifth quintile mortality rate	2·03 (1·94–2·11)	1·99 (1·91–2·08)	2·06 (1·92–2·20)
Difference in first and fifth quintile mortality rate	72·0 (67·7–76·5)	57·4 (53·9–61·1)	33·2 (29·9–37·6)

highest wealth quintiles has reduced from 72 in 1990 to 33.2 deaths per 1,000 live births in 2016; however, it remains the case that around twice as many of the poorest children in a country die under the age of 5 than do the richest children.

16.3 The Global Burden of Disease

There have been rapid falls in mortality and overall improvements in health globally in the last half century, but many low- and low-middle-income countries (collectively referred to as LMICs in this chapter) have not shared in these benefits. The number of people living in extreme poverty (currently measured as the equivalent of less than US$1.90 per day) fell from 1.8 billion in 1990 to 689 million in 2017. However, the rate of decline in poverty is slowing down and has been adversely affected by the COVID-19 pandemic. Africa has had the highest rates of extreme poverty since the mid-1990s with the slowest rates of poverty decline, while East Asia has experienced a rapid reduction in extreme poverty [4] (see Figure 16.1). Multidimensional poverty measures provide more detailed analysis of trends in multiple aspects of poverty [5].

Poverty and ill health are closely linked. The premature deaths and preventable ill health of millions of poor people present a major contemporary challenge. To

Figure 16.1 Global and regional poverty trends, 1990–2019, World Bank (shown as percentage of the population in poverty, at US$1.90 poverty line) [4]. © World Bank. Available at: https://blogs.worldbank.org/opendata/april-2022-global-poverty-update-world-bank License: CC BY 4.0.

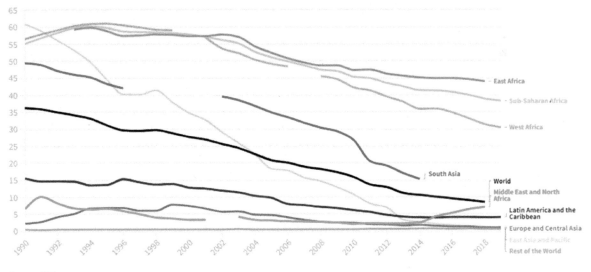

Source: PIP •

Regional and global poverty estimates are reported if the available survey data account for at least 50% of the population within a three-year window of the reference year. In addition, the global estimate is only reported if at least 50% of the population in low- and lower-middle-income countries is covered.

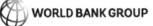

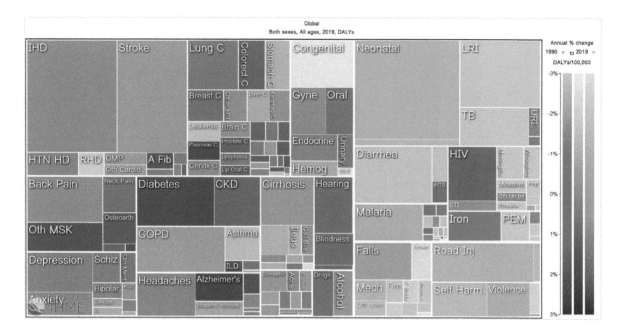

understand the challenge, it is important to note how these are commonly measured. As discussed in Chapter 2, the disability-adjusted life year (DALY) is a measure of the burden of ill health that takes into account both reduced life expectancy and quality of life. It is widely used internationally despite limitations. Values vary according to the weighting used for different age groups. Relatively poor data are available for some countries and conditions, but no better alternative measure has been agreed as yet, and it is this measure that helps us understand the major causes of illness and death and how these are changing over time and between countries.

Significant progress has been made against communicable diseases since 1990, and in all regions of the world non-communicable diseases now account for the greatest burden of disease (see Figure 16.2). Recent research has shown that among the poorest billion people, 65% of DALYs are still lost due to communicable diseases, maternal and newborn mortality and nutritional diseases [6]. Lower respiratory infections, diarrhoeal disease, HIV, tuberculosis and malaria remain the most significant communicable diseases for these populations [6].

Other factors contributing to the changing pattern of disease include international migration, rapid rural-to-urban migration in most poor countries and changing family structures; also, climate change and emerging microbe and vector resistance to drugs and insecticides, which are further discussed in Chapter 17. New pandemic communicable diseases described in Chapter 10, such as COVID-19 and its variants, have emerged and others are likely to follow.

Population growth is a major issue, particularly in the face of climate-change impacts and resource scarcity. The total global population exceeds 8 billion.

Growth is fastest in some of the poorest countries – for example, Nigeria's population is projected to rise from 201 million in 2019 to 733 million in 2100, Pakistan from 217 to 403 million, Malawi from 19 to 67 million and Tanzania from 58 to 286 million over the same period [7].

16.4 Key Health Issues and Effective Interventions

16.4.1 Preventable Illness and Deaths among Children

Despite population growth, the number of deaths in children under 5 worldwide declined from 12.6 million in 1990 to 5.0 million in 2020 – a fall in the mortality rate from 93 to 37 per 1,000 live births [8]. A total of 90% of the deaths occurred in only 41 countries. In these countries, serious illnesses commonly occur sequentially or concurrently before death. For example, measles is often complicated by pneumonia or diarrhoea [9]. Underweight and micronutrient deficiencies decrease host defences, and malnutrition is estimated to contribute to over 45% of avoidable childhood deaths [10]. A total of 149 million children under 5 are stunted (low weight for height) due to chronic undernourishment, resulting from the combined effects of dietary insufficiency, including micronutrient deficiency, and related infections. This will limit their cognitive as well as physical development if not addressed in the first 2 to 3 years of life. The extent and impact of undernutrition remains a silent emergency, which often only becomes visible when exacerbated by acute famine.

The interventions to prevent these deaths are well researched and, with improved coverage, could save many lives. The interventions that have the highest impact on deaths are:

- management of labour and delivery;
- care of pre-term births;
- treatment of pneumonia, diarrhoea, malaria and neonatal sepsis;
- childhood immunisation; and
- management of severe acute malnutrition.

It is estimated that over 3 million lives could be saved annually if 90% of mothers and children had access to these interventions (based on 2015 rates of birth and child mortality) [11]. Providing sustained access to these interventions for the poorest people remains a major challenge, due primarily to the health system and wider public health challenges outlined through the rest of this chapter.

16.5 Maternal Health

A total of 94% of deaths in pregnancy and childbirth occur in low- or lower-middle-income countries, and over two-thirds in 13 countries: Nigeria, India, Democratic Republic of Congo (DRC), Ethiopia, Tanzania, Indonesia, Pakistan, Afghanistan, Chad, Uganda, Cote d'Ivoire, Bangladesh and Niger [13] (see Table 16.2).

Table 16.2 Estimates of maternal mortality ratio (MMR, maternal deaths per 100,000 live births), number of maternal deaths, lifetime risk and proportion of deaths among women of reproductive age that are due to maternal causes (PM), by UN SDG region, sub-region and other grouping, 2017 [13]

SDG region	MMR point estimate and range of uncertainty interval (UI: 80%)			Number of maternal deaths	Lifetime risk of maternal death	PM* (%)
	Lower UI	MMR point estimate	Upper UI			
World	199	211	243	295,000	190	9.2
Sub-Saharan Africa	498	542	649	196,000	37	18.2
Northern Africa and Western Asia	73	84	104	9,700	380	5.9
Central and Southern Asia	131	151	181	58,000	260	6.6
Eastern and South-Eastern Asia	61	69	85	21,000	790	3.3
Latin America and the Caribbean	70	74	81	7,800	630	3.8
Oceania	34	60	120	400	690	4.1
Europe and Northern America	12	12	14	1,500	4,800	0.6
Least developed countries	396	415	477	130,000	56	17.5

* The number of maternal deaths in a given time period divided by the total deaths among women aged 15–49 years.
MMR and lifetime risk rounded according to the following scheme: <100, no rounding; 100–999, rounded to nearest 10; and >1,000, rounded to nearest 100. The numbers of maternal deaths have been rounded as follows: <1,000, rounded to nearest 10; 1,000–9,999, rounded to nearest 100; and >10,000 rounded to nearest 1,000.

Overall, the lifetime risk of maternal death for a woman in high-income countries is 1 in 5,400; in low-income countries it is 1 in 45. This is the largest disparity in health outcomes between the richest and poorest countries. Almost all of these deaths could be prevented if known, cost-effective interventions were available to all women.

Maternal and child health are linked, but there are fundamental differences in effective approaches to addressing them. While evidence-based, successful approaches to improving child health involve delivering services as close to the community as possible, the reduction of maternal mortality requires access to hospital-based interventions to deal with life-threatening complications, which mostly develop around the time of delivery. Good maternal health requires functioning health services at community, clinic and hospital levels, and effective referral systems between them, and is therefore considered an important marker of a functioning health system [12]. The reduction of neonatal deaths is closely linked to improving maternal health.

16.6 Reproductive Health

Concern at the rapid population growth in the second half of the twentieth century often resulted in population policies focusing on controlling demographic growth, at the expense of the needs and rights of individuals. At the landmark International Conference on Population and Development held in Cairo in 1994, more than 170 countries agreed that reproductive health services should be available without coercion to all those who need them, and the conference set out a clear action plan. It defined comprehensive reproductive health-care as:

- voluntary contraceptive and family planning services;
- antenatal care, safe abortion, delivery, post-partum and post-abortion services (or safe motherhood services); and
- services for the prevention, detection and treatment of sexually transmitted infections, including HIV.

It was recognised that many of the issues which impact on reproductive health, including women's empowerment, literacy, poverty and lack of access to health services, could not be resolved quickly, and would require new policies and, in some cases, new legislation. There has been considerable progress in many countries, but about half of pregnancies worldwide each year, approximately 121 million, are unintended. Globally, 257 million women who want to delay or avoid pregnancy are not using an effective method of family planning [14]. There are on-going concerns about how to ensure the future supply of contraceptive methods to those who need them. These concerns are exacerbated when political choices restrict access to reproductive health services within countries, or restrict funding to key organisations that increase access to contraceptive products and services.

16.7 Communicable Diseases

Communicable diseases remain a major cause of ill health and death for the poorest, despite advances in vaccine development, diagnosis and available treatment. Most of this disease burden is from malaria, HIV, TB, diarrhoeal and respiratory diseases (see Figure 16.2), and from neglected tropical diseases, including leishmaniasis, trypanosomiasis, Chaga's disease, lymphatic filariasis, onchocerciasis (river blindness), schistosomiasis, dracunculiasis, soil-transmitted helminth infections, leprosy and trachoma (which causes nearly 2 million people to go blind or become visually impaired each year). Globally, in 2020, there were: 1.5 million deaths from TB; 627,000 from malaria (mostly children in Africa), together with a huge morbidity; and 680,000 deaths due to HIV-related causes, mostly in Africa. Table 16.3 summarises health-care interventions that address the 'big three' and should be considered in conjunction with Chapter 10 and general measures for controlling the spread of communicable disease.

Table 16.3 Summary of effective health-care interventions for reducing illness and death from HIV and AIDS, TB and malaria

Goal	Health-care preventive intervention	Treatment
Prevent and reduce burden of HIV and AIDS	Safe sex, including use of male (and female) condoms; injecting drug users have clean needles and oral substitution therapy; safe, screened blood supplies; antiretroviral drugs to prevent mother-to-child transmission; male circumcision.	Prompt treatment of opportunistic infections, including TB; cotrimoxazole prophylaxis; highly active antiretroviral therapy; palliative care and support.
Prevent and reduce burden of TB	Directly observed treatment of infectious cases to reduce transmission and emergence of drug-resistant strains; testing of people with AIDS for early diagnosis of TB; preventive isoniazid therapy; BCG (Bacille Calmette Guérin) to reduce childhood TB.	Directly observed treatment to cure symptomatic cases; second-line therapies for multiple drug-resistant cases.
Prevent and reduce burden of malaria	Use of insecticide-treated bed-nets; in epidemic-prone areas indoor residual spraying and intermittent presumptive treatment of pregnant women; prompt identification of drug-resistant strains.	Rapid diagnosis and treatment of cases with locally effective medicines, depending on drug resistance. Increasing use of artemisin combination treatments (ACTs), and effective parenteral drugs for severe malaria.

16.7.1 HIV and AIDS

Human immunodeficiency virus was first reported in the early 1980s, and became the first pandemic since that of influenza in 1918. As described in Chapter 10, it has stabilised and the number of new infections has been declining since the late 1990s, and there are fewer deaths due to the scale-up of antiretroviral therapy. An estimated 38.4 million people are currently living with HIV and 1.5 million people worldwide became newly infected in 2021, fewer than half the peak of 3.1 million in 1999. Sub-Saharan Africa has 14% of the world's population and two-thirds of all those living with HIV. Women are disproportionately affected, especially in sub-Saharan Africa, where three women are affected for every two men. People infected with HIV are particularly susceptible to TB and co-infection is very common. Africa remains the global epicentre and even though new infections are decreasing, the time lag between infection and death means the burden of disease will remain high for years to come [15].

16.7.2 COVID-19

As discussed in Chapter 10, during the COVID-19 global pandemic, the lack of vaccines and treatments throughout 2020 meant that non-pharmaceutical interventions had to be implemented in most countries to prevent its spread. National measures such as lockdowns of various durations and closing national borders had significant negative impacts on the economies of households and nations and disrupted service delivery, including at health facilities and in schools. While the direct effects of the COVID-19 pandemic in low-income countries were typically not as severe as in wealthier countries (partly due to their populations being younger), the indirect effects were significant; the case study in Chapter 11 describes the impacts on children and young people, for example. As of July 2022, more than 6 million deaths worldwide have been attributed to COVID-19, 4.8 million of which have been reported in Europe or the Americas [16]. However, there will have been many indirect deaths due to the impacts of health-service interruptions, reduced financing for health services, food insecurity and lower household incomes. One study in 18 low- or low-middle-income countries estimated that there would be 2.6 maternal or child deaths for every reported COVID-19 death, based on data on reductions in health facility utilisation [17].

16.8 Non-Communicable Diseases

Figure 16.2 illustrates that two-thirds of the global burden of ill health is from non-communicable diseases (everything to the left of the vertical line starting at 'neo-natal') or injuries (the boxes below and to the right of 'malaria') and that DALYs due to these have increased significantly since 1990 (darker shading). Projections to the year 2030 suggest that ischaemic heart disease, stroke, smoking-related cancers, respiratory problems and road traffic accidents will cause proportionately more deaths, although AIDS will remain a significant cause globally [18]. Deaths due to injury and violence are likely to increase further following conflicts in Afghanistan and Ukraine since 2021, in addition to on-going conflicts elsewhere.

As is specifically explored in Chapters 8 and 14, robust public health measures in sectors other than health are required to address the key risk factors of nutrition, smoking, unsafe sex and the growing epidemic of injury and death from road traffic accidents [19]. Around 5% of the disease burden globally is due to mental health disorders, mostly chronically disabling depression and other common disorders, alcohol and substance disorders, and psychoses; these also increase the risk of physical illness [20]. Many low-income countries lack policy or legislation for mental health, have very few trained mental health workers, little or no funding, and any available care is institutionally based. Sufferers are highly stigmatised. Scaling up access to an evidence-based package of interventions for core mental health problems would cost US$2 per person in low-income countries. There is growing evidence that many interventions can be delivered effectively in decentralised settings by people who are not mental health professionals [21].

16.9 Access to Medicines

Even when health services reach them, medicines are often not affordable for poor people, who frequently have to pay directly for them (referred to as 'out of pocket'). Nearly 2 billion people globally do not have access to essential medicines [22]. Barriers to accessing effective medicines in poor countries include: high prices; insufficient overall financing of health services and poor priority setting with too little money to fund supplies of essential drugs; inappropriate drug selection, weak procurement and distribution systems; and poor-quality or fake medicines. Some pharmaceutical companies are working in private–public partnerships to bring key medicines to poor people – for example, the ivermectin donation programme as part of the initiative to eradicate onchocerciasis in Africa [23].

The World Trade Organization agreement on trade-related aspects of intellectual property rights (TRIPS) gives countries the right, under the Doha TRIPS and public health decision of 2003 [24], to protect public health (e.g. by importing copies of patented medicines) if their own pharmaceutical industry has insufficient capacity to produce them. International trade policy is important to increase poor people's access to medicines.

There are a number of public–private product-development partnerships that develop medicines for diseases disproportionately affecting poor people. Advance market commitments (AMCs) for vaccines aim to create a competitive developing-country market for future vaccines that is sufficiently large and credible to stimulate private investment in research and development and manufacturing capacity, which otherwise would not take place [25]. AMCs through the Access to COVID-19 Tools accelerator (ACT-A) have ensured the development and manufacture of new technologies; the COVAX facility under ACT-A has been critical to ensuring access to vaccines for COVID-19 [26].

16.10 How Can Improvements in Health Be Delivered?

There is a complex inter-relationship between poverty and health which can be a virtuous cycle with a healthier population contributing to economic growth and prosperity, or a vicious cycle of worsening health, increasing indebtedness from health-care expenditure, marginalisation from the economy and slowing economic growth. Orthodox economic arguments highlight the need for macroeconomic growth to reduce levels of poverty, but not all growth benefits poor people, and there are increasing concerns about 'jobless' growth, with millions of poor people remaining at the margins of society. Debt relief, fairer trade with access to markets for poorer countries and communities are also key, and require action from rich-country governments. More predictable aid would enable low-income countries to fund sustainable 5- to 10-year health plans and invest in well-trained workforces, and

Box 16.1 Good governance

Good governance at governmental level can be summarised as:

- the capacity of the state to raise revenue, use resources and deliver services;
- responsiveness of public policies and institutions to the needs and rights of citizens; and
- accountability, including free media access to information and the opportunity to change leaders through democratic means.

greater domestic investment in health is necessary for the same reasons in middle-income countries. Greater investment in new technologies should yield better diagnostics, medicines and vaccines for communicable and other life-threatening diseases. However, none of these will make a significant difference without quality health services, accessible to poor people, staffed by well-trained, supervised, motivated and adequately rewarded health workers. In particular, investment in primary health-care is critical to ensuring an efficient and cost-effective use of financial resources.

Global knowledge of effective interventions alone is not sufficient to improve health. Governments have a key role, and where a government is unwilling or too weak to implement change, poverty and ill health prevail. The basic role of the state is to establish a foundation of law, maintain macroeconomic stability, invest in basic social services and infrastructure, protect the vulnerable and protect the environment [27] (see Box 16.1).

Much poor performance in terms of health-service delivery is due to weaknesses in institutions, budgeting and public-expenditure management, and the fact that governments are not accountable to their people [28]. The quality of private health-care providers ranges from excellent to dangerous, and is rarely adequately regulated. Governments should be held to account for maintaining fiscal discipline, ensuring resources are allocated and spent in line with stated priorities and not lost through corruption or mismanagement, and are used to achieve maximum impact on health outcomes (see also Chapter 5). Making information more accessible and promoting transparency in fees, budgets and expenditure enable corruption to be tackled more easily, but there are often strong forces at work to avoid such transparency [29]. Further discussions about ensuring quality of care are explored in Chapter 6.

Weak or corrupt states, engulfed in armed conflicts or run by repressive military regimes, will not have institutions capable of delivering health services. In such environments, creative, context-specific responses are needed. Donors may wish to work through UN bodies, non-governmental organisations (NGOs), faith-based organisations, for-profit providers and community-based providers to meet the humanitarian needs of the people, and support the long-term development of government institutions that can eventually take on responsibility for service delivery. Exceptional responses for humanitarian and other disasters such as earthquakes, hurricanes and floods need better coordination, and more should be invested in resilience and risk reduction, as referred to in Chapter 10.

16.11 Improving Health through Health-Care

16.11.1 Organising and Financing Health Systems

There are many ways to promote and sustain health outside the health sector, including housing, water and sanitation, food, security, education and employment. But timely access to a mix of promotion, prevention, treatment, rehabilitation and care is critical, and this needs a well-functioning health system.

One of the reasons for low health-service coverage and poor health outcomes is low per-capita expenditure on health. The World Bank Disease Control Priorities 3 (DCP3) identified the range of interventions necessary to progress towards Universal Health Coverage (UHC); a subset of these was identified as an essential UHC package and a smaller subset of the essential package was identified as the Highest Priority Package (see Figure 16.3). For low-income countries, these were assessed as costing (in 2012 US$) US$76 per capita for the essential UHC Package and US$42 per capita for the Highest Priority Package [30]. This would require an additional annual spend of US$23–48 billion and by 2030 would reduce by 1.6–2 million the expected 7.4 million premature deaths in that year.

The method of financing health services will influence whether poor people can access them. Tax-financed universal health-care is the most equitable, despite disproportionate use by the better-educated and well-off, but may also be subject to high administrative cost and poor governance. Widespread compulsory social health insurance can combine risk-pooling and distribute the financial burden according to ability to pay. Prepayment into a community financing scheme tailored to local needs, to pool risk, has to date delivered only limited coverage. Voluntary private insurance benefits those able to pay and will often exclude people with chronic conditions. Out-of-pocket payment at the time of illness is the most regressive form of financing, yet in many low-income countries it is the source of well over half of all financing for health-care. User charges levied by public and private providers of health-care have had mixed impact, but almost universally result in deterring access by poor people or impoverishing those on or near the poverty line [31].

Some countries are attaining measurably better levels of service coverage with lower levels of expenditure. Low-income countries where significant improvements have taken place in the health of the population without high or rapidly rising

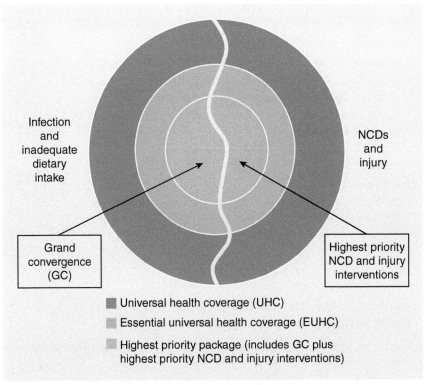

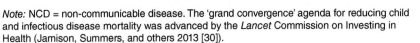

Note: NCD = non-communicable disease. The 'grand convergence' agenda for reducing child and infectious disease mortality was advanced by the *Lancet* Commission on Investing in Health (Jamison, Summers, and others 2013 [30]).

incomes include Bangladesh, Costa Rica, Cuba and Kerala State in India. Effective policies, well implemented, can greatly improve the health of poor people. The HIV epidemic, and the emergence of new diseases such as COVID-19, have highlighted the crucial role of governments in strengthening and maintaining core public health functions [32] (see Box 16.2).

To maximise their benefit, health resources must be re-allocated towards more cost-effective services, poorer geographical regions within countries and services that are used by poor people. DCP3 has provided guidance towards this from a technical perspective; however, the allocation and distribution of resources is an intensely political process, affected by power struggles between competing stakeholders (e.g. different parts of government, external agencies). The ability of the state to set priorities and negotiate the allocation of resources in a way which increases equity and meets the needs of stakeholders is a measure of the state's legitimacy and its commitment to procedural justice [33] (see Box 16.3 and Chapter 5).

Box 16.2 Core public health functions at a national level

Core public health functions include:

- collection and dissemination of evidence for public health policies;
- public health regulation and enforcement;
- pharmaceutical policy regulation and enforcement;
- epidemiological and, where appropriate, behavioural surveillance for risk factors of disease;
- prevention, surveillance and control of disease;
- health promotion;
- intersectoral action for improving health;
- monitoring and evaluation of public health policy; and
- development of human resources and capacity for public health.

Box 16.3 Critical issues in financing and organising of health services

- ensuring effective coverage of health-care services (i.e. bringing health-care benefits to those who are currently not accessing services of acceptable quality, including access to essential medicines);
- protecting people from unexpected large financial expenditures (risk protection);
- creating incentives for appropriate, cost-effective, quality health-care;
- strengthening core public health functions; and
- regulating and assuring the quality of service providers.

16.11.2 People-Centred or Disease-Specific Services – or Both?

Disease- or issue-specific vertical approaches tend to be top-down and controlled by experts. The eradication of smallpox was a success, but efforts to eradicate malaria since the 1960s have failed, and total eradication of malaria is not feasible with current tools. Current examples of vertical programmes include those addressing polio eradication, HIV/AIDS, TB and some childhood immunisation.

The Alma-Ata Declaration of 1978 [34] rejected such vertical approaches and called on governments to tackle common underlying causes of ill health, with the building of sustainable health-care systems, locally based and locally controlled. Emphasis was given to people's participation in health. In 2008, there was a renewed emphasis on the need for strong primary health-care services, close to the people they serve, and responsive to their needs [35].

Vertical programmes can raise the profile of and funding for specific diseases, and increase access to commodities such as insecticide-treated bed-nets for malaria, and affordable, quality medicines. They can often deliver short-term results against specific targets, but they can weaken the impact of other services, by distorting country priorities and diverting scarce trained staff [36]. A different focus on delivery systems for chronic conditions as well as acute episodes is needed in low-resource settings [37]. DCP3 has recognised this and considered the most cost-effective sets of services to make progress towards UHC. These include addressing key communicable diseases, non-communicable disease, sexual and reproductive health and other services and also highlight the provision that is required at community, health centre (primary), first level hospital and referral or specialist hospital, as well as those that need to be delivered population-wide (e.g. health-promoting activities).

In 2018, there were more than 200 global health partnerships and initiatives addressing disease or other specific health needs, many with private-public financing; this number has increased following the efforts to address COVID-19 and improve pandemic preparedness. These include the World Bank, Regional Development Banks, the World Health Organization and UN technical agencies, private entities such as the Bill and Melinda Gates Foundation, and many bilateral donors. There are concerns that this 'international health architecture' may be undermining poor countries' own capacity to deliver essential health services – multiple interventions and funding streams, and the reporting requirements that accompany them, create a burden for already fragile systems. International efforts must be better channelled, in line with evidence on the effectiveness of international aid [38]. China, India and other emerging donors in health are increasingly influential in low-income countries' health services.

16.11.3 What Else Hinders Access to Health-Care?

Cost is a major obstacle for individuals and families. Both formal and informal charges and transport costs will prevent poor people from using services, and may plunge them further into poverty if charges for drugs or treatments require selling assets or borrowing money at inflated rates. Other factors also prevent poor people from using health services. Complex social, cultural and political factors make it difficult to break intergenerational poverty, which affects hundreds of millions of people.

As described in Chapter 14, social exclusion is a process causing systematic disadvantage on the basis of factors such as ethnicity, religion, caste, descent, disability and HIV status (i.e. who you are and where you live). Excluded groups and individuals are denied equal rights and opportunities compared with others.

Some people may suffer multiple forms of exclusion (e.g. women with disabilities living in isolated rural areas) [39]. Gender inequalities are a manifestation of one form of exclusion. Sex disparities are higher in South Asia than anywhere else in the world. A girl in India is more than 32% more likely to die between her first and fifth birthday than is a boy. Child mortality would drop by 20% if girls had the same mortality rate as boys between the ages of 1 month and 5 years. The reasons for this are both environmental and behavioural. Girls are less likely to be brought for timely treatment and have less money spent on them when they are sick than boys [40].

16.11.4 Human Resources for Health

Adequate numbers of well-trained, motivated health workers are essential for effective service delivery. Many countries face a deep crisis in staffing their health services, resulting from chronic under-investment in staff and health systems. This is exacerbated by outward migration and, especially in southern African countries, by the impact of illness (most recently COVID-19, but previously HIV/AIDS) on health services and staff. Low-income countries are currently subsidising high-income ones by supplying them with trained staff. A study of nine sub-Saharan countries found that the collective investment loss for training doctors who were working abroad at the time of the study approached US$2.17 billion [41]. Changes to international recruitment practice may help to manage the flow of migrants, but migration is the result of low pay, lack of career prospects and poor working conditions in 'source' countries, as well as the inability of the high-income 'destination' countries to train and meet their own workforce requirements.

16.12 Measuring Progress, Increasing Success

The SDGs and targets collectively address the different dimensions of poverty. They succeeded the Millennium Development Goals (MDGs) in 2015 and their holistic nature means that whereas there were eight MDGs, three of which were focused directly on health outcomes, there are now 17 goals, one of which is focused on health. However, the goals are interconnected and have a stronger focus on issues such as transparency and accountability and on a wider set of rights than the MDGs had. The SDGs are set out in 'Transforming our world: The 2030 agenda for sustainable development' [42], which was adopted at the UN Sustainable Development Summit in New York in September 2015.

The SDGs have 169 targets and more than 200 indicators. An overarching principle is to 'leave no one behind' – an effort to address the inequities that marred the achievements of the MDGs.

Progress towards the health SDG and respective indicators is being monitored (more information on monitoring health data may be found in Chapter 2), but is limited by incomplete vital registration of births and deaths, and poor-quality data

[43]. The SDGs are also global, whereas the MDGs applied primarily to low- and low-middle-income countries. Reporting is voluntary and there is less focus on progress made than was apparent under the MDGs.

SDG 3 and some of its targets and indicators are shown in Table 16.4 to illustrate the type of metrics used to monitor progress.

There is an urgent need for better data systems to guide results-based performance monitoring, better disaggregation to allow analysis of equity and distributional issues, and improved capture of health-service quality measures. Governments and international organisations do not always use the same data sources or definitions. The demand for high-quality data grew in response to the need to monitor progress against the MDGs. It has since grown to monitor the impact of the global health initiatives and to monitor and evaluate health-system interventions, to show that increased funding is having the desired impact and delivering value for money, and to hold governments and international donors to account for the money spent on

Table 16.4 Sustainable Development Goal 3, selected targets and indicators

Goal: Ensure healthy lives and promote well-being for all at all ages

Target	Indicators
3.1 By 2030, reduce the global maternal mortality ratio to less than 70 per 100,000 live births	3.1.1 Maternal mortality ratio 3.1.2 Proportion of births attended by skilled health personnel
3.2 By 2030, end preventable deaths of newborns and children under 5 years of age: all countries aim to reduce neonatal mortality to 12 per 1,000 live births and under-5 mortality to 25 per 1,000 live births	3.2.1 Under-5 mortality rate 3.2.2 Neonatal mortality rate
3.3 By 2030, end the epidemics of AIDS, tuberculosis, malaria and neglected tropical diseases and combat hepatitis, water-borne diseases and other communicable diseases	3.3.1 Number of new HIV infections per 1,000 uninfected population, by sex, age and key populations 3.3.2 Tuberculosis incidence per 100,000 population 3.3.3 Malaria incidence per 1,000 population
3.4 By 2030, reduce by one-third premature mortality from non-communicable diseases through prevention and treatment and promote mental health and well-being	3.4.1 Mortality rate attributed to cardiovascular disease, cancer, diabetes or chronic respiratory disease
3.7 By 2030, ensure universal access to sexual and reproductive health-care services, including for family planning, information and education, and the integration of reproductive health into national strategies and programmes	3.7.1 Proportion of women of reproductive age (aged 15–49 years) who have their need for family planning satisfied with modern methods 3.7.2 Adolescent birth rate (aged 10–14 years; aged 15–19 years) per 1,000 women in that age group
3.8 Achieve universal health coverage, including financial risk protection, access to quality essential health-care services and access to safe, effective, quality and affordable essential medicines and vaccines for all	3.8.1 Coverage of essential health services 3.8.2 Proportion of population with large household expenditures on health as a share of total household expenditure or income

Source: https://unstats.un.org/sdgs/metadata.

health. Priorities include accurate reporting on mortality, morbidity, health status, service coverage and risk prevalence. For this to happen in a sustainable way, efforts must be made to strengthen poor countries' own capacity to collect and analyse data. Vital registration systems (of births and deaths), household surveys and analysis at sub-national level, wherever feasible, are priorities. The World Health Organization can play a key role in this.

16.13 Conclusions

Further research is needed into addressing the health problems that most affect poor people in LMICs. In addition to increased global investment, new ways of stimulating research into the diseases of poverty and the development of commodities, including vaccines, diagnostics and medicines, are required. Research is urgently needed on the best way of delivering health interventions, and more rigorous impact evaluations of new approaches to better understand what works, in which contexts and why.

REFERENCES

1. World Bank, Poverty overview online. Available at: www.worldbank.org/en/topic/poverty/overview#2https://unstats.un.org/sdgs/metadata
2. J. Sachs (chairman), Macroeconomics and health: Investing in health for economic development, Report of the Commission on Macroeconomics and Health, Geneva, World Health Organization, 2001.
3. F. Chao, D. You, J. Pedersen *et al.*, National and regional under-5 mortality rate by economic status for low-income and middle-income countries: A systematic assessment, *The Lancet Global Health* **6**(5), 2018, e535–47.
4. R. A. Castaneda Aguilar, A. Eilertsen, T. Fujs *et al.*, April 2022 global poverty update from the World Bank, 2022. Available at https://blogs.worldbank.org/opendata/april-2022-global-poverty-update-world-bank
5. S. Alkire and M. Santos, Acute multidimensional poverty: A new index for developing countries, OPHI Working Paper 38, July 2010.
6. M. M. Coates, M. Ezzati, G. Robles Aguilar *et al.*, Burden of disease among the world's poorest billion people: An expert-informed secondary analysis of Global Burden of Disease estimates, *PLoS One* **16**(8), 2021, e0253073.
7. UN Population Division, World population prospects 2019: Data booklet, United Nations, 2019.
8. World Health Organization, The Global Health Observatory, Child mortality and causes of death, 2022. Available at: www.who.int/data/gho/data/themes/topics/topic-details/GHO/child-mortality-and-causes-of-death
9. R. E. Black, S. S. Morris and J. Bryce, Where and why are 10 million children dying every year? *The Lancet* **361**(9376), 2003, 2226–34.
10. World Health Organization, Fact sheet: Malnutrition, 2021. Available at: www.who.int/news-room/fact-sheets/detail/malnutrition

11. R. E. Black, R. Laxminarayan, M. Temmerman and N. Walker (eds.), *Reproductive, Maternal, Newborn and Child Health, Disease Control Priorities*, 3rd ed., Washington, DC, World Bank, 2016, vol. 2.

12. UN Millennium Project Task Force on Child Health and Maternal Health, *Who's Got the Power? Transforming Health Systems for Women and Children*, London, Earthscan, 2005.

13. WHO, UNICEF, WHO, World Bank and UN Population Division, Trends in Maternal Mortality 2000–2017, World Health Organization, 2019.

14. UN Sexual and Reproductive Health Agency, The state of the world's population 2022: Seeing the unseen – the case for action in the neglected crisis of unintended pregnancy, United Nations, 2022.

15. World Health Organization, HIV and AIDS factsheet, 2022. Available at: www.who.int/newsroom/fact-sheets/detail/hiv-aids.

16. World Health Organization, Weekly epidemiological update on COVID-19, 20 July 2022. Available at: www.who.int

17. T. Ahmed, T. Roberton, Monitoring of Essential Health Services Team *et al.*, Indirect effects on maternal and child mortality from the COVID-19 pandemic: Evidence from disruptions in healthcare utilization in 18 low- and middle-income countries, *The Lancet*, 2021. Available at: https://ssrn.com/abstract=3916767

18. C. D. Mathers and D. Loncar, *Updated Projections of Global Mortality and Burden of Disease, 2002–2030: Data Sources, Methods and Results*, Geneva, World Health Organization, 2005.

19. Institute for Health Metrics and Evaluation, Global Burden of Disease (GBD). Available at: http://globalburden.org/design.html

20. GBD 2019 Mental Disorders Collaborators, Global, regional, and national burden of 12 mental disorders in 204 countries and territories, 1990–2019: A systematic analysis for the Global Burden of Disease Study 2019, *The Lancet Psychiatry* **9**(2), 2022, 137–50.

21. L. Eaton, L. McCay, M. Semrau *et al.*, Scale up of services for mental health in low-income and middle-income countries, *The Lancet* **378**(9802), 2011, 1592–603.

22. S. Ozawa, R. Shankar, C. Leopold and S. Orubu, Access to medicines through health systems in low- and middle-income countries, *Health Policy and Planning* **34**(3), 2019, iii1–iii3.

23. D. Molyneux, P. Hotez and A. Fenwick, 'Rapid-impact interventions': How a policy of integrated control for Africa's neglected tropical diseases could benefit the poor, *PLoS Medicine* **2**(11), 2005, 1064–70.

24. World Trade Organization, Implementation of paragraph 6 of the Doha Declaration on the TRIPS Agreement and public health, General Council WT/L/540 and Corr.1, 1 September 2003. Available at: www.wto.org/english/tratop_e/trips_e/implem_para6_e.htm

25. Bill and Melinda Gates Foundation, Vaccine development and surveillance. Available at: www.gatesfoundation.org/our-work/programs/global-health/vaccine-development-and-surveillance

26. World Health Organization, COVAX: Working for global equitable access for COVID-19 vaccines. Available at: www.who.int/initiatives/act-accelerator/covax

27. World Bank, *World Development Report 1997: The State in a Changing World*, Washington, DC, World Bank, 1997.

28. M. Grindle, *Good Enough Governance: Poverty Reduction and Reform in Developing Countries*, Cambridge, MA, Kennedy School of Government, Harvard University, 2002.

29. Commission for Africa, Our common interest, Report of the Commission for Africa, March 2005. Available at: www.bris.ac.uk/poverty/downloads/keyofficialdocuments/Commission%20for%20Africa%20report.pdf

30. World Bank Group, *Disease Control Priorities: Improving Health and Reducing Poverty*, 3rd ed., Washington, DC, World Bank, 2017, vol. 9.

31. N. Palmer, D. Mueller, L. Gilson *et al.*, Health financing to promote access in low income settings – how much do we know? *The Lancet* **364**(9442), 2004, 1365–70.

32. World Health Organization, *World Health Report: Health Systems Financing: The Path to Universal Coverage*, Geneva, WHO, 2010.

33. A. Wagstaff and M. Claeson, *The Millennium Development Goals for Health, Rising to the Challenges*, Washington, DC, World Bank, 2004.

34. World Health Organization, Primary health care, Report of the International Conference on Primary Health Care, Alma-Ata, USSR, 6–12 September, Geneva, WHO, 1978.

35. World Health Organization, Global health report, 2008.

36. WHO Maximising Positive Synergies Collaborative Group, An assessment of interactions between global health initiatives and country health systems, *The Lancet* **373**(9681), 2009, 2137–69.

37. P. Allotey, D. Reidpath, S. Yasin *et al.,* Rethinking health-care systems: A focus on chronicity, *The Lancet* **377**(9764), 2011, 450–1.

38. R. Manning, *Organisation for Economic Co-operation and Development (OECD) Development Co-operation Report 2005*, Paris, OECD, 2005.

39. N. Kabeer, Poverty, social exclusion and the MDGs: The challenge of 'durable inequalities' in the Asian context, *IDS Bulletin* **37**(3), 2006, 64–78.

40. C. Z. Guilmoto, N. Saikia, V. Tamrakar and J. K. Bora, Excess under-5 female mortality across India: A spatial analysis using 2011 census data, *The Lancet Global Health* **6**(6), 2018, e650–58.

41. E. J. Mills, S. Kanters, A. Hagopian *et al.,* The financial cost of doctors emigrating from sub-Saharan Africa: Human capital analysis, *British Medical Journal* **343**, 2011, d7031.

42. United Nations, Transforming our world: The Sustainable Development Goals, 2015. Available at: https://sdgs.un.org/2030agenda

43. J. Waage, R. Banerji, O. Campbell *et al.* for the Lancet and London International Development Centre Commission, The Millennium Development Goals: A cross-sectoral analysis and principles for goal setting after 2015, *The Lancet* **376**(9745), 2010, 991–1023.

17

Planetary Health

James Smith

Key points

- Planetary health addresses human disruptions to the Earth's natural systems on which life depends.
- Environmental injustice cannot be separated from issues of racism, sexism, coloniality and economic injustice.
- The climate emergency is an unprecedented threat to health and climate action is an unprecedented opportunity for health improvement and social justice.
- Everyone can and must take urgent action to address planetary health.

17.1 Introduction

The world has greatly changed in the 10 years since the previous edition of this book. The COVID-19 pandemic has demonstrated the interconnectedness of the modern world and reminded us that human health and the natural world are inextricably linked. The ever-worsening climate crisis is driving extreme weather around the world. Droughts, floods, hurricanes and typhoons, and food and water shortages are becoming tragically commonplace. In the summer of 2022, the UK experienced an unprecedented heat wave, with temperatures topping 40 degrees Celsius for the first time. Fires raged across Western Europe. China's megacities suffered record-breaking temperatures.

The gross injustice of environmental change, with those who have polluted the least suffering the biggest consequences, is becoming more apparent. Society is not responding at the scale and pace required to avoid catastrophic loss of life, but from courtrooms to the streets, changes are emerging. In this context, public health is now practised. Public health skills, knowledge and attitudes are essential to create a more sustainable and fairer world.

This chapter defines key terms, describes some of the most important environmental transitions, challenges and opportunities, and considers what our public health response to these can be. It seeks to equip the reader with some basic knowledge and all-important motivation for becoming a more effective agent for change at a time when planetary health must become everyone's business.

17.2 Planetary Health

If another (more) intelligent life form were to circle our planet and could see what we are doing, they might be struck by two strange things. Firstly, despite being a 'global village', there are huge variations in opportunity, empowerment and health around the world: differences that harm us all [1]. Secondly, most of us are consuming resources with a dangerous and selfish lack of consideration for the consequences. The way most people, particularly those in wealthy countries, live is unsustainable. In recent years, planetary health has come to the fore as a way of understanding how global environmental challenges impact on health and shape society.

Planetary health has been defined as 'a solutions-oriented, transdisciplinary field and social movement focused on analyzing and addressing the impacts of human disruptions to Earth's natural systems on human health and all life on Earth' [2]. These disruptions include climate change, biodiversity loss, ocean acidification, and pollution of air, rivers and oceans. Human health depends on the stability of these environmental systems, and it is this stability which is being lost. Earth's natural systems do not behave in simple linear ways and scientists are trying to identify at what point various systems might tip into a new state. These so-called planetary boundaries are thresholds which we should avoid crossing. Unfortunately, it is thought we have already crossed the boundaries related to climate change, land use, nitrogen and phosphorus cycles, novel entities such as plastics and extinction of species [3].

One way of understanding how environmental and social factors can be brought together is presented in 'Doughnut Economics', which combines environmental planetary boundaries as an ecological ceiling with a social foundation to create 'a safe and just space for humanity' (see Figure 17.1) [4]. A planetary health approach recognises the complexity of the environmental and social systems on which health depends. Simpler cause and effect understandings, widespread in much of medical and public health practice, will not be sufficient to address global issues. A systems thinking approach is required, which requires appreciation for the complexity and inter-relatedness of each system.

'One Health' is another integrated approach to bring together planetary health concerns, endorsed by the World Health Organization [5]. It is often conceived as a triumvirate of human health, animal health and the environment, so is valuable for

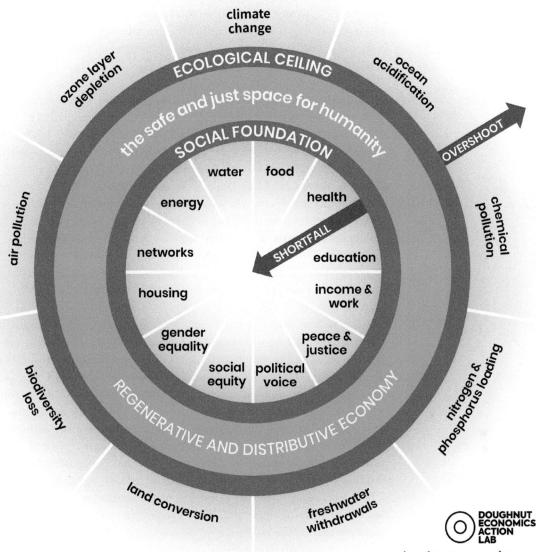

Figure 17.1 The doughnut of social and planetary boundaries. Credit: Kate Raworth and Christian Guthier, CC-BY-SA 4.0.

understanding issues such as zoonotic diseases or antimicrobial resistance and working with colleagues across other disciplines such as agriculture.

Sustainable development describes a way of thinking and acting that improves the lives and welfare of people and populations today, but which avoids prejudicing the lives and welfare of future generations; a whole-system approach to prosperity and equity without unsustainable material growth [6]. This is the essence of Gro Harem

Brundtland's definition: 'development that meets the needs of the present . . . without compromising the ability of future generations to meet their own needs' [7]. For public health practitioners, who think in terms of both time and space, the definition can be usefully expanded to development that meets the needs of the present . . . without compromising the ability of *others elsewhere and* future generations to meet their own needs.

Sustainability is commonly considered in three interlinked domains: economic or financial, social and environmental. As described in Chapter 16, the UN Sustainable Development Goals (SDGs) consist of 17 goals supported by 169 targets [8], adopted by all UN member states in 2015. In the same year, the Paris Climate Agreement was agreed, with the goal of keeping the mean global temperature rise since pre-industrial times to well below 2 degrees C and to pursue a 1.5 degree C target, with each country being expected to submit a nationally determined contribution every 5 years [9]. Unfortunately, since then, global carbon emissions and temperatures have continued to rise [10]. The Sendai Framework for Disaster Risk Reduction was also agreed in 2015 [11]. This aimed to substantially reduce loss in lives, livelihood, health and assets globally and set out priorities for action to achieve this. In 2021, 123 countries reported that they had a national disaster risk reduction strategy, an improvement on the 55 countries which reported having plans in 2015 [12].

For those working in public health, it is important to understand why more progress has not been made in pursuit of these global goals. Planetary health cannot be understood as a purely scientific or environmental challenge. It is at its heart a social challenge. There are huge institutional and cultural barriers to change. Power is not fairly distributed in society; a few people and organisations hold disproportionate amounts of power. These power structures often work against the goal of improving public health or reducing injustice. There are many social narratives which have been constructed and encouraged by those with vested interests in slowing progress towards these global goals. This practice of profiting from delaying progress (e.g. on reducing greenhouse gas emissions), and in so doing harming others, is known as 'predatory delay'. The narratives used by the fossil fuel industry are a good example of this [13]. Understanding the narratives which exist around climate action enables us to avoid blindly accepting propaganda promoted by those with vested interests. It also helps us to consider our own communication and to tailor our approach to the communities we are working with. The Oxford-based Climate Outreach is an example of an organisation which generates relevant learning in this sphere [14].

A significant criticism of previous public health work on climate change is that it can reflect historic and colonial power structures and overlook the traditional knowledge of Indigenous peoples. This traditional knowledge is 'collective, holistic, community-based, land-informed ways of knowing that are inherently interconnected with people and environment' [15]. They cannot be easily fitted into a

Western scientific perspective. They bring together a range of determinants of planetary health, including respect for the feminine, ancestral legal personhood designation, interconnectedness with nature, Indigenous languages, land rights and health. They place great emphasis on ancestors and descendants which are typically absent from other discourses.

Planetary health, One Health, sustainable development and Indigenous knowledge are all valuable as we seek to understand and act in response to the planetary crises in the twenty-first century.

17.3 Disruptions to Environmental Systems

This section focuses on three important disruptions to climate, air pollution and biodiversity, and the relationship of these to health. Climate change and biodiversity have been selected as they are critical for all life on Earth. Air pollution, as a more local issue, is a highly effective entry point to engage colleagues, policy-makers and the public in planetary health. For all environmental disruptions, it is important to recognise that impacts are not evenly distributed through society. Their distribution is shaped by structural injustices such as those related to race, gender, disability, wealth, class and coloniality.

17.3.1 Climate Change

Climate change is currently the most obvious and directly life-threatening disruption to the environmental systems we depend on. There are many terms used for climate change: climate disruption, climate emergency, climate chaos, global warming and global heating. The terms used refer to a process of changing climate driven by greenhouse gas emissions. Climate change depends on the balance between greenhouse gas emissions and carbon sinks, which can be natural or potentially man made. Our climate will only stop worsening after so-called 'net zero' has been achieved – when carbon sinks are equal or greater to emissions. Greenhouse gases, including carbon dioxide, methane, nitrous oxide and fluorinated gases (F-gases), are generated by many human activities, notably burning fossil fuels, cement production, food production and changes to land use.

The warming impact of increased atmospheric carbon dioxide lasts for several thousand years and so at human timescales it is the cumulative emissions and the area under the curve of emissions against time that determine the resultant climate change. For this reason, addressing climate change is a highly time-dependent problem. Every day we keep burning fossil fuels is another day we move further away from stabilising the climate. As we continue to release greenhouse gases, we increase the risk of passing tipping points in natural systems, such as the melting of ice sheets or the drying out of rainforests. These are changes which cannot be reversed in the near term, or in the case of extinctions, once they have occurred

[16]. These environmental tipping points are another reason why urgent large-scale transformative action is the only sensible response to the climate crisis. A potential response to this urgent need for change is to trigger positive social tipping points, discussed further below.

The health impacts of climate change range from the obvious such as deaths in extreme weather events (including heat waves, hurricanes and floods) to changes in vector-borne disease such as dengue fever and malaria, to reducing the availability of food and water and the social consequences of this: migration, civil unrest and conflict. These are all interconnected. An example of this is that extreme weather events are associated with increased gender-based violence experienced by women, girls, and sexual and gender minorities [17]. This also illustrates how environmental injustice cannot be separated from other social injustice, racism, coloniality, sexism, homophobia and economic injustice.

This has led one expert to ask: 'Can we stop talking about the "health impacts of climate change" and just call it trauma embedding itself in the body when structural inequality meets the climate crisis?' [18].

We cannot properly understand planetary health unless we understand the distribution of the causes and effects of planetary challenges. Both within and between countries, climate impacts typically cause more harm to women, older people, people of colour and people with less income. Those with lower income, for example, are more likely to experience worse impacts of environmental change due to living in poorer quality housing or in communities poorly defended from flooding. They are less likely to have strong social networks which are protective when exposed to extreme events. But they are also likely to have contributed proportionally more of their income to policies to address environmental change while seeing proportionally less of the benefit of these policies [19]. Environmental change is a contributing factor to reduced availability and increased prices of vital resources, including food, water and homes. Lack of access to these is in turn making people more vulnerable to environmental extremes. The cost-of-living crisis and the planetary health crisis are inextricably linked.

Further description of the impacts of climate change can be found in the report of the Lancet Commission on Climate and Health (and subsequent Countdown reports). Because of the many health impacts of climate change, this report identified climate change as the 'greatest threat to health of the 21st century' [20].

Society urgently needs to be transformed to prevent ever-more climate change. 'Mitigation' is the term used to mean reducing greenhouse gas emissions, or levels in the atmosphere, to prevent ever-worsening climate change. The good news from a health perspective is that mitigation provides a huge opportunity for health improvement because many of the actions required are good for health. This is why the second Lancet Commission on Climate and Health identified climate action as potentially the greatest opportunity for improving health globally [21] (see Box 17.1). These opportunities are known as the health co-benefits of climate

Box 17.1 Examples of co-benefits of climate action

Changing how we move around

Car travel allows us to move around without moving our bodies [22]. Shifting to active modes of travel such as walking or cycling and multi-modal journeys centred on public transport can increase physical activity, reduce local air pollution, reduce road traffic incidents, free up space in cities for other uses – including much needed green space or cycling infrastructure, and improve social connectedness within communities. This in turn can reduce cardiovascular disease and respiratory disease, improve mental health and reduce injuries [23].

Changing what we eat

Meat and dairy foods have particularly high carbon footprints. Shifts to more plant-based diets can reduce carbon footprints while also reducing the risk of cardiovascular disease, diabetes and colorectal cancer [24]. To illustrate this, one study modelling dietary changes found a 19% and 22% reduction in premature mortality for flexitarian and vegan diets. With these diets, there were a wide range of environmental benefits: 54–87% reduction in greenhouse gas emissions, 23–25% reduction in nitrogen application, 18–21% reduction in phosphorus application, 8–11% reduction in cropland use and 2–11% reduction in freshwater use [25]. Over 77% of the world's agricultural land is used for meat and dairy production, including land for animal feed production, even though meat and dairy only provide 18% of global calories and 37% of global protein [26]. Changing diets to reduce consumption of meat and dairy products could have profound impacts on land use and ecosystems globally.

Changing how we power our lives

2.6 billion people globally do not have access to clean fuel for cooking. Use of wood or kerosene in low-income communities is associated with indoor air pollution. Indoor air pollutants in homes are associated with an annual estimated 2.31 million deaths globally. These risks are much higher for women and in some areas women are also exposed to higher risks of musculoskeletal injury and violence while collecting fuels [27]. Introduction of clean energy sources can help not only reduce these risks, but also allow other benefits, such as improving quality of life with electric lighting.

mitigation. In addition to mitigation, we also need to adapt to our worsening climate. Climate adaptation, preparing for and responding to our changing climate, is a critical public health need. It includes preventive measures and emergency planning in every part of our lives. It should not be seen as distinct from mitigation measures. Transformative action on climate needs both to shift the balance between emissions and sinks to zero and to prepare for and avert the worst impacts of climate change.

17.3.2 Air Pollution

Pollution to air, water and land threatens health across the globe. The Lancet Commission on Pollution and Health 2017 estimated that 9 million premature deaths per annum could be attributed to pollution in all its forms. This was three times as much as HIV, tuberculosis and malaria combined and much more than caused by violence and war [28]. A recent update to this work found that pollution remains responsible for approximately 9 million premature deaths, corresponding to one in six deaths worldwide [29]. The World Health Organization estimates that 6.7 million deaths are attributable to indoor and outdoor air pollution alone, with 99% of the world's population living in a place where air pollution levels exceed WHO guideline limits [30].

The major air pollutants causing local harm are particulate matter, often described by size as PM10 or PM2.5, nitrogen oxides, sulphur dioxide, ozone and carbon monoxide. These are commonly produced by the use of fossil fuels in the energy sector, particularly coal, transport-related emissions and fuel use in homes.

> ### Box 17.2 Example of the impact of air pollution
>
> Ella Adoo Kissi-Debrah was a 9-year-old girl who died from an exacerbation of severe asthma in 2013. She lived near a main road in London and had been admitted to hospital 27 times in the 3 years prior to her death. A coroner's investigation concluded in December 2020 that she had died from asthma contributed to by exposure to excessive air pollution. This was the first time air pollution had been listed as a cause of death in England. The coroner noted that during her illness she had been exposed to nitrogen dioxide and particulate matter levels in excess of WHO guidelines and that traffic emissions were the principal source of this exposure. The temporal association between air pollution episodes and her admissions was central to the coroner's verdict. Ella's mother had not been informed by health professionals about the risk of air pollution and its potential to exacerbate asthma.
>
> The coroner identified three area of concern:
>
> - national limits which were higher than WHO guidelines which themselves should be seen as minimum requirements;
> - low public awareness about air pollution; and
> - health professionals not communicating the adverse effects of air pollution to patients [31].

Agricultural practices and natural sources can also be responsible for significant air pollutants. Particulate matter is associated with respiratory disease, cardiovascular disease and lung cancer, with emerging evidence showing impacts on diabetes and birth weight. Nitrogen dioxide has been associated with asthma, diabetes, lung cancer, dementia and low birth weight. Box 17.2 describes a tragic example of the consequences of air pollution in London.

17.3.3 Biodiversity Loss

We are not just in the midst of a climate emergency; we are also in the midst of an ecological emergency, with species becoming extinct at such a rate that this has been described as 'the sixth extinction' [32]. The previous extinction period, the Cretaceous-Tertiary extinction, was about 65 million years ago and wiped out the dinosaurs. It occurred over a span of 1 to 2.5 million years. This is much slower than the current extinction rate caused by humans, which is happening over decades.

Biodiversity loss is also about loss of the complex web of ecological interactions which provide the basis for many of the benefits we have unknowingly received from nature. Economists sometimes refer to these as ecosystem products and services. They include availability of fresh water, food and fuel. There are direct impacts from biodiversity loss on health, such as the emergence of zoonotic diseases, which occurs when human–animal contact is increased (e.g. in zones of deforestation). The COVID-19 pandemic is a recent example of this, but Ebola and HIV are previous examples of emergent infectious diseases which continue to have devastating global impacts.

Loss of biodiversity also reduces potential sources of novel medicines. An example of this is cone snails, of which there are thought to be approximately 700 species, each with 100 to 200 unique peptides poisons which are highly potent and receptor-specific. These could provide a source of novel analgesics if they do not become extinct, with the destruction of their coral reef homes due to climate change and ocean acidification [33].

There is growing evidence that access to green spaces and nature can have a beneficial impact on health, particularly on mental well-being [34]. As with all planetary disruptions, those who most suffer due to loss of biodiversity are not the ones who profit from the destruction leading to its loss. As farming and food production have become increasingly industrialised, harms to the environment have escalated. Global corporations and international relationships drive the exploitation of the natural world and the economic, gender and race inequalities which determine who is most affected. These corporate, political, economic and legal structures reflect on-going coloniality, the sustained relationships resulting from the exploitation and domination of peoples by colonialism. It is important for public health professionals to recognise the power structures in which they are working, challenge on-going injustices resulting from coloniality, and work with those who have been exploited to protect the natural environment on which we all depend.

Unfortunately, in the modern era, there are too many environmental disruptions to include in a single chapter. The focus here has been on three of the most important: climate change, air pollution and biodiversity loss. This is not to diminish the importance of other threats to health. Clean water is a fundamental requirement of health. Ocean acidification threatens ecosystems on which millions depend for food. Plastics are found throughout natural environments and in animal and human bodies across the world. Planetary health encompasses all these threats and more. It is relevant in every sector from agriculture to urban planning – and to every public health professional wherever you are.

17.4 Decarbonising Health-Care: A Case Study of the NHS in England

Health-care is estimated to be responsible for approximately 5% of the global carbon footprint [35]. Since 2008, the National Health Service (NHS) in England has been developing policy, instigating research and engaging policy-makers, clinicians and other staff in how a health service should take seriously its responsibility for high-quality health-care, both now and in the future. In 2020, the Greener NHS team, building on years of work by the NHS Sustainable Development Unit, released its Delivering a Net Zero Health Service report [36]. In doing so, it became the first national health system anywhere in the world to commit to reaching net zero. This set out a net zero target of 2040 for the emissions it controls, 10 years ahead of the national 2050 target of the UK Climate Change Act. Box 17.3 shows the main areas of action identified by the NHS in England.

Box 17.3 NHS in England Delivery Net Zero Health Service report [36]

The Delivering a Net Zero Health Service identified four areas for direct intervention:

- estates and facilities;
- travel and transport;
- supply chains; and
- medicines, specifically inhalers and anaesthetic gases.

It also identified four areas of work:

- sustainable models of care, including digital transformation;
- workforce, networks and leadership;
- funding and financial mechanisms; and
- data and monitoring.

In addition, research and innovation has been identified as vital to reaching net zero.

A key focus of the work of the NHS Sustainable Development Unit and more recently the Greener NHS team was engaging with clinicians in recognition that much of the carbon footprint of health-care depends on decisions made by clinicians. A good example is inhaler prescribing. Inhalers for asthma and chronic obstructive pulmonary disease come in several forms: metered dose inhalers, dry powder inhalers and soft mist inhalers. Metered dose inhalers use hydrofluorocarbon propellants which are highly potent greenhouse gases, whereas dry powder and soft mist inhalers do not use these, so have a much lower carbon footprint. In the UK, a much higher proportion of inhalers prescribed are metered dose inhalers compared to other Northern European countries [37]. Differences can also be seen between different parts of England. These are not driven by differing clinical need. Changing prescribing patterns is therefore a social challenge requiring an understanding of professional cultures and patient beliefs. Education is needed so that patients and prescribers understand their options. Financial incentives were introduced in 2022 to incentivise general practices to use more dry powder inhalers and reduce the carbon footprint of the inhalers they prescribe. This example illustrates how what may appear to be a relatively simple change in clinical practice is remarkably complex.

Public health professionals are ideally placed to bring together scientific understanding, skills relating to institutional and social change, and values-based leadership to create sustainable health-care systems.

17.5 Public Health Is Planetary Health

There is no future which is not radically different from the present day. The planet on which civilisation developed and which older generations have enjoyed as children is no longer stable. This is apparent not just from the extremes of weather we are experiencing, but also from the realisation that our targets for decarbonising our lives are rapidly approaching. There can be no public health without planetary health. Challenges do not get more complex than these. New ways of thinking and working are required to address them.

How do we take action on planetary health? A simple structured way to organise action is to consider it as personal, professional and political (see Box 17.4), which also links back to the Pencheon and Bradley model of driving forces of health (see Figure 8.3). These are overlapping and dependent on individual context and privileges. Personal actions may be quantitatively small compared to the impact a public health professional can have in their broader role, but are mentioned here because they are often an individual's starting point for action. Taking personal action can also help reduce cognitive dissonance and create a valuable feeling of self-consistency. Personal actions give credibility to efforts to lead professional or political actions.

Box 17.4 Taking action on planetary health

- **Personal** – making changes to one's own life, such as in travel, diet and home.
- **Professional** – working on projects which improve planetary health, such as QI projects in health-care or sector-specific strategies in public health, such as in transport or food systems.
- **Political** – using one's voice to advocate for change, such as campaigns for clean air, fossil fuel divestment or a Green New Deal, and amplifying the voices of those who have been exploited, particularly Indigenous communities.

It is through professional *and* political actions that public health professionals can have the greatest impact on planetary health. To do this, it is necessary to work with others, bringing together scientific knowledge, leadership skills and personal values, to develop meaningful projects or campaigns. Public health professionals can integrate planetary health into whatever domain of public health they work in. For example, when working on local housing policy, they can ensure the environmental harms of housing development or renovations are minimised, that buildings are prepared for our future climate and that communities are engaged with effectively so that equity is improved. It is not just in policy such as housing, transport and food and land use that planetary health can be integrated. It is possible to integrate it into public health services (e.g. when commissioning smoking or sexual health services). For example, it is helpful to consider what are the environmental and wider social implications of the proposed services? Similarly, health protection services should not solely focus on responding to the local consequences of planetary changes, but can look to prevent future harms both through mitigation and adaptation planning (e.g. when developing local, regional and national heat wave or flooding plans).

Whatever policy or intervention is being developed, a planetary health approach demands attention to the distribution of anticipated benefits and harms and to the inclusion of the voices of those most affected. For any of the illustrative actions described above, whether related to the wider determinants of health, health protection or the health-care system, they all have the potential to widen or reduce inequalities.

With their expert knowledge and skills, public health professionals have a powerful voice advocating for change. Central to this advocacy is to make clear the urgency and scale of action needed. This also links to Chapter 7, and the role of public health practitioners as leaders of change, deploying skills for advocacy and ensuring expertise and evidence influence action. The co-benefits outlined above mean that they will also be advocating for changes which can dramatically improve the local health outcomes which they are tasked with improving. Sharing this understanding with senior civil servants and politicians at local, regional or national levels is one of the most important things which public health professionals can do. All sectors of government are affected by both the threats and the substantial benefits of action.

In public health, and especially when reflecting on planetary health, it is also important to acknowledge our own position and perspective, and appreciate that we are inevitably biased by our own world view and experiences and privileges: understanding this potential bias and seeking out others with differing perspectives and world views is necessary to understand and take effective action on planetary health.

Some of these perspectives were captured in a framework for planetary health education [38], which identifies five domains for learning: the Anthropocene and health, movement building and system change, interconnection with nature, equity and social justice, and systems thinking and complexity (see Figure 17.2).

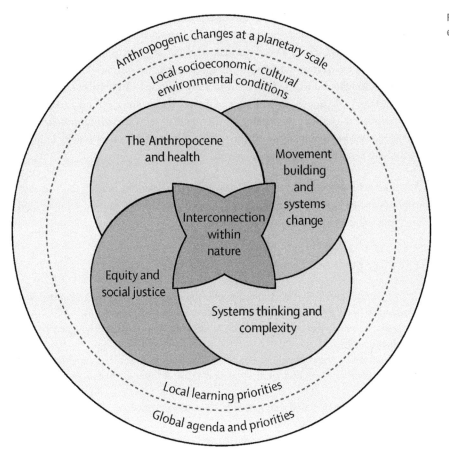

Figure 17.2 The planetary health education framework [38].

At the core of the framework are the five planetary health education domains represented in an intertwined figure, similar to the threads of a rope. Although the model separates each domain, the reality of planetary health requires an understanding of the interdependent and interconnected nature of each domain [38].

Readers are encouraged, informed by their own position, interests and priorities, to build on the learning from this chapter by exploring domains of this framework. Think carefully about whose voices you are listening to and the extent to which these are embedded in current power structures and reinforce or challenge the dominant thinking which has led to the current planetary health crisis.

17.6 Conclusions

This chapter has offered a brief overview of some of the fundamental challenges threatening planetary health and offered my own perspective. I strongly encourage readers to seek perspectives from around the world and read more widely on this most pressing of issues. This chapter has discussed some of the potential opportunities for action and emphasises the urgency of this mandate and call to action: we must all take responsibility and take action now to play our part as individuals, and in public health as advocates, to effect meaningful change.

One final thought and word of advice: planetary health work is very challenging. It can be traumatic to acknowledge the state of the planet on which our futures depend and an important element of working in this field is self-care. Without caring for yourself, you will be unable to contribute to humanity's effort to turn society around. It is in taking action that hope can be found.

* With acknowledgement and thanks to David Pencheon for authoring the previous sustainable development chapter and providing comments on this chapter and Peter Bradley for comments on the chapter.

REFERENCES

1. R. G. Wilkinson and K. E. Pickett, Income inequality and population health: A review and explanation of the evidence, *Social Science & Medicine* **62**(7), 2006, 1768–84.
2. Planetary Health Alliance, Planetary health. Available at: www.planetaryhealthalliance.org/planetary-health
3. L. Persson, B. M. Carney Almroth, C. D. Collins *et al.*, Outside the safe operating space of the planetary boundary for novel entities, *Environmental Science & Technology* **56**(3), 2022, 1510–21.
4. K. Raworth, *Doughnut Economics: 7 Ways to Think Like a 21st-Century Economist*, London, Chelsea Green Publishing, 2017.
5. Centers for Disease Control and Prevention, One Health basics. Available at: www.cdc.gov/onehealth/basics/index.html

6. T. Jackson, *Prosperity without Growth: Economics for a Finite Planet*, Washington, DC and London, Earthscan, 2009.

7. G. Brundtland, Report of the World Commission on Environment and Development: Our common future, Oxford Paper, 1987.

8. United Nations, Transforming our world: The 2030 agenda for sustainable development, New York, NY, 2015. Available at: https://sdgs.un.org/2030agenda

9. UN Framework Convention on Climate Change, Paris Agreement, Bonn, 2015.

10. P. Friedlingstein, M. O'Sullivan, M. W. Jones *et al.*, Global carbon budget 2022, *Earth System Science Data* **14**(11), 2022, 4811–900.

11. UN Office for Disaster Risk Reduction, Sendai framework for disaster risk reduction 2015-2030, Geneva, 2015. Available at: www.undrr.org/publication/sendai-framework-disaster-risk-reduction-2015-2030

12. UN Office for Disaster Risk Reduction, Annual report, Geneva, 2021.

13. W. F. Lamb, G. Mattioli, S. Levi *et al.*, Discourses of climate delay, *Global Sustainability* **3**, 2020, e17.

14. Climate Outreach. Available at: https://climateoutreach.org

15. N. Redvers, Y. Celidwen, C. Schultz *et al.*, The determinants of planetary health: an Indigenous consensus perspective, *The Lancet Planetary Health* **6**(2), 2022, e156–63.

16. T. M. Lenton, J. Rockström, O. Gaffney *et al.*, Climate tipping points – too risky to bet against, *Nature* **575**(7784), 2019, 592–5.

17. K. R. van Daalen, S. S. Kallesøe, F. Davey *et al.*, Extreme events and gender-based violence: A mixed-methods systematic review, *The Lancet Planetary Health* **6**(6), 2022, e504–23.

18. G. K. Bola, Tweet by @guppikb, Twitter, 2022. Available at: https://twitter.com/guppikb/status/1519390154410143747

19. I. Preston, N. Banks, K. Hargreaves *et al.*, Climate change and social justice: An evidence review, York, Joseph Rowntree Foundation, 2014. Available at: www.jrf.org.uk/sites/default/files/jrf/migrated/files/climate-change-social-justice-full.pdf

20. A. Costello, M. Abbas, A. Allen *et al.*, Managing the health effects of climate change, *The Lancet* **373**(9676), 2009, 1693–733.

21. N. Watts, W. N. Adger, P. Agnolucci *et al.*, Health and climate change: Policy responses to protect public health, *The Lancet* **386**(10006), 2015, 1861–914.

22. I. Roberts and P. Edwards, *The Energy Glut*, London and New York, NY, Zed Books, 2010.

23. J. Woodcock, P. Edwards, C. Tonne *et al.*, Public health benefits of strategies to reduce greenhouse-gas emissions: Urban land transport, *The Lancet* **374**(9705), 2009, 1930–43.

24. W. Willett, J. Rockström, B. Loken *et al.*, Food in the Anthropocene: The EAT-Lancet Commission on healthy diets from sustainable food systems, *The Lancet* **393**(10170), 2019, 447–92.

25. M. Springmann, K. Wiebe, D. Mason-D'Croz *et al.*, Health and nutritional aspects of sustainable diet strategies and their association with environmental impacts: A global modelling analysis with country-level detail, *The Lancet Planetary Health* **2**(10), 2018, e451–61.

26. H. Ritchie, Half of the world's habitable land is used for agriculture, Our World in Data, 2019. Available at: https://ourworldindata.org/global-land-for-agriculture

27. M. Romanello, A. McGushin, C. Di Napoli *et al.*, The 2021 report of the Lancet Countdown on health and climate change: Code red for a healthy future, *The Lancet* **398**(10311), 2021, 1619–62.

28. P. J. Landrigan, R. Fuller, N. J. R. Acosta *et al.*, The Lancet Commission on pollution and health, *The Lancet* **391**(10119), 2018, 462–512.

29. R. Fuller, P. J. Landrigan, K. Balakrishnan *et al.*, Pollution and health: A progress update, *The Lancet Planetary Health* **6**(6), 2022, e535–47.

30. World Health Organization, Air pollution data portal, 2023. Available at: www.who.int/data/gho/data/themes/air-pollution.

31. P. Barlow, Regulation 28: Report to prevent future deaths, Ella Kissi-Debrah, 2021. Available at: www.judiciary.uk/wp-content/uploads/2021/04/Ella-Kissi-Debrah-2021-0113-1.pdf

32. G. Ceballos, P. R. Ehrlich, A. D. Barnosky *et al.*, Accelerated modern human-induced species losses: Entering the sixth mass extinction, *Science Advances* **1**(5), 2015, e1400253.

33. E. Chivian, Why doctors and their organisations must help tackle climate change: An essay by Eric Chivian, *British Medical Journal* **348**, 2014, g2407.

34. B. W. Wheeler, R. Lovell, S. L. Higgins *et al.*, Beyond greenspace: An ecological study of population general health and indicators of natural environment type and quality, *International Journal of Health Geographics* **14**(1), 2015, article 17.

35. Health Care Without Harm, Health care climate footprint report, 2019.

36. The NHS Net Zero Expert Panel, Delivering a 'net zero' National Health Service (2022 update), London, NHS, 2020. Available at: www.england.nhs.uk/greenernhs/wp-content/uploads/sites/51/2022/07/B1728-delivering-a-net-zero-nhs-july-2022.pdf.

37. F. Lavorini, C. J. Corrigan, P. J. Barnes *et al.*, Retail sales of inhalation devices in European countries: So much for a global policy, *Respiratory Medicine* **105**(7), 2011, 1099–103.

38. C. A. F. Guzmán, A. A. Aguirre, B. Astle *et al.*, A framework to guide planetary health education, *The Lancet Planetary Health* **5**(5), 2021, e253–5.

Absolute risk reduction (ARR)   The difference in the absolute risk (rates of adverse events) between study and control populations, in the case when risk is lower in the study population. In the case where the risk is higher in the study population, the absolute risk increase (ARI) is used instead.

Absolute risk   The observed or calculated probability of an event in the population under study.

Acquired immunity   Resistance acquired by a host to a pathogen as a result of previous exposure from natural infection or immunisation. It is the result of the production of antibodies (immunoglobulins) targeted to specific antigens.

Adjustment   A summarising procedure for a statistical measure in which the effects of differences in composition of the populations being compared have been minimised by statistical methods.

Aetiology   The study of the causes of disease.

Agent (of disease)   A term used to imply the organism that causes a disease.

Antibody   Protein molecule formed in response to a foreign substance (antigen). It has the capacity to bind to the antigen to allow its removal or destruction.

Antigen   A foreign molecule which elicits an antibody response.

Association   Statistical dependence between two or more events, characteristics or other variables. An apparent association may come about due to chance or may be produced by various other circumstances; the presence of an association does not necessarily imply a causal relationship.

Attributable risk   The proportion of the risk of a disease which can be attributed to a named causal factor.

Audit (clinical)   A planned assessment of a clinical process against predefined standards.

Bias (syn: systematic error)   Deviation of results or inferences from the true value in the underlying population of interest, or processes leading to such deviation. See also selection bias.

Blind(ed) study (syn: masked study)   A study in which observer(s) and/or subjects are kept ignorant of the group to which the subjects are assigned, as in an experimental study, or of the population from which the subjects come, as in a nonexperimental or observational study. Where both observer and subjects are kept ignorant, the study is termed a double-blind study. If the statistical analysis is also done in ignorance of the group to which subjects belong, the study is sometimes described as triple blind. The purpose of 'blinding' is to eliminate sources of bias.

Carriage/carrier   When a host is infected but shows no signs of disease it is termed a carrier. It may transmit infection, so is a potential source of infection.

Case fatality rate   The proportion of people with a disease who die within a defined period from diagnosis.

Case-control study   Retrospective comparison of exposures of persons with disease (cases) with those of persons without the disease (controls) – see retrospective study.

Case series   Report of a number of cases of disease.

Causality   The relating of causes to the effects they produce. Most of epidemiology concerns causality and several types of causes can be distinguished. It must be emphasised, however, that epidemiological evidence by itself is insufficient to establish causality, although it can provide powerful circumstantial evidence.

Clinical governance   The framework through which NHS organisations and their staff are accountable for the quality of patient care.

Cohort study   Follow-up of exposed and non-exposed defined groups, with a comparison of disease rates (or rates of some other outcome of interest) during the time covered.

Commensalism   A neutral relationship between host and another organism. Often used to describe the bacteria which live in the human gut harmlessly.

Co-morbidity   Co-existence of a disease or diseases in a study participant in addition to the index condition that is the subject of study.

Comparison group   Any group to which the index group is compared. Usually synonymous with control group.

Confidence interval (CI)   An interval we generate from the data which gives a measure of our uncertainty about the effect size. Typically, 95% confidence intervals are used. If we were to repeatedly sample the population, 95% of the 95% confidence intervals produced would contain the true value. Confidence intervals indicate the strength of evidence; where confidence intervals are wide, they indicate more uncertainty, and so give less-precise estimates of effect. As a study's sample size increases, we gain more certainty about the true effect size, and so the confidence interval becomes narrow and the 'precision' of the study's estimate is increased. In a 'positive finding' study, the lower boundary of the confidence interval, or lower confidence limit, should still remain important or clinically significant if the results are to be accepted. In a 'negative finding' study, the upper boundary of the confidence interval should not be clinically significant if you are to accept this result confidently.

Confounding variable, confounder   A variable which is associated with both the exposure being studied and the outcome of interest. The presence of confounders can lead to bias. If a confounding variable is not properly controlled for, this can lead to a spurious association between exposure and outcome and it may not be possible to distinguish the effects of a confounder from the effects of the exposure(s) being studied.

Contamination   The presence of an infectious agent on the body of a host or on inanimate articles. A contaminated host does not always become infected, but may be a possible source of infection for others.

Demography   The study of human populations.

Determinant   Any definable factor that effects a change in a health condition or other characteristic.

Disability   In the context of health experience, a disability is any restriction or lack (resulting from an impairment) of ability to perform an activity in the manner or within the range considered normal for a human being.

Disability-adjusted life year (DALY)   A method of calculating the health impact of a disease in terms of the cases of premature death, disability and days of infirmity due to illness from a specific disease or condition.

Dose-response relationship   A relationship in which change in amount, intensity or duration of exposure is associated with a change – either an increase or a decrease – in risk of a specified outcome.

Dynamic population   A population in which there is turnover of membership during the study period.

Effectiveness   A measure of the benefit resulting from an intervention for a given health problem under usual conditions of clinical care for a particular group; this form of evaluation considers both the efficacy of an intervention and its acceptance by those to whom it is offered, answering the question, 'Does the practice do more good than harm to people to whom it is offered?' See intention-to-treat analysis.

Efficacy   A measure of the benefit resulting from an intervention for a given health problem under the ideal conditions of an investigation; it answers the question, 'Does the practice do more good than harm to people who fully comply with the recommendations?'

Endemic   The constant presence of a disease or infectious agent within a given geographic area or population group.

Environmental health   The theory and practice of assessing, correcting, controlling and preventing those factors in the environment that can potentially affect adversely the health of present and future generations.

Epidemic   The occurrence of disease at higher than expected levels. This could be an endemic disease at higher than usual levels or non-endemic disease at any level.

Epidemiology   The study of the distribution and determinants of health-related states or events in specified populations, and the application of this study to control of health problems.

Evaluation   A process that attempts to determine as systematically and objectively as possible the relevance, effectiveness and impact of activities in the light of their objectives.

Evidence-based health-care/medicine/public health   Systematic use of evidence derived from published research and other sources for management and practice.

Exclusion criteria   Conditions which preclude entrance of candidates into an investigation even if they meet the inclusion criteria.

Fertility   The childbearing capability of a woman, couple or population.

Follow-up   Observation over a period of time of an individual, group or initially defined population whose relevant characteristics have been assessed in order to observe changes in health status or health-related variables.

Gold standard   A method, procedure or measurement that is widely accepted as being the best available.

Handicap   In the context of health experience, a handicap is a disadvantage for a given individual, resulting from an impairment or a disability, that limits or prevents the fulfilment of a role that is normal (depending on age, sex and social and cultural factors) for that individual.

Health   The extent to which an individual or a group is able to realise aspirations and satisfy needs, and to change or cope with the environment. Health is a resource for everyday life, not the objective of living; it is a positive concept, emphasising social and personal resources as well as physical capabilities. Your health is related to how much you feel your potential to be a meaningful part of the society in which you find yourself is adequately realised.

Health equity audit   A technique to identify how fairly services or other resources are distributed in relation to the health needs of different population groups or geographical areas.

Health improvement   The theory and practice of promoting the health of populations by influencing lifestyle and socioeconomic, physical and cultural environment through methods of health promotion, directed towards populations, communities and individuals.

Health inequality   Differences observed between groups due to one group experiencing an advantage over the other group rather than to any innate differences between them.

Health inequity   The presence of unfair and avoidable or remedial differences in health among populations or groups defined socially.

Health promotion   The process of enabling people to exert control over and improve their health. As well as covering actions aimed at strengthening people's skills and capabilities, it also includes actions directed towards changing social and environmental conditions, to prevent or to improve their impact on individual and public health.

High-risk strategy   This targets preventive interventions at people most at risk of a disease.

Host   A living organism on or in which an infectious agent can subsist.

Impairment   In the context of health experience, an impairment is any loss or abnormality of psychological, physiological or anatomical structure or function.

Incidence   The number of new cases of illness commencing, or of persons falling ill, during a specified time period in a given population. See also prevalence.

Incidence rate   The rate at which new cases occur in a population.

Incubation period   The interval from exposure to onset of clinical disease.

Index case   The first case identified in an outbreak.

Infant mortality   The proportion of live births that die up to 1 year of age.

Infection (colonisation)   This occurs when an organism enters the body and multiplies. It may be termed infection when damage is caused and colonisation when no damage is caused to the host. Acute infection implies a short-lived infection with a short period of infectivity. Chronic infection refers to a persistent condition with on-going replication of the organism. Latent infection refers to a persistent infection with intermittent replication of the organism.

Infectivity   The proportion of exposed, susceptible persons who become infected (for a given number of organisms).

Intention-to-treat analysis   A method for data analysis in a randomised clinical trial in which individual outcomes are analysed according to the group to which they have been randomised, even if they never received the treatment they were assigned. By simulating practical experience, it provides a better measure of effectiveness (versus efficacy). It also prevents attrition from acting as a confounding variable.

Interviewer bias   Systematic error due to the interviewer's subconscious or conscious gathering of selective data.

Koch's (Henle-Koch's) postulates   These postulates should be met before a causal relationship can be inferred between an organism and a disease:
1. The agent must be shown to be present in every case of the disease by isolation in pure culture.
2. The agent must not be found in cases of other disease.
3. Once isolated, the agent must be able to reproduce disease in experimental animals.
4. The agent must be recovered from this experimental disease.

Lead time bias   If prognosis study patients are not all enrolled at similar, well-defined points in the course of their disease, differences in outcome over time may merely reflect differences in duration of illness. Lead time bias occurs when detection by screening seems to increase disease-free survival, but this is only because disease has been detected earlier and not because screening is delaying death or disease.

Length time bias   Length time bias occurs if a screening programme is better at picking up milder forms of the disease. This means that people who develop a disease that progresses more quickly or is more likely to be fatal are less likely to be picked up by screening and their outcomes may not be included in evaluations of the programme. Thus, the programme looks to be more effective than it is.

Life expectancy   The average number of additional years a person could expect to live if current mortality trends were to continue for the rest of that person's life. Generally given as a life expectancy from birth.

Likelihood ratio   Ratio of the probability that a given diagnostic test result will be expected for a patient with the target disorder rather than for a patient without the disorder.

Maternal mortality ratio   The number of deaths during pregnancy and up to 42 days after delivery, per 1,000 live births.

Morbidity   The impact of a disease which is not death. Measures of morbidity include incidence and prevalence rates.

Mortality (rate)   The number of deaths in an area as a proportion of the number of people in that area.

Needs   These may be expressed by action (e.g. visiting a doctor), or felt needs (e.g. what people consider and/or say they need). The need for health-care is often defined as the capacity to benefit from that care.

Negative predictive value (of a diagnostic or screening test)   The proportion of persons testing negative for a disease who, as measured by the gold standard, are identified as non-diseased.

Neonatal mortality   The proportion of live births who die within the first 28 days.

Non-specific immunity   This is the natural barriers a host has to pathogens. It includes mechanical barriers, body secretions, physical removal of organisms, phagocytosis and inflammatory response.

Normal distribution   Many biological variables show a normal distribution of ranges between individuals within a population. A probability density graph of the normal distributions takes the shape of a bell-shaped curve.

Number needed to treat (NNT)   The number of patients who must be exposed to an intervention before the clinical outcome of interest occurred; for example, the number of patients needed to treat to prevent one adverse outcome. In the case where an exposure or intervention is harmful, we instead calculate the number needed to harm (NNH).

Odds   A proportion in which the numerator contains the number of times an event occurs and the denominator includes the number of times the event does not occur.

Odds Ratio   A measure of the degree of association; for example, the odds of exposure among the cases compared with the odds of exposure among the controls.

Outbreak   A localised epidemic. Health-protection professionals often look for two or more cases linked in time and place.

P value   The probability of seeing something at least as extreme as the data we have just observed, if the null hypothesis, H0, were true. If the p-value is high (typically >0.05 for a single test), we do not reject the null hypothesis. If the p-value is low (typically <0.05 for a single test), we reject the null hypothesis.

Pandemic   A global epidemic. This term is sometimes used for a very large-scale epidemic.

Perinatal mortality   The proportion of all births that die before birth or in the first week.

Placebo   A substance that has no therapeutic effect, used as a control in interventional studies.

Policy   An overall statement of the aims of an organisation within a particular context.

Population strategy   Targets preventive interventions at the whole population.

Positive predictive value (of a diagnostic or screening test)   The proportion of persons testing positive for a disease who, as measured by the gold standard, are identified as diseased.

Poverty   Absolute poverty – a family's ability to purchase essential goods (such as housing, heating, food, clothing and transport). Relative poverty – poverty in relation to the average income in a particular population (such as below 50% of the national average).

Precision   A measure of how close a series of estimators are to one another.

Predictive value   In screening and diagnostic tests, the probability that a person
with a positive test is a true positive (i.e. does have the disease) or that a person with
a negative test truly does not have the disease. The predictive value of a screening
test is determined by the sensitivity and specificity of the test, and by the prevalence
of the condition for which the test is used.

Prevalence   The proportion of persons with a particular disease within a given
population at a given time. Point prevalence is the prevalence at one single point in
time. Period prevalence is the proportion of persons with a particular disease over a
specified period of time.

Prevention   Primary prevention – actions designed to prevent the occurrence of the
problem (e.g. health education, immunization).
Secondary prevention – actions designed to detect and treat the occurrence of a
problem before symptoms have developed (e.g. screening, early diagnosis).
Tertiary prevention – actions designed to limit disability once a condition is manifest
(e.g. limitation of disability, rehabilitation).

Prevention paradox   Preventive measures bringing large benefits to the community
offer little to each participating individual.

Primary health-care   First-contact care provided by a range of health-care
professionals: general practitioners, nurses, dentists, pharmacists, optometrists and
complementary therapists working in the community.

Prognosis   The possible outcomes of a disease or condition and the likelihood that
each one will occur.

Prognostic factor   Demographic, disease-specific or co-morbid characteristics
associated strongly enough with a condition's outcomes to predict accurately the
eventual development of those outcomes. Compare with risk factors. Neither
prognostic nor risk factors necessarily imply a cause-and-effect relationship.

Prospective study   Study design where one or more groups (cohorts) of individuals,
who have not yet had the outcome event in question, are monitored for the number
of such events which occur over time.

Public health   The science and art of preventing disease, prolonging life and
promoting health through the organised efforts and informed choices of society,
organisations, public and private, communities and individuals. Public health
practice is the emphasis in this book, while public health may also be considered as a
discipline or a social institution.

Public health practitioner   In this book, includes anyone working in the broad field of public health, neither defined by formal qualifications nor restricted to a professional group.

Quality-adjusted life year (QALY)   A health measure which combines the quantity and quality of life. It takes 1 year of perfect-health life expectancy to be worth 1 and regards 1 year of less than perfect life expectancy as less than 1.

Randomised controlled trial   Study design where treatments, interventions or enrolment into different study groups are assigned by random allocation rather than by conscious decisions of clinicians or patients. If the sample size is large enough, this study design avoids problems of bias and confounding variables by assuring that both known and unknown determinants of outcome are evenly distributed between treatment and control groups.

Recall bias   Systematic error due to the differences in accuracy or completeness of recall to memory of past events or experiences.

Relative risk   The ratio of the probability of developing, in a specified period of time, an outcome among those receiving the treatment of interest or exposed to a risk factor, compared with the probability of developing the outcome if the risk factor or intervention is not present.

Reproducibility (repeatability, reliability)   The results of a test or measure are identical or closely similar each time it is conducted.

Retrospective study   Study design in which cases where individuals who had an outcome event in question are collected and analysed after the outcomes have occurred (see also case-control study).

Risk   The number of cases of a disease that occur in a defined period of time as a proportion of the number of people in the population at the beginning of the period.

Risk factor   Patient characteristics or factors associated with an increased probability of developing a condition or disease in the first place. Compare with prognostic factors. Neither risk nor prognostic factors necessarily imply a cause-and-effect relationship.

Screening   A public health service in which members of a defined population, who do not necessarily perceive they are at risk of, or are already affected by, a disease or its complications, are asked a question or offered a test. The aim is to identify those individuals who are more likely to be helped than harmed by further tests or treatment to reduce the risk of a disease or its complications.

Secular trend   A trend over time, also termed temporal trend.

Selection bias   A bias in assignment or a confounding variable that arises from study design rather than by chance. These can occur when the study and control groups are chosen so that they differ from each other by one or more factors that may affect the outcome of the study. In screening, selection bias occurs when the screening programme attracts people who are more or less likely to have the condition being screened for than the general population.

Sensitivity (of a diagnostic or screening test)   The proportion of truly diseased persons, as measured by the gold standard, who are identified as diseased by the test under study.

Social capital   Networks, together with shared norms, values and understandings, which facilitate cooperation within or among groups and which may thereby improve health.

Specificity (of a diagnostic or screening test)   The proportion of truly non-diseased persons, as measured by the gold standard, who are identified as non-diseased by the test under study.

Strategy   A plan of action designed to achieve a series of objectives.

Stratification   Division into groups. Stratification may also refer to a process to control for differences in confounding variables, by making separate estimates for groups of individuals who have the same values for the confounding variable.

Strength of inference   The likelihood that an observed difference between groups within a study represents a real difference rather than mere chance or the influence of confounding factors. This can be quantified by the calculation of P values or confidence intervals. Strength of inference is weakened by various forms of bias and by small sample sizes.

Surveillance   The on-going, systematic collection, collation and analysis of data and the prompt dissemination of the resulting information to those who need to know so that an action can result.

Survival curve   A graph of the number of events occurring over time or the chance of being free of these events over time. The events must be discrete and the time at which they occur must be precisely known. In most clinical situations, the chance of an outcome changes with time. In most survival curves, the earlier follow-up periods usually include results from more patients than the later periods and are therefore more precise.

Sustainability   Requires the reconciliation of environmental, social and economic demands. Sustainable development meets the needs of the present without compromising the ability of future generations to meet their own needs.

Validity   The extent to which a variable or intervention measures what it is supposed to measure or accomplishes what it is supposed to accomplish. The internal validity of a study refers to the integrity of the experimental design. The external validity (generalisability) of a study refers to the appropriateness by which its results can be applied to non-study patients or populations.

Years of life lost (YLL)   Years of potential life relate to the average age at which deaths occur and the expected life span of the population. Therefore, this is a measure of how many potential years are lost due to early death and provides a measure of the relative importance of conditions in causing mortality.

Index

absolute risk increase (ARI), 60
absolute risk reduction (ARR), 60
Acheson Inquiry 1998 (NHS), 284
action-centred leadership, 127
advance market commitments (AMCs), 312
adverse child experiences (ACEs), 225
age standardisation
   direct, 32
   indirect, 32
agent (infection), 186
air pollution and planetary health
   deaths attributed to, 330
   impact, 331
   main sources of, 330-1
Alma-Ata Declaration (1978), 316
alternative hypothesis, 74
analytic studies (epidemiology)
   defined, 66, 67
   interventional, 70, 72
   observational, 67-8
attributable risk, 62
audit cycle (UK), 116
authentic leadership, 127

Beauchamp and Childress principles of
   bio-medical ethics, 104
bedside rationing, 106
behavioural science and infection
   containment, 193
behavioural science model (public health),
   149-50
bias
   screening programme evaluation, 179-80,
   181
   unconscious, 283
bias (epidemiology result)
   information bias, 76
   overview, 75-6
   selection bias, 75-6
bio-medical model (population health
   improvement), 146-9
Black Report 1980 (UK), 298
bounded rationality (public health policy), 292
British Doctors' Study, 62-4

cancer
   global rates of, 233

policy implications (UK), 234-5
   risk factors, 233
cancer prevention
   primary, 234
   secondary, 234
   tertiary, 234
cardiovascular disease
   economic cost of, 235
   leading cause of UK mortality, 235
   mortality inequalities, 235
   policy implications (UK), 236-7
   prevention measures, 235-6
   risk factors, 235-6
Carstairs deprivation index, 42, 43
case fatality (epidemiology), 57
case reports (epidemiology), 66
case series (epidemiology), 66
case-controlled study design (epidemiology),
   59-65
change models (organisational behaviour)
   commitment enrolment and compliance
     model, 140
   diffusion of innovation, 139
   eight-step model for leading change,
     140
   forcefield analysis, 136
   PESTLE analysis, 138
   SWOT analysis, 137
   transition model, 139
child mortality
   demographics, 217
   economics and, 217-18
   global improvements, 218
   international, 304, 307
   international COVID-19, 310-11
   public health challenges, 219
children's public health
   child demographics, 216-17
   child early development critical
     importance, 212-14
   child mortality, 217-18
   features, 211-12
   health promotion, 218-20
   Healthy Child Programme, 212
   importance, 210
   inequality recognition, 215
   professional collaboration, 220

351